T0138342

THE MODULATED SCREAM

THE MODULATED SCREAM

Pain in Late Medieval Culture

ESTHER COHEN

THE UNIVERSITY OF CHICAGO PRESS

CHICAGO AND LONDON

ESTHER COHEN is a research fellow at the Scholion Center and professor of medieval history at the Hebrew University of Jerusalem. She is the author of three books, most recently of *Peaceable Domain, Certain Justice: Crime and Society in Fifteenth-Century Paris* (1996), and coeditor of *Medieval Transformations: Texts, Power, and Gifts in Context* (2001).

The University of Chicago Press, Chicago 60637
The University of Chicago Press, Ltd., London
© 2010 by The University of Chicago
All rights reserved. Published 2009
Printed in the United States of America

19 18 17 16 15 14 13 12 11 10   1 2 3 4 5

ISBN-13: 978-0-226-11267-1 (cloth)
ISBN-10: 0-226-11267-5   (cloth)

Library of Congress Cataloging-in-Publication Data

Cohen, Esther, 1947 Dec. 21–
    The modulated scream : pain in late medieval culture / Esther
Cohen.
        p. cm.
    Summary: This book provides an integral, readable account of changing attitudes toward pain in late medieval Europe. Since pain itself cannot be known, the book looks at pain by chronicling what people wrote about it, and what they did with and about that.
    Includes bibliographical references and index.
    ISBN-13: 978-0-226-11267-1 (cloth : alk. paper)
    ISBN-10: 0-226-11267-5 (cloth : alk. paper)
    1. Pain in literature. 2. Pain—History—To 1500. 3. Suffering—History—To 1500. 4. Torture—History—To 1500. 5. Pain—Religious aspects—Christianity. 6. Suffering—Religious aspects—Christianity. 7. Literature, Medieval—History and criticism. 8. Middle Ages. I. Title.
PN682.P25C64 2010
809'.93353—dc22

                                        2010004793

⊗ The paper used in this publication meets the minimum requirements of the American National Standard for Information Sciences—Permanence of Paper for Printed Library Materials, ANSI Z39.48-1992.

IN MEMORY OF YA'AKOV MEIR
MAGISTER

CONTENTS

FIGURES

ACKNOWLEDGMENTS

This book owes its existence first and foremost to those blessed havens of research, the institutes of advanced studies where scholars are free to devote time to their real passion. The original idea for the book was born as a glimmer in 1989 while I was at the Netherlands Institute for Advanced Studies in the Humanities and Social Sciences (NIAS), working on a totally different project. A sabbatical year at Clare Hall, Cambridge (1999–2000), allowed me to research the subject in depth, using the wonderful Cambridge University Library, and a year at the National Humanities Center in North Carolina (2003–4) saw the birth of the book's first version. The final version owes its existence to the Scholion Interdisciplinary Research Center in Jewish Studies, the Hebrew of University of Jerusalem (2007–10). To the helpful directors and staff of all these institutes I owe my thanks. I also thank the Hebrew University of Jerusalem for sabbatical and research funds over the years. The help of the interlibrary loan librarians of the National Humanities Center and the Hebrew University—Betsy Dain, Jean Houston, Elizabeth Robertson, and Gila Emanuel—was essential to my work. The final version could not have been produced without the support of the staff and assistants of Scholion, especially Asya Bereznyak, Adam Farkash, and Lotem Pinchover.

Portions of chapters 2, 5, and 8 were previously published in the following articles: "Naming Pains: Physicians Facing Sensations," in *Benjamin Z. Kedar Festschrift Volume,* edited by Jonathan Riley-Smith, Iris Shagrir, and Ronnie Ellenblum (London, 2006), 245–62; "Sacred, Secular, and Impure: The Contextuality of Sensations," in *Sacred and Secular in Medieval and Early Modern Cultures: New Essays,* edited by Lawrence Besserman (London, 2006), 123–33, 210–13; and "The Vocabularies of Pain: A Disharmony of Different Voices," in *Piacere e dolore: Materiali per una storia delle passioni nel Medioevo,* edited by Carla Casagrande and Sylvana Vecchio, Micrologus Library (Florence, 2009), 11–28. I acknowledge with thanks the permission granted by the publishers to reproduce these sections within the book.

People are even more important than environment. The two godparents of my book, Barbara Rosenwein and Moshe Sluhovsky, made me rethink its entire structure and provided arguments, thoughts, and ideas throughout the years. Both were coparticipants in the formation of the book and deserve more thanks than can be expressed here. Both read the entire manuscript carefully and corrected as many of my errors as they could find. Those that remain are my own. Many others have contributed throughout the years, including John Arnold, Caroline W. Bynum, Carla Casagrande, Rita Copeland, Chiara Crisciani, Marilynn Desmond, Dyan Elliott, Michael R. McVaugh, Gianna Pomata, Miri Rubin, Pamela Sheingorn, Randolph Starn, Ian P. Wei, Ulrike Wiethaus, Israel J. Yuval, Joseph Ziegler, and the members of our Scholion research group: Michal Altbauer, Naama Cohen-Hanegbi, Manuela Consonni, Otniel E. Dror, Omri Herzog, Noa Shashar, and Leona Toker. This is only a minimal list of the people whose ideas (and responses to mine) have contributed to the book. To all those whose comments enriched the book and whose names do not appear due to my forgetfulness of names, not of ideas, I tender my thanks. Over the years, I have lectured at various fora about the book's contents, and to all those who commented and critiqued my talks, I offer many thanks for their ideas.

It is customary at this point to thank one's family for either helping or not interfering with the book's progress. Neither my sons nor my daughters-in-law nor my granddaughters have had anything to do with the book. All the same, their existence is the meaning of life. May they never know the meaning of pain.

ABBREVIATIONS

AASS	J. Bollandus and G. Henschenius. *Acta sanctorum . . . editio novissima.* Edited by J. Carnandet et al. Paris, 1863–.
BFSMA	Bibliotheca Franciscana scholastica Medii Aevi.
CCCM	Corpus Christianorum continuatio mediaeualis.
CCSL	Corpus Christianorum series Latina.
Cod.	*Codex.* In *Corpus iuris civilis,* edited by Paul Krueger, Theodore Mommsen, and Rudolph Scholl. Translated by Alan Watson. 3 vols. Berlin, 1884–95. Reprint, Philadelphia, 1985.
CSEL	Corpus scriptorum ecclesiasticorum Latinorum.
Dig.	*Digest.* In *Corpus iuris civilis,* edited by Paul Krueger, Theodore Mommsen, and Rudolph Scholl. Translated by Alan Watson. 3 vols. Berlin, 1884–95. Reprint, Philadelphia, 1985.
MGH, SS	Monumenta Germaniae historica, Scriptores.
MGH, SSRG	Monumenta Germaniae historica, Scriptores rerum Germanicarum.
MGH, SSRM	Monumenta Germaniae Historica, Scriptores rerum Merovingicarum.
PL	Patrologiae cursus completus: Series Latina. Edited by J.-P. Migne. 221 vols. Paris, 1857–64.
ST	Thomas Aquinas. *Summa theologiae.* Edited by Roberto Busa. 7 vols. Sancti Thomae Aquinatis opera omnia 2. Stuttgart, 1980.
TSMA	Typologie des sources du Moyen Âge occidental.

INTRODUCTION

Pain is the sensation of our own decay.
—Augustine, *De libero arbitrio*

Pain is the shrinking from those things that happen to us against our will.
—Alexander of Hales, *Glossa in quatuor libri sententiarum Petri Lombardi*, misquoting Augustine

Pain is the rupture of continuity.
—Alexander of Hales, *Glossa in quatuor libri sententiarum Petri Lombardi*, citing Aristotle (unverifiable)

Pain is the feeling of a rupture in continuity.
—Matthew of Acquasparta, *Quaestiones disputatae*

Real pain emerges purely from apprehension.
—Henry of Ghent, *Quotlibeta magistri Henrici Goethals a Gandavo*

Pain is specifically a passion, and a quality of the sensitive appetite, caused by the sensitive apprehension and not by the object apprehended by the senses.
—John Duns Scotus, *Quaestiones in tertium librum sententiarum*, citing William of Ockham

The two types of pain are a sudden change of temperament and a rupture of continuity.
—Galen, *Opera omnia*

Pain is the sensing of a contrary thing. All pains are subsumed into two
types, that is the quick change of complexion . . . and the rupture of
continuity.
—Avicenna, *Liber canonis Avicenne*

Pain: An unpleasant sensory and emotional experience associated
with actual or potential tissue damage, or described in terms of such
damage.
—U. Lindblom et al., "Pain Terms"

The wealth of incongruous and incommensurate definitions of pain from
antiquity to the late twentieth century is proof of a very simple fact:
though almost everybody knows what pain feels like, general definitions
are difficult and unsatisfactory. No one has succeeded in providing a definition of bodily pain that is in any way helpful in understanding it. The
definitions cited above fail to convey the essence or meaning of pain. They
are discipline bound, either scholastic or medical: they explain the phenomenon but do not convey a meaning.

Nevertheless, these definitions have a few things in common. None of
the scholastic definitions dissociates physical pain from the human soul
and emotions. Many of them cite (or invent) ancient sources for their definitions. In contrast, the medical definitions are purely functional: they indicate the causes of pain rather than try to define it. In fact, they achieve
the dignity of definition simply because all medieval medical authorities
repeated ancient authorities on the subject, as though the listing of causes
were a sufficient definition. Even the modern medical definition hinges
upon causality, albeit in a more subtle fashion. Physical pain, then, was and
is almost impossible to define and inexorably attached to emotional precedents or responses. And yet, it is and has always been known to humans.

Pain has been a constant companion of humankind from the beginnings
of time. It is not a phenomenon which pertains to any specific era, yet different societies at different times have evinced different codes of behavior and
sensitivity around pain. This has misled some historians into wondering
whether some people in the past suffered less than we do, merely because
those people had neglected to leave recorded expressions of their suffering.
Pain appears and disappears from historical sources like a landscape mo-
mentarily floodlit by a revolving light, only to vanish again in darkness. The
later Middle Ages are a time when the sources starkly outline the landscape
of pain. All modes of cultural expression were harnessed to the effort of

articulation, explanation, and display of pain in the most extravagant possible manner. Not only sufferers but professionals—doctors, theologians, and lawyers—wrote their own versions of pain. Thus, an intrinsically individual feeling became a social, religious, and cultural phenomenon.

This book is not about pain in the Middle Ages, for pain itself cannot be known;[1] it is about what people thought and did about pain, how they conceptualized it, how they explained it to themselves and to others. By "people," I mean mainly those who have left a record behind. The multitude of sufferers whose voices we cannot hear across the chasm of the ages can be perceived only through the writings of those who told them how to behave, what to believe, how to relieve pain, and how to suffer it in an appropriate manner. Most importantly, the same authorities told people *how* and *what* to feel. Professionals of pain management and interpretation—preachers, scholars, physicians, and jurists—told sufferers that they could trace their pain back to Eve, the first human who gave birth in pain; through Christ, who undertook pain willingly for the redemption of humanity; through martyrs, who withstood pain and manifested faith; to their own gallstones and headaches and future in purgatory or, worse yet, in hell. Some people left letters and autobiographical writings as a testimony to their pain. For most, we have only secondhand evidence of observers, compassionate or indifferent, sympathetic or disgusted. Sometimes observers took the liberty of penetrating the sufferers' emotional universe and describing and inventing their pain at secondhand. The wealth of evidence from the later Middle Ages is an index of the interest and compassion, as well as the prurient curiosity and cruelty, which pervaded that society. A sensation worth expressing and recording rather than suppressing and eradicating stood a good chance of leaving its imprint upon the legacy of the period, and pain in the later Middle Ages did just that.

Why did this outpouring take place? One standard answer is that there were more causes for suffering in an era plagued with the Black Death, famines, and wars than at any earlier time. To anyone familiar with earlier medieval chronicles, which occasionally state dryly that there had been a great famine or another disaster in this or that year, this answer is not convincing. Alternatively, it could be argued that the late medieval cultural expressivity of pain was merely part of a cultural trend toward emotive sensitivity that had begun in the eleventh century and probably culminated in Baroque culture—in other words, that late medieval expressivity was merely part of a long-term trend. I would argue rather that the culture of pain from the thirteenth to the fifteenth century was unique in many ways. It was not merely that behavioral norms in the face of pain changed. Late medieval pain culture was characterized by the multifarious ways in which pain was treated—even in fields of thought that we might consider irrelevant—and the tremendous *positive* significance identified in pain. Suffering was not to be dismissed, vanquished, or transcended: suffering was to be felt with an ever-deepening intensity.

The growing interest in pain was manifested in medicine, law, and theology, and the scholastic framework that provided a matrix for all three disciplines enabled mutual enrichment and feedback between fields of knowledge. Mostly, thinkers and meditators of pain sought (though did not always find) understanding of the purpose of a sensation that one automatically recoiled from. The use and application of pain were not merely an ungovernable emotional preoccupation but were considered aspects of a teleological, all-embracing civilizing process. By approaching what one wished to avoid, argued medieval thinkers, one could perfect one's self. In all fairness, though, I must admit that physicians found only the usefulness of specific painful procedures, but not of pain in and of itself. They fit my paradigm only because they saw little virtue in analgesia and anesthesia.

Two paradoxes stood at the basis of the pain phenomenon. The first was the tension between the natural human recoiling from one's own pain and the preachers' ubiquitous message that pain was morally beneficial for human virtue. The paradox is summed up in William of Auvergne's (bishop of Paris; d. 1249) claim that pain is good because it is bad, beneficent because destructive. The second paradox was between experience and expectation. Exempla, sermons, stories about impassible martyrs, and tales of sufferers who were miraculously cured existed in constant contradiction with a harsh reality where there was no effective cure for pain. But such stories could work only for listeners who did know what pain was, so that they could appreciate how wonderful relief, or utter lack of pain, was. People may have become used to smells or noises, but not to chronic pain, and its ubiquitous presence was the constant jarring accompaniment to existence. No wonder, then, that in many cases pain behavior was construed as madness. The uncontrollable body language of both sufferers and mad people could be understood as one and the same. Significantly, such descriptions usually occur only when the narrator is dealing with "bad pain" that the saint or healer will presently vanquish. Few sufferers from the heavenly gift of pain ever acted like mad persons.

Modern Western medicalized cultures, as a rule, deal with pain as an enemy that must be defeated. Late medieval society, rather than trying to exterminate the beast, domesticated it in a number of ways. It provided pain with a constructive meaning: pain was useful; it was a key to unlock secrets of the human mind and body. The materials for this interpretation could be found in biblical and patristic writings, and during the later Middle Ages the subject of suffering was a favorite. It was no accident that Gregory the Great's commentary on the Book of Job was highly popular in the later Middle Ages and that it merited translations into several vernacular languages.

On the basis of this tradition came the use of pain. Inquisitors ordered suspects to be tortured in order to elicit their true confession. Physicians questioned patients as to the type of pain they felt in order to decipher their symptoms and diagnose their diseases. Devout people inflicted pain upon themselves in order to gain firsthand comprehension of the Crucifixion. Involuntary sufferers could interpret and diagnose their own illnesses as punishment, as a sign of divine favor, or as a nuisance and a cause for seeking a cure at the hands of physicians or saints. When we read of someone in severe pain, yet bravely hiding it, we must query the statement. If the camouflage of pain was so very perfectly opaque, how did the recorder of the hidden pain know about it? Since many (good) people in the Middle Ages are described as bravely hiding their pain, the secret must have been an open one. There must have been approved and recognized methods of bravely hiding pain that nonetheless demonstrated that one was indeed bravely hiding pain. Not showing pain was in and of itself a performance. All pain had meanings available for decoding, reading, interpreting, and understanding.

The belief that the purpose of pain could be understood led to the perception of its many uses. These can be divided for convenience into two general categories: pain as a tool and pain as a sign. The usefulness of pain made it a multipurpose tool. When parish priests wanted to dissuade their flock from sinning, they sometimes recommended physical mortification as part of active penitence. When virtuous people sought a way to rid themselves of temptations, pain was a usefully chastising discipline of mind and body. When preachers tried to instill virtue in their listeners, they spoke of the pains awaiting sinners in hell in the most realistic and frightening terms possible. At the same time, judges interrogating suspects threatened them with torture, a most efficient tool for extracting confessions, while physicians queried patients' types of pain in order to diagnose their disorders.

This use attributed to pain also meant a slow change in norms of behavior. While there were different standards for different people on different occasions, the valorization of most types of pain did lead to new norms of pain expression. The positive value of pain in specific situations meant that sufferers were occasionally expected to give voice to pain. It was inconceivable to late medieval burghers that flagellants parading through their streets, whipping themselves and their colleagues, should act as though the lashes of the corded whip were no more than a caressing breeze. They were expected to cry out loudly under the whip. Within a small conventual community, a nun who ceaselessly complained of her pains first earned her sisters' contempt, but when her reputation for saintliness spread beyond the convent's confines, her screams were tolerated and honored. Unless pain was articulated, the louder the better, its meaning was lost. Overt norms of pain expression in turn affected attitudes toward the suffering self, other sufferings, and perhaps even other sufferers. If empathy—*com-passio*—was to be reserved for meditations on Christ, sympathy for the pain of others could grow out of one's own acknowledged experience.

Awareness of pain could maintain not only the body human but also the body politic. Judicial systems perceived pain as an indispensable tool of justice and government. Pain became one of the cornerstones of hierarchic society: just as God maintained hell for sinners, so kings must maintain dungeons as well as palaces. The ultimate power belonged to the afterlife, and preachers continually shouted the threat of posthumous pains beyond all human imagination before the people. But this authoritative power, when relegated to human hands, carried with it shades of ancient defiance. Both the public and the secret pain of judicial activities undoubtedly sustained the state, but did the state necessarily sustain the public Good? In the thirteenth century the stories of suffering martyrs were clothed in a new glory. Though the martyrs were heroes in an ancient mold that was the stuff of legends, they were entirely human. Did the tortured martyrs control their pain bravely, or did they feel no pain? Unlike the ambiguous narratives of late antiquity, late medieval versions came down squarely on the side of the martyrs' suffering and endurance. In contrast, late medieval and early modern criminals were occasionally credited with the power to block out pain. Both martyr and criminal defied the system that caused them pain by refusing to break down and confess what was required of them. The parallel between the two was to sit most uncomfortably with lawyers and writers.

In addition to being a tool, pain was also a multivalent sign. This, too, was obviously not new. When physicians wanted to diagnose an illness, one of the things they queried was the associated pain. What type of pain was it? Where was it located? How strong was it? Was the pain a symptom or the illness itself? Eliciting from sufferers the exact nature of their symptoms could lead to a correct diagnosis, and thus to the proper treatment. Most importantly, pain manifested the inherent logic of the entire human destiny. From original sin to Crucifixion, and thence to the Apocalypse, pain was a primary herald of a change from one era to the next: the Fall signaled the incipient human vulnerability to pain; the Crucifixion redefined divine pain as the instrument of human salvation. At the end of time, the ultimate division of humanity would be between those who were destined to suffer forever and those destined to eternal deliverance from pain.

These truths were basic assumptions in late medieval society. Pain was therefore not a force one could, or would wish to, totally eradicate. No pain stands naked without a context. Every sufferer or observer who recorded her memories imbued pain situations with specific meanings, be they theological, moral, legal, or medical. Those meanings were invariably articulated within a dualistic value system, which leant itself equally to the performance or to the silencing of pain. Pain was either good or bad; it signified either virtue or vice; sufferers were shown as behaving according to these values. It was not a straightforward value system: martyrs could die in terrible pain while singing hymns, good kings could die in terrible pain while hiding it bravely, bad kings could die in terrible pain, writhing and screaming, and holy people screamed during empathy with Christ. To add to the complexity, virtuous sufferers could be described as writhing and screaming at a saint's shrine until cured, while others, of whose moral standing we know nothing, could describe their pain to the treating physician and gain relief through payment of his bill. The subtle construction of each case included the sufferer, the context, the observer/recorder, and the moral of the story. The observer, often a professional dealer in pain, was responsible for the interpretation. A headache could mean an upset stomach or an oncoming divine vision, depending upon the sufferer's unique physical and spiritual attributes.

Despite the immense variety of cases and modes of behavior, the professional literature of pain shows a certain coherence. All disciplines assumed the usefulness of pain. All scholastic disciplines were based upon Aristotelian thought and physiology, even when the discussion concerned Christ's body. Both medicine and law adopted ideas and structures from scholastic theology. Even devotional literature showed traces of a uniform basis of learning. While each discipline had its viewpoints, much of what was written and said came down to the basic paradoxes I have stated earlier. Pain was useful because it incapacitated; it was good because it was bad.

This brief argument must stand both as a justification for the existence of this book and as the basis and structure for the ensuing analyses. I intend above all to look at pain as medieval writers did and, I hope, through their eyes. For anybody before the mid–nineteenth century, physical pain was a given reality. For late medieval thinkers, pain had purposes. As I shall show further on, my central argument is that in this period the valuation of pain depended upon its utility. This usefulness could be as a sign, as a present force, or as a prophecy for future human destinies. While interpretation belonged to a rarified elite, probably the most basic method of confronting pain was to harness it to moral, legal, or social purposes. Beginning with the uses of pain, I shall explore what different professionals, who observed and controlled human behavior, had to say about it. Chapter 1 is an overview of the uses of pain in various fields: as an inducement to a moral life, as a punishment (in this life and the afterlife), and as a healing procedure. The following two chapters are devoted to the professional manipulators of pain. Chapter 2 deals with the overt use of coercive pain in judicial torture. Jurists used either present or imagined pain as their tools, coupling fear and intimidation with actual infliction of pain. Chapter 3 moves into the field of pain management and alleviation: it was—or so physicians claimed— their proper realm, and indeed, they had a great deal to say about the subject. Chapter 4 deals with the manipulation of pain as a social signal by all orders and genders of society. Here, I enter the realm of socialized pain in its formatted, scripted form and attempt to deduce actual pain management from licit, approved descriptions of "proper" institutionalized behavior by analyzing writings that shaped the contours of a biographical subject, who used pain and pain expression as part of the construction of virtue or vice.

Using pain and deciphering pain are intimately tied together, and in part II of the book I survey those who tried to elicit knowledge from pain. A physician diagnosing an incipient aposteme (abscess), shall we say, by the type of pain the subject reported in the affected organ (e.g., a throbbing, concentrated, hot pain of the left foot) used pain as a signifier that required learned decoding. Torturers or, rather, authors of torture tractates were equally careful observers and connoisseurs of pain. The ways in which physicians and jurists named and categorized pains, assigning different meanings to different types, are the subject matter of chapter 5. The vocabulary of pain and the shifting meanings attached to old words played a central role in the professional perceptions of pain. Theologians, too, constructed a general human theory of pain in order to explain human history: creation, paradise, the Fall, and postlapsarian humanity. The Christian history of humanity is the subject of chapter 6, though preachers also shared the stage with theologians. If a common person suffered a painful illness, it could mean remission of a few millennia in purgatory. If such a sufferer appeared in a relative's dream later on, complaining of the purgatorial pain, it could mean that loving relatives must do all in their power to shorten further the punitive period. If a sinner's soul suffered eternally in hell, it meant divine retribution. The interpretation of pain as a prognostic for future existence in afterlife belongs here.

All of human suffering was no more than a foundation for understanding Christ's pain. Christ had suffered on the cross (and he continued suffering for human sins every day) and his pain meant human salvation. Theologians devoted a great deal of thought and discussion to understanding the typology, intensity, and characteristics of Christ's pain. Their analyses, discussed in chapter 7, were no less painstaking than those of present-day neurologists. While it might be argued that Christ's role was so pivotal in medieval cultural perceptions of pain that his sufferings ought to dominate my discussion throughout the book, I have opted to place Christ's pain within the context of encryption and decoding, for that is how medieval scholars viewed it: a matter for argument, discussion, and elucidation. Though the Crucifixion was the utter cosmological use of pain, no ordinary mortal could copy it with any degree of exactitude, and all were reduced to contemplating it.

Decoding is also the topic of chapter 8. Here, I deal with the attempts to understand painlessness under extremely painful conditions and confront two opposite categories: martyrs and criminals under torture. Whether martyrs were enduring pain and hiding it bravely like medieval kings or were feeling nothing at all could never be clearly resolved. Whether criminals who slept through tortures were simply well-trained professionals or dealers in dark magic, however, did not long remain in doubt. By the end of the period under review, martyrs were diagnosed as passible and endurable, while impassible criminals resorted to witchcraft and spells. Between the late antique martyr facing a pagan judge and the late medieval suspected criminal facing a Christian judge, even impassibility stood revealed as ambiguous, amenable to opposite interpretations.

Probably from the very beginning of human history, pain has been managed, used, interpreted, and defied. Several contradictory attitudes concerning pain were prevalent in the later Middle Ages. Although there was no one consistent statement about pain, there were consistent ways of dealing with it, using it, and interpreting it. In the following, I shall attempt, not to unravel the tangle of conflicts, but to reweave them into a more coherent picture of a worldview.

Finally, a word of caution and apology is necessary. I have excluded from this book any systematic treatment of visual art, theater, and literature. The reason is not because they are unimportant: to the contrary, they are far too important to be appended to the dry bones of scholasticism, medicine, and law. Unlike the fields I analyze, art and literature have already generated a vast corpus of research on expressions of pain within them, and I am not qualified to add to it. Gragnolati, Mills, and Merback have in recent years contributed significantly to artistic and literary analyses of pain, and my work is simply another side of the same phenomenon, analyzed with different tools.[2]

SETTING THE STAGE

A book on pain draws inevitably upon a bewildering range of sources. From private letters to medicine, from rigid scholastic questions to narratives of miracles—any written document surviving from the Middle Ages became grist for my mill. To complicate matters further, the book is arranged, not by source, but by topic. Preachers and surgeons share sections and chapters cheek by jowl, as do lay mystics and duchesses. Lest readers find themselves bewildered by the crowd of unknown names, all jostling for recognition and none of them familiar to scholars from different disciplines, I have found it necessary to begin by introducing the discussants of pain. Often they wrote at cross-purposes; personal views of subjective experience informed their insights.

Writers who were part of a tradition were in the grip of past wisdom. No university-trained medieval professional could write without citing ancient authority, for those authorities were the axiomatic basis of each discipline. This is not to say that ancient roots shaped later views; as a rule, medieval writers picked and chose among the wealth of ancient wisdom what suited their purposes, using their past mostly as a validating authority.

To begin with the most impressive corpus of writers and sources, I shall first deal with scholasticism as a formative discipline to all university learning. One of the richest sources of pain theory in the later Middle Ages lies in the capacious writings of scholastics and theologians. They were the intellectuals who built the edifice of medieval Western thought. It is impossible, though, to speak of scholastic writing without seeing its background or, rather, backgrounds. Twelfth-century scholars were already heirs to a long tradition of theological scholarship, and their thirteenth- and fourteenth-century successors received an even richer influx of traditions.

Since all scholastics relied upon patristic authorities as their justification, one must begin with the church fathers. Church fathers developed their
doctrines very much in reaction to contemporary problems and divergences
in belief. How any specific father viewed pain depended very much on what
his adversaries thought and upon his need to place those adversaries in the
heretics' seat. What survived for use in later centuries was whatever ended
up being classified as orthodox. The most influential of church fathers remained Augustine of Hippo (354–430). In fighting Manichaeism, Donatism,
and Pelagianism, he established the tenets of future scholastic opinions
concerning the body, the soul, and the role of sensations. Augustine was
strongly imbued with Aristotelian ideas of the soul. Though the names of
all church fathers proliferate in scholastic references, none of them formed
scholastic anthropology to the extent that the bishop of Hippo did.

There was, however, a small trend of Neoplatonist ideas, going from
John Scotus Eriugena (ca. 815–77) to Honorius Augustodunensis (d. ca.
1115).[1] The ideas of these thinkers concerning human sensations were
naturally different from those of Aristotelian thinkers; whereas Neoplatonists tended to attach sensations to the body, Aristotelians assumed they
belonged with the soul. Neither position contradicted Christian tenets, but
each demanded a different interpretation of some of the most crucial points
of Christianity: the role of the Crucifixion in the economy of salvation and
the nature of afterlife punishment for human beings.

Twelfth-century theologians were not yet bound by scholastic schemata
of argumentation. Anselm of Canterbury (d. 1109), Hugh of Saint Victor
(1096–1141), and Bernard of Clairvaux (1090-1153) could still write their
arguments without resorting to counterarguments and imaginary debates.
Though bound by rules of logic and tradition, their argumentation is largely
straightforward. But by the middle of the twelfth century the model of the
quaestio began coalescing, and by the thirteenth century it became obligatory in almost all scholastic theological writing. As a rule, topics were first
posed as questions and then disputed between opposing teams, who finally
reached a *determinatio*, which established the required opinion and refuted
the contrary arguments.[2] With the ensuing influx of Aristotelian writing
and thinking, another formal rule came to dominate scholastic thinking:
the need for taxonomy. Topics could no longer be treated pell-mell but had
to be fitted into a clear-cut conceptual scheme and then broken down into
subcategories, each one to be analyzed apart. The first thing one did with
a question was to divide it into its logical constituent elements, each to be
treated separately.

The adversarial nature of the *quaestio* was born in the milieu of public disputations. Much of scholastic literature is the written version of oral disputations. The *quaestio disputata* was a standard scholastic exercise in which a master made a statement and his students offered opposing views. Later, a respondent was added to the team. Though there were also private disputations, the public ones are the most famous. In some public debates, men in the audience could hurl any question they wished at a debater, and the latter was allowed a day in which to construct an answer to the *quaestio quodlibeta*. The answer, when it came, was bound by the same rigid rules of argumentation as any preconceived question was.[3]

Somewhat later, vernacular theology developed without the rigid framework of scholasticism. Of a more devotional nature than pure scholastic theology, vernacular theology covered a vast field. Lives of Christ, meditations, liturgy, and the cult of saints played a much greater role in this type of writing than in scholastic debates. Domenico Cavalca's (ca. 1270–1342) *Lo specchio della croce* and the *Myroure of Oure Ladye* (fifteenth–sixteenth centuries), employed by the nuns of the Syon Convent, are excellent examples.[4]

Preachers' manuals constituted another genre that became extremely popular among clergy and mendicants.[5] Preaching had always been part of clerical duty, but in the thirteenth century the growing competition between episcopal and parochial clergy, on the one hand, and mendicants, on the other, forced all preachers to enrich their sermons with exempla, to embellish them with learned quotations, and to organize them according to the rules of sermon writing. Preachers' manuals are among the first encyclopedic works to be organized by alphabetical order: any preacher who wished to speak of the evils of riches had only to look in John Bromyard's *Summa praedicantium* (early fourteenth century) under the letter *D* (*divitia*) to find all the material he needed. The Dominican tradition in this field was especially notable, going back to the middle of the thirteenth century with Stephen of Bourbon (1190/95–1261), Humbert de Romans (d. 1277), and, later, Arnold of Liège (d. 1345).[6] Collections of exempla, useful for enlivening any sermon, increased as well.[7]

At the same time, many preachers were editing and publishing their sermons for circulation by others. Jacobus de Voragine's (ca. 1230–98) work is probably the best known. Both his *Golden Legend* (conveniently arranged according to the liturgical calendar) and his sermons, written concurrently, were much copied and used.[8] Occasionally sermon writers were inspired to add their own insights to whatever subject or saint they were writing about. Assuming that the written sermons, best-sellers in the fifteenth and sixteenth centuries, indeed served as bases for countless oral deliveries, their impact must have been considerable.[9] Finally, the later Middle Ages were also known for the number of charismatic and controversial preachers who attracted audiences in Italy, France, Spain, and Germany. Bernardino of Siena (1380–1444), Vincent Ferrer (1350–1419), and Girolamo Savonarola (1452–98) are only the best-known ones.

The written sources on pain that were available to preachers and laity varied along a wide spectrum, ranging from the learned, scholastically based Latin texts instructing preachers, to sermons, to individual meditations, and to vernacular, unofficial literature. Even within the realm of hortatory literature, the differences in emotional pitch between theological writings, handbooks, model sermons, and spoken sermons are remarkable, and personal experiences set a totally new standard of emotivity. I have quite arbitrarily divided the literature into preachers' manuals, sermons (model sermons, written sermons, and *reportatae* of live ones), biographies (whether of Christ or of martyrs), meditations, and mystical visions. This categorization does not do justice to the intermingling of genres that is typical of the entire theme. Much of the literature drew its form and contents from scholastic debates; university theologians, like Jean Gerson (1363–1429) and Gabriel Biel (ca. 1425–95), wrote and preached sermons, both Latin and vernacular. They often transposed their own materials from one genre to another. Some visionaries (at least, the men among them) also taught in schools of mendicant orders and universities. The meditations and accounts of visions they produced were popular reading for all literate society. In fact, the very act of writing them down was done in order to disseminate the record of the experience. Some of those mystics, like Heinrich Suso (1295/97–1366), were in touch with women visionaries and encouraged them to put in writing their visions and experiences. Thus, visionary literature written by women also became available. The line between the didactic and the individual record is extremely blurred, motifs seeping from one type of writing to another, changing form and content in the process. What one author of a preachers' manual recommended as a sermon subject might turn up in a sermon, be heard by an imaginative listener, and reappear in a vision. The vision might then be recorded in the vernacular (and sometimes translated into Latin) and achieve once more the dignity of the written word, becoming matter for further meditations and devotional practices.

Nevertheless, there were differences scripted in the different genres. Thus, preachers' manuals were usually sober and dry, listing topics according to some logical order and paying little attention to the reification of pain. Thomas of Chobham (d. 1233–36) employed the seven virtues as the guiding principle of his manual; John Bromyard (d. ca. 1390) simply adopted an alphabetical order.[10] Model sermons, naturally, followed the tripartite division of all sermon collections: saints' days (*sermones de sanctis*), time (the liturgical year, including Christmas and Easter, *sermones de tempore*), and special occasions (weddings, funerals, etc., *de occasione*).[11] Their style was sometimes just as dry and factual as that of the manuals, and their debt to scholastic writing is evident in their content as well as form. However, interspersed between theological points, one finds the exempla for entertaining and instructing the audience. Conversely, live sermons were exciting, full of imaginative leaps and rhetorical tricks. Spoken sermons put flesh and life on the dry bones of the models and manuals.

Meditations are an equally rich lode to mine for pain.[12] Whether genuine meditations were indeed reading material for aspiring mystics remains an open question. Nevertheless, meditations were read, known, and extensively copied. From the fourteenth century onward, the prescriptive meditation became a very popular genre. In the fourteenth century Ludolph of Saxony (d. 1378), a Carthusian, and John of Caulibus, a Franciscan, wrote detailed meditations, amounting in fact to biographies, upon the life of Christ. The latter meditation, falsely attributed to Bonaventure, was translated into several vernacular languages. As a basis for sermons, meditations, and visions, the lives of Christ were an essential source in all that concerned the Crucifixion.

Visions of the Crucifixion abound during the later Middle Ages, many of them, possibly a majority, experienced by women. While we know mostly about those whose visions received the stamp of ecclesiastical approval, there may have been far more visionaries who never recorded their experiences. Though often written in the vernacular, these visions rarely had much impact at the time. They are extremely important, though, as historical, eloquent testimony to the private practice of feeling pain with Christ. The authors of personal meditations and visions reached for the inaudible pitch of the incommunicable experience. Often, they used such terms as "a sweetness that cannot be described" or "a pain beyond description." Having exhausted all superlatives, they opted for a silence that goes beyond all expression of sensation.

The testimony of the laity, however, is not uniformly devout and pain seeking. To the contrary, there is a vast literature that stands as evidence for the human wish for surcease. This literature, however, belongs, not to the realm of medicine, but to that of thaumaturgic miracles, in which the power of saints is evinced precisely by ridding people of pain. As of the twelfth century, the greater part of the miracles recorded as taking place at saints' shrines were thaumaturgic. The manner in which the seekers for health were recorded to have behaved is an excellent indicator of norms.

People could and did approach physicians for less spectacular healing. Though it had existed from time immemorial, the medical profession was late in gaining admission to the scholastic world. Medicine as an academic field taught at universities became a general phenomenon only in the thirteenth century. Until then, most physicians (barring the graduates of the school of Salerno) had no university background.

Medicine, however, had a somewhat disreputable sister discipline in surgery. The two were distinct professions, with most physicians considering surgeons as little better than barbers and butchers. While some surgeons may indeed have practiced those two trades, there were surgeons who not only had a university education but also wrote handbooks and supervised the health of the mighty. Henri de Mondeville (1260–1320) was surgeon to the king of France; Guy de Chauliac (ca. 1300–1368) was the pope's surgeon. Both wrote compendia of surgery as loaded with quotations as those of any physician. They were part of a tradition of learned surgery that existed side by side, not always amicably, with contemporary medicine.[13]

Medical intellectual genealogy differs from those of law and scholasticism in its wide-ranging basis. The authorities that medieval physicians quoted were either the great physicians of the Greco-Latin past or the Persian-Arab tradition. The main authorities quoted by scholastic physicians and surgeons were Galen of Pergamon (ca. 129–ca. 211) and Avicenna (980–1037), both in Latin translation. The medical authors in the present book range from professors of medicine and royal surgeons to anonymous compilers of recipe collections. Among all genres of medical writing, the *consilia*, adopted as a method of writing from law, stand out as the one indicator of actual clinical medicine. Nevertheless, we know that medical *consilia* often concerned putative, rather than real, cases.[14]

If physicians aimed to diagnose, interpret, and heal pain, jurists were their opposite. They, too, were scholastically trained professionals, and they wrote *consilia* before physicians had even dreamed of them. Unlike physicians, however, their roots lay firmly in the study of Roman law. It was there that they found justification for torture and a basis for the literature of torture. The subject of torture in legal literature usually crops up within treatises and *consilia* that specifically deal with torture. In general, treatises on penal law avoided discussion of torture, which was conceived as a truth-finding mechanism, not a punishment. The treatises on torture are remarkably repetitive, concentrating upon the evidence necessary for torture.

The number of jurists who devoted treatises and opinions to torture and related topics is remarkable. *Consilia* treating specific cases are more cautious, warning against abuses of torture. Medieval jurists, practicing both as university law teachers and as private advocates or judges, invented the genre of writing up specific cases parallel with general treatises. Presumably, *consilia* were born out of the need of specific clients for a learned opinion that would argue their cases in such a manner as to convince judges to exonerate them. Consequently, the judicial *consilium* analyzed a personal case from all points of view, usually ending up with resounding proof that, according to all precedents in law, the client ought to be declared innocent. By the fourteenth century producing a volume of *consilia* became the badge of recognition for the well-known lawyer and jurist. Often, a jurist wishing to make a point would write a *consilium* that fitted the exact putative situation he had in mind.

The last type of sources I wish to discuss is hard to name. Rudolf Dekker has coined the term "ego-documents" for autobiographies, diaries, and letters.[15] I would like to add the category of "alter-documents" for all other sources describing the behavior of someone in pain. Essentially, such sources include any narrative that tells of people's sensations. Since almost all the autobiographical texts speaking of pain were written by people of religion and in connection with their religion, for the most part we must seek descriptions of sensations in other types of sources: chronicles, biographies, letters, and any other type of writing medieval history has left behind.

One of the most clearly scripted genres is anachronistically named "biography." In fact, a biography could be one of at least two genres. Hagiography was different from laudatory lives of the good and the great, but both dealt with how their subjects faced pain. In addition, one finds minibiographies of villains embedded within chronicles, if only to tell of their dread final destiny. Letters were just as strictly scripted texts, governed by the *ars dictaminis*. As literacy grew in the later Middle Ages, norms became less rigid, and different groups of society began using correspondence as a means of contact. Thus, under the heading of letters we have the literary masterpieces of Petrarch and the simple communications of Margaret Paston. Like biographies, their inclusion of pain was a matter of changing norms.

The materials of this book are an unapologetic hodgepodge of sources. There is no predefined corpus of materials that provides the basis of this study. On the contrary, my method has been to search for any mention of sensory pain and then examine the context. Although each source will be treated according to its own type and in its own place, they all share one thing: they all speak of the human condition and of human pain.

Manipulating Pain

Part I of this book quite deliberately deals with a purely medieval view of pain. While any contemporary clinical study of pain would discuss means of diagnosing, treating, or coping with intractable pain,[1] late medieval attitudes toward the phenomenon of pain were different. Certainly, there were attempts to vanquish pain, but the most common attitude, in practical terms, was to make use of it. The assumption was that pain was to a large extent ineradicable, and therefore, coping with it meant making the best of it. Consequently, various practical disciplines of life turned perceptions around by claiming that pain, rather than being destructive, was constructive in more than one sense: on the purely moral plane, as a harbinger of hell it helped fend off temptations and purify the soul; at the same time, it was a recompense for sins committed and led one to contrition. In other words, it was a salvific instrument of great power. This view was shared by devout ascetics, who undertook self-inflicted pain as a regular discipline, and preachers, who tried to make sense of involuntary pain to their audiences.

Other than moral uses, pain possessed several other applications. With the exception of England, all European legal systems from the thirteenth century onward used physical pain to extract confessions (assumed to be the truth) from criminal suspects. The connection between pain and truth was one of the basic tenets of the inquisitorial system of justice, despite constant criticism of its value. At the same time, the use of physical punishment for crimes kept increasing throughout the later Middle Ages; it was viewed as salutary both for the culprit and for society as a whole. Finally, medicine too considered the application of painful procedures as a standard mode of healing, though pain in itself carried no salutary value in medicine. Pain was thus viewed as a practically useful tool for body, soul, society, and state: not despite its harshness but because of it. The basic view underlying this practice was categorically opposed to the modern view: humans were not meant to strive for freedom from pain; they were to use pain as a ladder to climb toward salvation. Salvation would indeed include freedom from pain, even pleasure, but that vision lay outside human reality. To reach heaven, one had to climb through pain all the way up.

The discussion of the interpretation and understanding of pain as a signifier and a historical force belongs in later sections of the book, but it is impossible to understand the uses of pain for soul and body without some apprehension of the matter of which human beings, both female and male, were made. Nemesius of Emesa's fourth-century work *Concerning the Nature of Man* was translated into Latin by the mid–twelfth century and became the standard description of human creation. According to Nemesius, though the soul was infused into the body after the body's creation, it had existed already in God's mind and was coeval with the body. At no point was the human body an insensate clay figurine. On this basis pain could be explained as an integral part of both soul and body. Though he had little to say about pain, Nemesius had laid the foundation for linking body and soul in theology and medicine: pain was not a passion of the soul (i.e., a reaction to external forces) but the sensation of the passion. Indeed, sadness was literally sensed as pain in the abdomen's mouth (*os ventris*).[2] Given these axiomatic beliefs about the human frame and the indisputable fact of death, scholars and preachers could proceed from there to the interpretation of pain throughout human history.

All the uses made of pain were grounded in the perception of the malleability of the human body, and all the metaphors used for flesh, bones, and blood were of malleable substances, crafted by human forces. The malleability of the human frame through painful procedures lay at the basis of all uses of pain. Far from being a philosophical or theological question, it is one of those basic conceptions that dictate all further explanations. At the most basic level, different substances responded to different forces in different ways. Rocks could be eroded or broken, liquids flowed, and clay could be shaped into different forms and then burned in a kiln to preserve those forms. Viewing the human body even metaphorically as part of physical nature granted certain unique insights to those who considered its lesions and pain.

Even taking into account the change humanity underwent with the Fall, the best way to begin is at the beginning. Thinkers turned to the book of Genesis, especially as seen through Augustine's literal exegesis. The biblical stories of creation are somewhat contradictory. According to the first version (in Genesis 1), God created humans (both male and female) in his image and likeness, with no distinct stages for the body and the soul.[3] The second version (Genesis 2), however, does distinguish different stages of creation. First, God made man (later named Adam) out of mud (often transmuted into clay in exegesis). Next, he blew life into him. Finally, after the creation of paradise, God created Eve, both body and soul, from Adam's rib.

Two ideas shine clearly through the different accounts of creation: first, there was, according to all exegetes, the element of God's preceding intentionality (expressed for no other creation) to make a creature intended to rule the world in his image and likeness. Second, according to Genesis 2, neither Adam nor Eve was created out of new matter, or *ex nihilo*. Humans were not created but fashioned. In each case, God took something already existent—clay or a rib—and shaped it into a living being. Alone of all creation, humans were made of something else. The substance of which the human body was made was therefore central to understanding sensations. No matter how much thinkers stressed that sensations, pain among them, were part of the soul, they shared in a very embodied soul, a sensory and sensual soul. And creation from matter thus affected some of the views concerning the substance of the body.[4]

Later apocryphal sources added other elements to Adam's creation. The *Life of Adam and Eve*, originally written during the early Middle Ages, probably in Greek, and subsequently translated into several vernacular (mostly Eastern) languages, depicts Adam as formed of eight elements:

> It must be known that the body of Adam was formed of eight parts. The first part was of the dust of the earth, from which was made his flesh, and thereby he was sluggish. The next part was of the sea, from which was made his blood, and thereby he was aimless and fleeing. The third part was of the stones of the earth, from which his bones were made, and thereby he was hard and covetous. The fourth part was of the clouds, from which were made his thoughts, and thereby he was immoderate. The fifth part was of the wind, from which was made his breath, and thereby he was fickle. The sixth part was of the sun, from which were made his eyes, and thereby he was handsome and beautiful. The seventh part was of the light of the world, from which he was made pleasing, and thereby he had knowledge. The eighth part was of the Holy Spirit, from which was made his soul, and thereby are the bishops, priests, and all the saints and elect of God. It must also be known that God made and formed Adam in that place where Jesus was born, that is, in the city of Bethlehem, which is in the center of the earth. There Adam was made from the four corners of the earth, when angels brought some of the dust

of the earth from its parts, viz. Michael, Gabriel, Raphael, and Uriel.
This earth was white and pure like the sun and it was gathered together
from the four rivers, that is, the Geon, Phison, Tigris, and Euphrates.
Man was made in the image of God, and he blew into his face the breath
of life, which is the soul. For just as he was gathered from the four rivers,
thus from the four winds he received his breath.[5]

The formation of Adam began with components of the physical world—
earth, water, stones, clouds, and wind—all of which generated his negative
traits. His flesh, blood, bones, breath, and—surprisingly—thoughts, all came
from a wide spectrum of natural elements.[6] Progressing from the terrestrial
to the ethereal and the heavenly, Adam gradually became imbued with the
positive qualities of the higher world—beauty, knowledge, and holiness.
Both Adam's body and personality were thus a compound of various cosmic
elements. Adam was made in the image and likeness of God, and his body,
unlike the bodies of animals, had been intentionally created out of preexistent matter. This matter, culled by archangels from the four corners of the
earth, was no mere mud but was the finest earth in the world.[7] Thus, though
humanity was made of mundane matter, it was the best mundane matter
available. The extent to which this tradition was familiar to Western scholars and theologians cannot be determined,[8] but it accords with the Genesis
versions and their exegesis in the uniqueness of fashioning from preexistent
creation. What does surface in the West, through the metaphors and similes
of twelfth- and thirteenth-century thinkers, is the view of the human body
as "made up" of elements symbolizing human characteristics.

   Of all the elements that went into Adam's making, the most central was
the earth, or clay, as it became in later exegesis. Clay was a good metaphor
to think with precisely because it was ubiquitous, plain, and vitally essential to civilization. To begin with, it was a compound of earth and water,
soft and malleable. Fashioned and dried, it became rigid and unalterable.
Tempered in the kiln of pain, it hardened into impermeability. Hit too hard,
it shattered irremediably. Clay vessels were favorite metaphors also in the
arguments concerning the resurrection of the body, for the shards of a clay
vessel could not be remade into a whole.[9] When Dante Alighieri visualized
hell, he saw the bodies of gluttons retransmuted into earth, slowly melting
into mud.[10]

   Other substances also served as metaphors for the human body. Jerome
spoke of impassibility as a rocklike characteristic, alien to malleable humans.[11] Conversely, martyrs who withstood torture without reacting assumed a remarkable similarity to rocks in their *vitae*.[12] Even rocks, though,

could be swept along by the waters of tribulation that God sent to punish sinning humanity. Unlike rocks, which represented either superhuman or inhuman impassivity in the face of pain, metals (especially gold) were malleable when subjected to fire, as most humans were when subjected to pain. Moreover, like humans, they were cleansed of dross by fire. Purification, mostly through the actions of fire or water, was the aim of all these forces that affected the human frame.

Earth, clay, rock, metal, water, fire. So common were these metaphors that audiences and readers must have encountered them with a sense of recognition that disempowered their imaginative force. At some point, the metaphor must have lost its transcendent meaning and become a synonym: earth and clay were almost synonymous with human matter; fire and water, with pain.

All these metaphors pointed to change and decay. None of them referred to immutable substances, and all stressed the vulnerability of human matter. Created out of preexistent nature, humanity was affected by natural (and unnatural) forces, buffeted and susceptible to passions and pain. Though the biblical story stressed that pain came only with the Fall, the elements coalescing in the human frame already predicated the human ability to suffer.

The Galenic medical tradition, accepted throughout the Middle Ages, accorded with the religious narrative in one point: the human body and some of its sensations were created out of preexistent matter and forces. The fourfold scheme claimed that humanity was compounded of four humors: blood, yellow bile, black bile, and phlegm. They were closely related to heat and cold, dryness and humidity. These, the natural forces of the body, were connected to the four seasons, the four points of the compass, and the four elements composing the world (fire, water, air, and earth); while the different permutations and combinations of these elements created different human conditions, the basic elements bore a remarkable similarity to those of the religious tradition. The main difference lay in the assumption that the basic building blocks of the human physique—the humors—were inherent within the human frame, not borrowed from preexistent matter. Nevertheless, the forces that affected humanity extended to the entire cosmos.[13] Furthermore, human beings were affected by external forces: physicians counted six nonnatural forces and several forces that acted against nature. The nonnatural forces were those neutral elements (neither benevolent nor maleficent) affecting health: air, motion and rest, sleeping and waking, diet, evacuation and retention, and, finally, the "accidents of the soul," or passions.[14] Forces acting against nature were maleficent and hurtful and obviously needed no listing.[15] The same tradition permeated the world of Christian thought. Hildegard of Bingen summed up the homogeneity between humans and world, which was common knowledge in her time: "the elements are fire, air, earth, and water, and their forces work in him . . . fire is in the brain and the marrow of man [and also in the five senses]. Air is in the breath and rationality of man . . . water is in the humors and in blood . . . earth is in the flesh and bones."[16]

The fourfold scheme of the human temperament—Galen's term for a condition of the body—remained unchallenged and unchanged until well into modern times. It provided an alternative answer to what people were made of, and there is little doubt that those very basic medical ideas became part of a much wider perception. Literary mentions of the humors alone would prove this point. The assumption that people could be melancholic, sanguine, choleric, or phlegmatic was part and parcel of Renaissance non-medical writing.[17] I am not aware of any discord arising from two different, albeit fairly similar, narratives. They seem to have coexisted in relative amity. The connection was unquestionably the assumption that there was a close tie between the building blocks of humanity and the surrounding world. The concept of the human microcosm was grounded in both narratives and remained the basis of all interpretations of sensations, especially pain.

CHAPTER ONE

The Uses of Suffering

Given the usefulness of pain and the malleability of the human frame, how far was one to go in embracing it? The answer covered the entire spectrum from resignation to active self-infliction of pain. Depending upon the person in question and the circumstances (illness, martyrdom, or punishment), one could adopt a variety of attitudes. Given the varieties of painful experience, the human will played a crucial role in the different applications of pain. There were those who sought pain out, there were those who accepted it, and there were those who made their pain worse by fighting it. The guiding will, therefore, will guide the structure of this chapter. I will begin with the moral uses of pain as a deterrent to sin and as an integral part of penitence and then proceed to examine the uses jurists and physicians—the manipulators of pain—made of the sensation, if at all. Finally, I shall attempt to find a common denominator among all thinkers concerning the uses of pain.

"Waters of Tribulation": The Moral Uses of Suffering

Self-infliction and Asceticism

Shall I go to Cybele's fair grove of pines?
The lad unmanned because of her foul lust forbids,
Who by a shameful mutilation saved himself
From that immoral goddess' passionate embrace,
A eunuch by the Mother mourned in many rites.
—Prudentius, *Peristefanon*

St. Romanus, undoubtedly the most invincibly garrulous of martyrs in Prudentius's *Peristephanon*, defended Christian ascetic practices by pointing to the devotees of Cybele, who castrated themselves in ecstasy for her sake.[1] This, he ascertained, was an immoral practice. The point that emerges from Romanus's words is that ascetic practices and self-inflicted pain (though two clearly distinct disciplines of the body) belonged in many religious universes and were not specific to Christianity. Indeed, there is little indication of extreme asceticism in early Christianity. Origen, who did castrate himself, was condemned by many other church fathers; Jerome was practically exiled from Rome for advocating chastity. But, even before Jerome's trenchant advocacy of virginity, desert monasticism set new standards of fasting, vigils, and self-flagellation.[2] Moreover, the heroic tales of martyrs, who clearly had welcomed their torture and martyrdom and did nothing to evade it, branded Christianity as a religion whose holy men and women sought pain as a badge of faith and courage.[3] Both martyrs and famous ascetics are remembered in their Lives as athletes who had exercised their bodily virtues in the arena of God and won in his name.

The search for martyrdom in a Christian universe promoted some unusual cases. In the eighth century, St. Emmeram, thirsting for martyrdom, undertook a mission to the Bavarians in the hope of being martyred. As it turned out, the Bavarians welcomed him politely and allowed his missionary activities; it was not until Emmeram had succeeded in getting himself (falsely) accused of seducing the duke's daughter that he achieved his desire, in a detailed and gruesome manner.[4] Still, the frustrated search by a few for martyrdom did not lead to an alternative monastic severity. Early medieval monastic authorities were not unanimous on the subject of voluntary austerities. Though the rule of St. Benedict did ordain physical punishment in extreme cases, it avoided what was considered unbridled excesses. Conversely, monastic foundations deriving from Irish roots stressed ascetic practices far more strongly than the Benedictines did. With the enforcement of Benedictine rules in the ninth century, self-mortification ostensibly became a rarity in the West, and it even carried the faint taint of dualist heresy. When one ardent ascetic set himself up on a pillar, in imitation of the great Eastern pillar saints, the local bishop promptly ordered him down and had the pillar destroyed.[5]

The trend against extreme asceticism was reversed by the eleventh century. Holy people found self-mortification to be a substitute for martyrdom. From the north Italian eremitic communities of the eleventh century onward there is a record of increasingly severe monastic practices, not foisted upon resistant monastic communities but, to the contrary, at their insistence.[6] Figures such as the Camaldolese monk Dominic Loricatus, who wore metal plates on his body and practiced self-flagellation and difficult prayer positions, once more were viewed as heroes. Peter Damian himself wrote the *vita* of Dominic, describing in detail all his austerities. With such backing, no wonder self-mortification became a laudable form of piety. From the times of St. Francis (1181–1226), voluntary suffering and voluntarily undertaken self-inflicted suffering became part and parcel of spirituality, lay as well as clerical and monastic. Practically all the holy women of the later Middle Ages, nuns as well as Beguines and laywomen, practiced the self-infliction of pain and welcomed divinely inflicted sufferings. Men were equally zealous, with extreme cases such as Heinrich Suso, who carved a cross in his own flesh.[7] During the thirteenth century, collective flagellant processions began appearing in Europe, initiating a movement of communal self-mortification.[8] By the fourteenth century, physical suffering had become the landmark of living sanctity.[9]

There is little point in listing the various means of self-torture. Giles Constable has succinctly surveyed the list of practices, and a detailing of self-mortification methods does not explain the trend.[10] There are, however, some common traits to these practices that do need to be mentioned. First, in sharp contrast to the extravagant austerities of earlier Syrian holy men, most of these practices were performed in private.[11] Second, they were usually not one-time events but a discipline undertaken on a regular basis. Be they hair shirts, self-flagellation, or fasting, they formed part of an order of life that accompanied the practitioner for a lifetime. Unlike stigmata, a God-given gift, these practices resulted from conscious decisions. True, there are exceptions, such as the flagellant processions of the later Middle Ages, which were both public and one-time affairs, but even those processions tended to go from city to city in penitential repetition. Finally, none of the self-mortificatory disciplines involved self-mutilation. Marring divine creation was simply not a virtuous manner of ridding oneself of importunate urges. Though secular rulers used mutilation as a standard punishment for specific offenses, none of the minutely described self-disciplines were carried to this point.

One ought to ask why late medieval Christianity came to valorize and glorify so ubiquitous a phenomenon as physical pain. After all, there was sufficient physical suffering in medieval life without adding to it. A modern person, usually intent upon avoiding pain, might think self-infliction supererogatory. Nevertheless, I would argue the contrary. Just as Caroline

Bynum has shown that fasting was one way for women, preparers of food, to demonstrate their mastery over their bodies and their world, I claim that embracing pain was a way to dominate it. Rather than being enslaved by a ferocious force that could dehumanize people, ascetics and self-inflictors became masters of pain, embracing it freely and using their sensations to reach new levels of spirituality. Adopting pain as a regular discipline had several rationales, but none of them had to do with gratuitous suffering. Self-inflicted suffering was never gratuitous: it could be penitential, saving the sufferer further pains in purgatory. At the same time, for those intent upon a religious life, it had a specific Christian context: it was the most common form of *imitatio Christi* in the later Middle Ages.[12] While one could imitate Christ at any stage of life or divinity, late medieval religious sought mostly to imitate the Passion and Crucifixion of Christ. By the fourteenth century, the theme of a God who had died blameless for the sake of humanity in the most shameful and painful manner imaginable was central to Western Christian religiosity. Empathizing with Christ's pain and feeling it, even having it stamped upon one's body in the form of stigmata, was the ultimate accolade for mystics. Many of these sensations were a gift from heaven rather than a self-imposed discipline, but there are numerous records of self-inflicted pain not as a mode of penitence or as an athletic, martyrological exercise but as a form of identification with Christ.

The Christian self-infliction of pain was thus not simply part of a universal trend of spiritual people seeking to mortify the body in order to raise their souls to new heights. It was deeply tied to the most basic narrative of Christianity: the Crucifixion.[13] While the tradition of self-inflicted pain in Western Christianity was taken to new extremes during the later Middle Ages, it remained tied to practices of the body that stressed a voluntary choice, constant discipline, the privacy of one's own individual body, and respect for the wholeness of the same.

Penitence as Pain

Penitence was perhaps the most salutary of pains, inflicted by one's own self upon oneself in remittance of sin. Lest we dismiss penitence as a purely psychological, internal process, we must see how penitence appeared in the words of preachers and their guides. Already Bernard of Clairvaux had compared contrition to a caustic salve that causes stabbing pain.[14] His successors went farther in their efforts to construct penitence as pain straddling both body and soul. When William of Auvergne discussed penitence, he included under contrition the visceral passions (*motus*) of fear, shame, pain, anger, indignation, abomination, expulsion (*vomitus*) of horror, hatred, execration, and detestation (of sin, of course).[15] William was thus aware of the role of emotional pain within contrition, but he also included somatic elements within his description. This instinctive recoiling was one of the mixtures of emotions and sensations that led people to genuine penitence. He was not the only one to view true penitence as pain, and the entire tradition of penitential literature deliberately did not differentiate between physical and emotional pain in this context. Two centuries later Pelbart of Themeswar (d. 1504) conflated the two in his sermons. Penitential sermons naturally belonged in the penitential season of Lent, and Pelbart let loose the full arsenal of penitential emotion for the Sundays of Lent. He deplored the fact that people wept for the death of a friend or child or at the loss of a fortune but shed not a single drop in regret for their sins. Genuine penitence was not the clear-headed decision to avoid doing wrong; it was emotional suffering of the most agonizing kind, of the sort that ought to bring out rivers of weeping.[16] Tears were the road to salvation and were, in the words of Jacobus de Voragine, the witnesses of pain, wounding the sinner's heart.[17] The preacher deliberately elided any distinction between sensory and emotional pain, using the term *dolor intensus*—a term any physician might have employed to describe physical suffering—to blur any irrelevant differences.

Confession of sins, of one type or another, had existed in Christianity since late antiquity. It was not, however, a religious duty that laypeople regularly fulfilled. The big change in lay confession began with the interiorized religion of the twelfth century. Abelard was the first to insist that all must confess their sins and that confession was primarily an internal process, to be followed only later by the verbal act. Confession was about the recognition of sin for what it was, repentance, and its rejection—all essentially interior processes. These theories became practical when the Fourth Lateran Council (1215) ordered all believers to confess at least once a year, at Easter, and then take communion. By then, mendicant orders and their preaching had begun to hammer into their audiences the urgent need to confess only to an ordained priest, at any time, because nobody knew when their end would come.[18] Numerous exempla told of people who had died unconfessed and unshriven, thus ending up in purgatory or, worse, in hell. In some stories, the dead were miraculously resuscitated for a few minutes, only to confess and receive the sacrament of penitence.[19]

How were penitence—and penance—presented to the laity in hortatory literature and sermons? The presentation, despite the wealth of exempla, was extremely sophisticated. Confession and preaching handbooks continued to stress the interior dimension of penitence, the fact that oral confession formed only a small part of the process, and the utter importance of perseverance in contrition. Though the confessor was viewed as a healer of the sick, contrition—*contritio in corde seu gemitus*, as Abelard had defined it—was the essential basis for any moral conversion.[20] Late medieval handbooks of penance, however, viewed contrition, not as a cerebral decision, but as an emotionally overwhelming crisis. The penitent was to feel deep remorse and express it in weeping. Tears were the visible manifestation of contrition. Stephen of Bourbon listed the fourteen ways in which the penitent was to weep: like those who were disinherited, despoiled, widowed, orphaned and bereft, wounded, made captive, unjustly accused, besieged, jailed, charged with debt, oppressed, giving birth, being sentenced to death, and in great danger. The very grief of contrition and the weeping often erase the sinner's guilt, without having performed any active penance. In general, the virtuous had many good reasons to weep, for themselves as for others, and their tears were of great healing value.[21] Those who did succeed in weeping for their own sins, said Pelbart, were in reality sensing the greatest of terrestrial pains. Those on the threshold of death ought to weep not only with their eyes but also with their souls.[22] If Stephen stressed the first, internal stage of penitence, John Bromyard stressed the last one: the firm perseverance of the penitent not to fall into sin again.[23] He began by distinguishing between certain, dubious, and false penitence. Most of Bromyard's rather-disillusioned comments on penitence have nothing to do with affliction, but with decision. All his exempla come down to the same moral: those who repent only when sick or in danger and those who do not remain firm in their penitential decisions are cheating God.

Neither Stephen nor Bromyard recommended any physical penance. Stephen concentrated upon fasting as a discreet penance that would save the penitent embarrassment, and pilgrimage as the overt penitence.[24] Bromyard prescribed no penalties at all, either dictated by the confessor or self-imposed. He did mention penitential practices, but only as an illustration for an argument against dubious penitents: those who fast when the food is bad, who avoid wine when not thirsty, who keep a [hair] shirt on in cold weather, who give to charity when they have no other uses for the money, and who pray in church when they have nobody to gossip with.[25] Both authors insisted that what mattered most was the will to repent and that the penance was of lesser importance. The pain of the heart, they said, was greater than the pain of the body. Stephen of Bourbon tells the exemplum of a knight who had wished to do penance but rejected all of the bishop's suggestions. The bishop therefore asked him what he loved most, and the knight answered that his favorite activity was feasting, whereupon the bishop strictly forbade the knight to undertake any servile activity. Perversely, the next day the knight found himself plowing, though he had never done so before. The knight returned to the bishop, telling him of his failure to observe the imposed penance, and the bishop asked him what food he hated most. The knight responded that he most disliked raw leeks, which the bishop then forbade him from eating. Inevitably, the knight found himself eating raw leeks, and this time he realized the virtue of obedience, and submitted himself to the bishop's prescribed penance.[26] We can glimpse, beyond the obvious moral of the story, the bishop's utter tolerance toward a willful and stubborn penitent and a genuine attempt to bring him to repentance without using coercion.

Sermons inclined even further toward contrition and grief rather than punishment. Penitence was closely tied to the figure of Mary Magdalene, presumed since the sixth century to have been also the anonymous sinner of the Gospels. Indeed, the Magdalene was "preternaturally disposed towards weeping" as Katherine Jansen puts it. Late medieval mendicant preachers, especially the Franciscans among them, depicted her as actually melting into a puddle of tears, liquefied by lachrymosity.[27] Parisian thirteenth-century preachers dwelled upon the blessings of suffering, using, among others, the recurring images of fire purifying gold or cleansing liquids.[28] Jacobus de Voragine spoke quite openly of the emotional pain of regret and penitence.[29]

Penitence was thus clearly distinct from penance. In clear contrast to practices of self-infliction of pain undertaken by the heroically devout, what preachers advised for most people was not self-flagellation but genuine remorse. Nor did preachers prescribe physical penalties for their communities. Was this caution simply a policy geared to attracting penitents? I rather think that preachers had a different reason for avoiding physical penalties. Sensory pain was not considered a harsher penalty than continence; a whipping was a one-time punishment, not a manner of beginning a new life free of sin, and was therefore probably viewed as a lighter penalty than a conversion to a virtuous life.

In conclusion, penitence was pain, though one would be hard put to class it as either sensory or spiritual. It straddled both categories: genuine remorse was manifested in genuine weeping that drowned both soul and eyes in tears. The pain of penitence also included the renunciation of vices and the adoption of austerity. Most of all, it was supposed to be genuine, heartfelt regret, and such regret was undoubtedly painful.

"Illness Is Christ's Messenger"

One of the numerous *artes moriendi* of the fifteenth century, the *Prohemium de arte bene moriendi*[30] counted the pains of terminal illness as a danger rather than a blessing. Men are beset by temptations when dying, one of them being the despair resulting from the sharp pangs of terminal illness, "probably a fever or an aposteme," that drive them mad and induce despair. The way to avoid despair was to accept these pains, renounce life, and welcome death.[31]

This text is a startling exception to the norm. Practically all late medieval religious texts dealing with pain counted it a blessing, not a danger. The idea that pain might distract people from concentrating upon salvation is extremely unusual. Both sermons and theoretical thinking on the uses of pain contained a great deal of material on involuntary pain, usually praising it. Illness and a lifetime of pain could easily be a fit subject for a sermon in several contexts. A text from the book of Job, a martyr's feast day, or simply a standard Sunday sermon could discuss how one could build one's hopes, fears, and understanding of life upon the irregular and abnormal that often became a regular part of life—illness and pain. Illness was a trial, a source of suffering, and a path to death, but it certainly had a positive role in Christian life. As Augustine had put it, pain is useful because it indicates life. It is better to have a painful wound than an insensitive gangrene, for the latter indicated the death of the affected organ.[32]

The paradoxical attitude to pain can best be seen in the approach of preachers to illness. Illness could be a punishment from heaven, a warning, or a sign of divine favor, but most often it was the latter. It was never accidental. Medieval Latin used the same word, *salus*, for "health" as for "salvation." In a world of the unsaved and uncondemned living, salvation and health swung like a cosmic pendulum back and forth. Physical illness was a bonus that might tilt the scales in favor of eventual salvation, for the pain it carried was payment in lieu of some of the years in purgatory. Hence, said the preachers, one should accept pain in life not only with resignation but gladly, for uninvited suffering was the greatest blessing God could bestow upon a human being. Neither a punishment nor the joke of inscrutable fate, it had a clear positive purpose. William of Auvergne's trenchant affirmation of the value of pain is perhaps the most strongly worded and the most richly imagined, but it is not unique.

Indeed, things that hurt, as you know, mortify and extinguish the con-cupiscence of desire, bodily and secular impulses. They mortify and di-vest men of those desires. You also know from others how harmful such desires are to men, because they capture, intoxicate, weaken, dissolve, blind, and madden people, body and soul, in all possible ways. Therefore, you can see how salvific pain is, extinguishing all of this and removing it; because it is powerful medicine, like absinthe destroying worms or like dangerous lye melting dirt. Because of these two—mortification and cleansing from vices—it is called waters of tribulation in the prophets' words. You must know that it uproots even avarice and pride with all their seeds, and just as the fire hardens and toughens the surfaces of clay dishes and makes them impregnable to water, and even to itself [i.e., fire], so that fired surfaces fear neither fire nor water, thus the pain of present tribulation arms and fortifies human souls, defending them like an armor.[33]

William of Auvergne's view of pain emerges through three metaphors. One, though unusually contextualized here, is the well-known image of fire. Fire is probably the most common metaphor for pain; both hell and purgatory are pervaded with various kinds of flames serving as punitive, pain-inflicting agents. Moreover, most martyrs were tried by fire at some point during their agonies. As fire in the crucible purifies gold, so fire in martyrdom purified saints. William perceived fire, not as an annihilating, all-consuming force, but as a cleansing, testing one. As it hardens earth-enware pots in a kiln, so it sets and materially alters human clay, mak-ing it impermeable to evil. And human beings were indeed made of clay, or earth, as the story of creation showed. Malleable at first, they become inflexibly virtuous once fired with pain.[34] The second metaphor, also con-cerned with processes of change, could almost have emerged from a labora-tory: a corrosive, slithery substance like absinthe or lye that gnaws away at vice, washing and cleansing the soul.[35] A liquid, often water (especially wa-ters of tribulation, to which William refers later), is the ultimate cleanser. As all could remember, God had once used the waters of tribulation—the Flood—to cleanse the earth of sinners.[36] But vice is too deeply embedded to be washed off, for it alters the very nature of mankind. To be removed, it must be destroyed, totally annihilated, even though the corrosive substance will also eat up the putrid flesh that hosts vice. Like a surgeon's knife, it re-moves the sickness with all that surrounds it. Pain is therefore destructive of vice and constructive of internal strength. Working inward, so to speak, it obliterates evil. Though its beneficent action may be directed from the outside, just like evil, it penetrates beneath the skin, materially altering the affected person's substance, making it impermeable to the trickles of temptation.

These statements are only the opening of an entire chapter devoted to the positive value of pain (*de bono doloris*).[37] Pain is a God-given medicine to cure human souls, granted out of the Creator's goodness. Any refusal to apply it or an attempt to circumvent it means refusing the remedy for the ill. The reader is left with the impression that physicians practicing anesthesia or analgesia of any sort are the devil's own collaborators. Any arguments claiming that pain originated with neutral, indifferent forces like disease or other people's malice were no more than empty sophistry. Forces other than divine intervention did cause pain from time to time (as Satan did to Job), but their agency was of trivial importance, for they were mere tools. Cruel people who caused unnecessary pain would eventually be punished by the appropriate (human) agencies, thus duly bearing the suffering too. But those who suffered at their hands would have in fact received a priceless gift from God: the gift of pain and its cleansing effects.

In the end, William returned to two of his original metaphors, the waters of tribulation and the cleansing fire. Fire and water are omnipresent in theological literature. Both are cleansers and agents of conversion and salvation, and both are agents of destruction and pain. At this point, both elements were far more than mere metaphors: "If indeed you wish to find out about the usefulness of pain and to count how often pain is called both water of tribulation and fire in holy, true writings, think about the action and operation of natural fire, and you will find the similarity and proportion of their actions and spiritual usefulness."[38]

This passage is unique in the literature about pain. It describes the usefulness of pain for generating human virtue in terms entirely divorced from heroic models: neither *imitatio Christi* nor martyrdom make any appearance in this text as models for constructive suffering. The salutary effect of suffering is stated simply and factually, as much a part of reality as the existence of devils or grass or any other part of the universe. Was the bishop of Paris trying to launch a call for universal asceticism and the banning of practical medicine? Far from it. Rather, his statements are a rueful acknowledgment that pain is there, unsought and unavoidable, just as rocks are there. Unlike rocks, however, it helps strengthen and shape people.

One would expect to find this flowery, fiery language in a sermon, an exhortation, or a piece of pastoral writing. Instead, it appears in an encyclopedia. *De universo*, though, is not an encyclopedic compendium in the manner of Hrabanus Maurus's ninth-century homonymous treatise. Ostensibly,

William's main arguments are with the writings of Avicenna (980–1037) and with his Aristotelian opinions concerning the eternity of the world. In fact, much of *De universo* is a polemic against the Cathar heresy, a combination of natural philosophy and pastoral guidance. The section on pain is a digression from discussing Avicenna's views of Providence.[39] "How and why does he allow the evil to flourish, to accumulate power, riches, and crimes? Similarly, for what purpose does he tolerate the afflictions of the good and their oppression by the evil, while those same evil ones rule the good?"[40] The only way to reconcile an ever-present Providence with the reality of triumphant evil was to make a virtue out of suffering.

Paradoxically, in William's sermons he rarely recounts the blessings of human suffering in such a forceful way. In one pre-Lenten sermon he did repeat that illness and tribulations were causes for glory, but when preaching, William sounded far more like a philosopher than he did when writing philosophy:

> First, because it is a virtue that heals the mind . . . tribulation of the body is like torture, which heals the mind.[41] . . . Torture is perceived as a wound or an illness, although it is health. By the same token, tribulation is seen as an illness, although it is health of mind. . . . Tribulation is the medicine of the Highest. . . . Thus, he who is sick of mind must rejoice when he is given tribulation as a hope for health, as if a physician had come to him. Second, tribulation pays our debts, and it is a great mercy of God to accept our present tribulations in place of future punishment. It is like he who is owed a gold or silver mark and accepts for them beans or pebbles and the account is settled. One bean, in relation to a silver mark, is more than present tribulation is in comparison to future pains. . . . Third, tribulation is a sign of divine love. . . . Fourth, tribulation teaches man. . . . Fifth, tribulation induces hatred of present life.[42]

In contrast with the impassioned tones of *De universo*, the sermon is written as an outline for preaching, enumerating virtues and citing biblical texts. It does not bear the style of a real, preached sermon, certainly not one delivered to a lay audience. The message, however, is the same: those who fall ill must count themselves blessed. Illness improves their mental health, diminishes the expected period of purgatorial suffering, and induces asceticism in the sufferers. Such is the mercy of God that he is willing to accept the beans of human suffering in exchange for the gold of the human debt.

William was ahead of his time in his praise of suffering and tribulation. The benefits of painful illness became increasingly dominant in devotional literature during the fifteenth century. With the proliferation of the *artes moriendi*, Jean Gerson (1363–1429) added another great benefit to sickness: it presaged death; it allowed the sick to prepare their souls, to give up the hope of bodily health, and to concentrate upon the health of the soul.[43]

Delivering a public sermon on pain and its value was perhaps conceivable only in the fifteenth century. A few decades after Gerson, the Dominican Johannes Herolt (d. 1468), whose model sermons were extremely popular for more than a century after his death, devoted one sermon to the subject.[44] While far less emotional than William of Auvergne's work, Herolt's sermon adduced even more reasons for embracing and welcoming illness, putting together all of the previous arguments. All sickness, even a headache or toothache, was a harbinger of death sent by Christ in order to encourage people to prepare for leaving the world. Furthermore, suffering purged people of previous sins (though not as drastically as William had envisaged), strengthening the soul at the body's expense. Thus, the sick find no pleasure in the vanities of life but concentrate on confession and penitence. It is God's special gift to some people and will shorten their stay in purgatory. Finally, and most importantly, it is a guarantee of eternal salvation, a door to heaven, and a form of *imitatio Christi.*

In praising sickness and pain, it was essential to acknowledge that sickness was salutary precisely because it made people suffer, which people did not wish to do. One way to make them accept illness was to point out the future advantages: any illness on earth would compensate in advance for much worse sufferings in the future. Illness thus stood for the sum of all earthly pains: its evil was good, its life was death. In trying to make sense out of a most common and prevalent phenomenon in contemporary life, late medieval preachers had found a way to valorize individual involuntary pain. They advised penitence and virtue; they did not advise the laity actively to seek pain. Flagellants and lay ascetics were more suspect than welcome to the clergy.

The similarity between William of Auvergne's and Johannes Herolt's approach to pain is obvious, but there is also a difference. William was careful not to interpret unsolicited pain as *imitatio Christi;* Herolt did so, granting the lay sick the dignity of being imitators of Christ. Two centuries of discussions and sermons about pain had produced a change: we find that personal suffering, voluntary or otherwise, came to be viewed as the imitation of Christ.

In conclusion, the discussion of pain in hortatory literature changed: pain had always been seen as a trial of fortitude, as the book of Job showed.

But from the thirteenth century onward human involuntary pain began to be equated with the voluntary pain of the saints: it was a God-given blessing, a purifier of souls and destroyer of vices and appetites. Those who had not chosen to afflict their bodies but had been granted affliction ought to count themselves blessed in every sense. By the fifteenth century, the terminally ill had almost been assimilated into the category of voluntary pain seekers. Even if one did not inflict pain upon oneself, it was just as useful when it came.

But the tale of the uses of pain, from voluntary self-infliction to involuntary illness, does not end here. Not every illness was mortal, and survivors carried with them the memory of pain and the attendant fear of recurrence.

"Take Away Pain and You Have Nothing to Fear": *Fear, Pain, and Memory*

Most humans familiar with pain carry the memory within them as a permanent mark and therefore fear its recurrence. At the same time, memory and fear magnify, and sometimes even cause pain. So close is the connection that the causality can easily be inverted with the claim that fear was the source of pain. Such an argument was not a matter for preachers but for theologians trying to explain how, in purgatory and hell, a virtual fire harmed the virtual bodies of real souls. One twelfth-century explanation came from the psychological realm. Souls were capable of feeling fear, and souls carried memories of pain:

> The force of pain is established not in the torment but in the feeling of the sufferer. . . . so why do you fear fire and flame unless because you fear to be burned? But if wounds and blows did not give pain, who would fear arms or weapons? Indeed, it is the fear that causes the pain: stones and blows do not hurt in themselves; it is the perception of torture that they imprint upon the soul that hurts.[45]

The words come from the stylus of Hugh of Saint Victor (1096–1141). Hugh had undoubtedly read and interiorized Augustine's famous words concerning the power of memory to re-create the past within the present. Augustine, however, had presented memory as a vast storehouse from which he could pick and choose at will, discarding all that was distasteful to him.[46] Hugh saw memory as a trigger of an ever-present looming force, impossible either to ignore or to resist. One did not choose which memory to carry. Memory, for Hugh, was the recollection of pain and fear of pain. Thus, fear served to create pain in a place where normal pain could not exist.

Basing sensations upon recollection and previous trauma, however, was not the way followed in later centuries. Other explanations of infernal sufferings replaced Hugh's psychological approach. The only other instance I know of recollection as a pain inducer comes, not surprisingly, from a fellow Victorine, Richard of Saint Victor (d. 1173). The power of pain to outlive the injury, for Richard, was closely connected with the observation that the sensation persisted long after the initial injury, and prolonged pain made a greater impact upon memory. His context was such that subsequent fear could have little place within his scheme of pain and memory. In a rather-gruesome passage, Richard of Saint Victor discusses the story of Shechem and Dina in Genesis 34. As the Vulgate tells it, Dina, Jacob's daughter, was raped by Shechem, who subsequently asked to marry her. Jacob agreed, provided Shechem and all his people were circumcised. But Dina's brothers Simon and Levi were not content with this solution. Waiting until the third day after the circumcision, "when the wound's pain was sharpest,"[47] they took their swords and killed all the people of Shechem in revenge for the rape. According to Richard, Simon and Levi waited until the third day because then the pain was at its worst. The reasons for this exacerbation were spiritual, not corporeal. On the first day, memory dwelt upon the loss of the beloved sexual customs, and this memory caused grave distress. On the second, the sentient soul discovered that through bodily damage it had also injured its mind, which aggravated the pain. On the third day, the soul realized that, though it had already suffered greatly through its decision, it must expect worse from divine judgment.[48] Thus, the cruelest pain of unanesthetized circumcision was the realization that pain was not over; an even worse pain awaited the sufferer. Given that Shechem and all his people were killed by Simon and Levi just as they had realized this, it seems that fear of further pain aggravated their sufferings only for a short while, though they undoubtedly continued suffering later in hell.

Perhaps the most interesting aspect of this discussion is that it does not take into account the very simple fact that all pain outlasts injury.[49] All causes prolonging and aggravating the corporeal pain of circumcision were attributed to the memory and the intellect.[50] Regret, puzzlement, guilt, and fear were the purely spiritual pain-causing factors. Extrapolating from the hapless Shechem and his people to all other injured humans, the Victorines traced pain as it traveled various roads, all within the mind and the soul.

The impact of pain covered past, present, and future. Mourning for past pleasure, coming to terms with present mental limitations, fearing worse in the future—all these caused and aggravated pain, says Richard. In his exegetical world, only minds, not knives, had the power to hurt.

Explanations of human suffering in hell—a problem that had puzzled theologians since Augustine's time—veered in the opposite direction in the thirteenth century. In the realist climate of the thirteenth century, recollections and fear of pain in the world assumed a new function: they were first-class deterrents for prospective sinners. The memory of pain and the fear of its recurrence, asseverated pastoral pain specialists, must be interiorized as part of one's own soul. The theme recurs among hortatory and philosophical writings; true pain, pain that "works," is not the blow, nor the lingering pain, but the image that one carries away in one's mind and senses after the bruise has disappeared. The marks left upon the soul need not be viewed as scars, for they do not harm the soul, but as an integral part of the person. Pain, they all said, was not felt at skin level, nor did it work to the person's benefit there. It seeped in, became part of one's memory and personality, and working from inside, it affected the entire person. Fear of pain carried inside the soul was the motive force that benefited people.

Still, one could not entirely divorce the body and sensations from pain by means of a theological interpretation. After all, even if pain was apprehended by the soul and resided there, it originated in physical sensations. It is therefore necessary first to see how medieval thinkers constructed the human physical entity. The understanding of pain invariably required the construction of human bodies, their substances and fluids, their architecture and connections. It was a question, not for healers only, but for any thinker who wished to consider the subject.

The theme came up in William of Auvergne's reflections upon *timor*, the useful passion that aided people in avoiding sin. In the treatise on *mores* (or, rather, virtues and vices) William sang the praises of fear:

I am mightily frightened of the enemy, of the jail of hell, of death, and of torture. So I turn the fire and sword against him [i.e., the devil] into the protection of a formidable and safe armor. In fact, I turn hell itself into an impregnable fortress. . . . I place hell in front of my eyes, and use that which would kill me as a shield. . . . Hell is a fear that deters evil persons who wish to commit evil deeds from carrying out their actions. It strikes servile fear into them and restrains their hands (but not their souls entirely). For, as Ambrose says, in men of this sort, the will to sin remains and the deed would follow if impunity could be expected.[51]

In other words, nothing served as well to dampen the fires of concupiscence as envisioning the fires of hell. Though William's fears centered upon the future, he considered the effects of present fear of the future as equivalent to those of present physical suffering. Passing easily from fire to other tribulations (such as water), he viewed them all as the teacher's rod or the washerwoman's laundry-beating stick (both geared to cleansing) or a bogeyman. Thus, he conflated the cause (pain) with the result (fear). This fear did not cause further pain; to the contrary, it prevented the horrible experience of hell. If one carried the knowledge of what pain felt like within oneself, one could envision a painful punitive future. Hence, he concentrated his praise of fear upon the bogeyman, harmless in reality but extremely efficient as a threat of pain because children attributed all sorts of horrible capacities to the frightening figure:

> [Hell] frightens the evil, for criminals, when speaking of the gallows (which, they say, is called *gibetum* in vernacular), call it, though tongue-in-cheek, "frightener" [elsewhere *expaventaculum*]. It is the same as what the people call *Malvesin*, that is *Barbualdus*, who is shown in order to frighten children, and mothers and nurses warn them that he will swallow them if they do this or that. *Barbualdus* in French is a terrifying figure or picture that mothers and nurses use to deter children.[52]

Pain and fear, then, had the same deterrent effect upon people. The very contemplation of future pain reified it, turning forebodings into either present tribulation or future remission. Suffering in this world, then, had a double salutary effect. Not only did it cancel out some of the time that was due to be spent in purgatory, but it also prevented people from accumulating more time in purgatory.

In general, William was careful to map the strands that connected emotions with sensations. In this emotional atmosphere fear assumed a personality and a clear form: "I [i.e., Fear] am the porter and guardian of the human heart. . . . I am the guardian of the two-bladed sword. . . . I [i.e., Tribulation] am a torturer, bent not upon killing but rather upon life."[53] The personification of fear and tribulation as the angel guarding the gates of paradise against a renewed human incursion, or as a good torturer,[54] underscores fear's duty to inflict suffering upon humanity.

William was writing these statements at a time when newly appointed inquisitors were battling Cathar heresies with a new legal tool—the inquisition of heretics, occasionally coupled with torture for extracting confessions. As we have seen, William devoted an important part of his work to confuting Cathar beliefs, and his manner of combating evil seems to have suited both questioning and torture. The difference between the inquisitors and the bishop of Paris is that he saw evil everywhere, also when free of heresy, and suggested that the same inquisitorial methods be applied also to his flock. After all, fear and pain were the best medicines against sin.

Frightening the faithful for their own good was an acceptable idea in the thirteenth century. Practically all preachers' manuals openly avowed the same aim: terrifying their audiences into obedience.[55] Thomas of Chobham (d. ca. 1233–36) wrote his handbook for preachers (a craft he practiced only rarely)[56] roughly during William of Auvergne's lifetime. Given that Thomas had studied in Paris, the similarity between the two is understandable. Thomas entitled his chapter on penalties for sin "Quomodo auditores abterrendi sunt": how to terrify listeners.[57] The answer was simple: speak of hell and its fires, of what pain does to the souls of the dead, and make the listeners fear this pain. Fear softened people, made them pliable, and made them repent. Though repentance born only of fear was insufficient, it was better than nothing. Pain was decidedly one of the things that frightened people most. But Thomas, true to the aim of his work, did not bother to praise fear as a deterrent; he merely recommended that preachers transmit the dread of pain in the afterlife to their audiences. Thomas did not allude to the possibility of divine retribution on earth. Though the Bible and saints' lives were full of stories of divine retribution, in reality the unjust rarely endured a bolt from heaven. Evidently, immediate divine vengeance was not a sufficiently credible threat. Such a penalty was chancy and vulnerable to contrary proof (as in Job's case), whereas purgatory and hell were an utter certainty.

A cleric writing or preaching about the terrors of hell was mapping out the grim possibilities of the afterworld while doing his best to scare his listeners into behaving themselves according to his lights. Because of sheer forgetfulness, whether intentional or not, it was difficult for people constantly to bear in mind what might await them after death; dwelling upon it constantly, exciting the auditors' imagination and fears, might actually save a few souls.[58] Sermons, visions, and meditations on purgatory and hell reached an unprecedented level of popularity in the later Middle Ages. But one did not have to wait until death to encounter pain. It was present in life, every day and every hour. The shepherds of Christian thought and behavior also put pain suffered during life into their writings. The aim was twofold:

first, to make sense out of pain and give it a purpose and, second, to use it as fear had been used—as the schoolmaster's rod, both deterrent and punishment. Pain and fear of pain were both useful.

The Legal Infliction of Pain

From pain as an autonomous force we pass to the infliction of pain. The following sections treat of topics that will recur in other contexts further on. At this point, I concentrate purely upon the uses of torture and bodily punishment. The interpretation of pain inflicted in punishment belongs below, in chapter 6.

While to modern eyes the two procedures, namely torture and punishment, seem almost indistinguishable, in medieval legal systems they belonged to two totally different parts of the law. Torture belonged to the law of proof and was the preferred method of eliciting confessions from criminal suspects from the thirteenth century onward in most of continental Europe. The infliction of torture was predicated upon the certainty, not that the suspect was guilty, but that there were sufficient grounds for assuming guilt. The use of torture lay in bringing to conclusion trials in which no certain proof of guilt existed barring the culprit's confession.

Those found guilty of a crime were punished. The idea of punishment inherently assumes the existence of a superior, ruling force that can evaluate, legislate, judge, condemn, and execute the sentence. Punishments were deemed to be useful as far back as human memory went. The punishment might outlast existence, as the punishment of the damned after doomsday, but physical penalties meted out by secular authorities—even death penalties—were still considered useful, because existence continued after death.

Torture

"Torture is an inquiry performed in order to elicit the truth by means of torments and bodily pain."[59] This definition recurred, with some variations, in all legal treatises discussing torture. The very definition of torture contains the use of inflicted pain. It stresses the nature of the result: truth.

There is written evidence of the torture of crime suspects in Continental courts beginning in the early twelfth century. The legal literature concerning torture is massive, consisting mainly of repetitive treatises, *consilia*, and court records. None of it, however, says anything about the useful results of torture. Conversely, much of the literature contains warnings against unrestricted use of torture and its possibly lethal results. The very basic assumptions of the practice—that torture was useful for eliciting confessions and that those confessions were true—never needed to be stated or defended and thus were never even discussed.

These axiomatic assumptions were not limited to lawyers and judges. They permeated the literature of martyrdom, which is wholly based upon Roman torture. For a successful martyrdom one needed first a brutal prefect/governor to extensively and imaginatively torture the heroic Christian. Had humane Roman judges refused to do so, a very great portion of the foundation narratives of Christianity would never have been written. Martyrdom, in fact, shows that torture was useful for more purposes than the law envisaged. Even if one discounts most martyrdom narratives as powerful myths, we are still left with Tertullian's (ca. 160–ca. 230) indignant complaint about the misuse of torture against Christians:

> And then, too, you do not in that case deal with us in the ordinary way of judicial proceedings against offenders; for, in the case of others denying, you apply the torture to make them confess. Christians alone you torture to make them deny; whereas, if we were guilty of any crime, we should be sure to deny it, and you with your tortures would force us to confession. Nor indeed should you hold that our crimes require no such investigation merely on the ground that you are convinced by our confession of the name that the deeds were done, you who are daily wont, though you know well enough what murder is, nonetheless to extract from the confessed murderer a full account of how the crime was perpetrated. So that with all the greater perversity you act, when, holding our crimes proved by our confession of the name of Christ, you drive us by torture to fall from our confession, that, repudiating the name, we may in like manner repudiate also the crimes with which, from that same confession, you had assumed that we were chargeable. . . . "I am a Christian," the man cries out. He tells you what he is; you wish to hear from him what he is not. Occupying your place of authority to extort the truth, you do your utmost to get lies from us. "I am," he says, "that which you ask me if I am. Why do you torture me to sin? I confess, and you put me to the rack. What would you do if I denied?" Certainly you give no ready credence to others when they deny. When we deny, you believe at once.[60]

Put in a slightly less rhetorical way, Tertullian claimed that torturing Christians was a travesty of the Roman legal system. They admitted their guilt at once and then were tortured to make them lie. There is no reason to disbelieve Tertullian's accusations, and what emerges is that in third-century Carthage (and perhaps in Rome too) torture was put to more uses and misuses than jurists had ever dreamed of.[61] In the writings of another, somewhat later Christian, one can still see how deeply ingrained torture was within Roman perceptions. In one of the basic narratives of martyrdom, Prudentius has a martyr posthumously exorcizing a demon by questioning and torturing it.[62]

This vision of torture as the fickle tyrant's instrument of abuse coexisted in late medieval Europe with intricate treatises on the correct uses of torture. For instance, when Angelo Clareno described the persecution of Spiritual Franciscans in the early fourteenth century, he put Tertullian's arguments into the mouth of an outraged rural castellan from southern Italy, revolted by inquisitorial interrogation tactics: "By my body, such justice will not be done in this town, that faithful Catholic men confess [their faith] and are tortured so that they deny it!"[63] The persecution of true believers had to be performed through the abuse of torture proceedings. This view of torture naturally undermined the belief in its effectiveness in producing truthfulness. Nevertheless, both positions saw torture as a useful tool, precisely because it was so flexible and amenable to different uses.

Corporal Punishment

The same rationale that dictated the praise of pain in hortatory literature lay at the basis of corporal punishment. "The aim of law is to correct the punished one, or that the punishment should improve others, or that, once evildoers are removed, the rest should live in greater safety." Thus proclaims the legend written beneath Pieter Breughel the Elder's famous engraving *Iustitia*. The artist presented his own ideas of how justice was to be meted out in the themes of the engraving: they are all different forms of capital execution, from decapitation to the wheel. In many senses, the engraving and its legend illustrate early modern views, when the vernacular words for "justice" (*faire justice* or *justicier* in French, *Hinrichtung* in German, *justiciar* in Castilian) all meant public capital execution. The trend of identifying justice with execution, though, had begun centuries earlier. In late medieval northern France the *droit de haute justice* meant the authority to pronounce and execute a capital sentence. The term "justice" therefore meant, not the abstract quality we tend to attach to it nowadays, but the political authority to pronounce over people's lives and deaths. Both law and justice were viewed as power, but power was supposed to be exercised for good, not evil.

Breughel's legend is also early modern in another sense. Medieval jurists considered the first purpose of law to be retribution, not correction. In the late thirteenth century, Philippe de Beaumanoir, standing so to speak at the cradle of state prosecution of crime, saw the state as taking revenge against malefactors, and thus merely replacing the private avenger. Later jurists no longer referred to punishment as revenge but as retribution, and later as correction—though the subjects of Breughel's engraving had no life left to correct and redeem.[64]

Throughout late medieval and early modern Europe, the subject of justice began assuming a markedly moral character.[65] Justice had a morally sanctioned purpose, and consequently, increasingly painful penalties for crime had a rationale. If the malefactor could no longer be corrected because justice had killed him already, the painful manner of his death would certainly count toward lessening his time in purgatory.[66] Furthermore, justice ensured both communal correction and peacekeeping. Consequently, most painful penalties were meted out in the public sphere in order to educate the public, while the payment of fines required no public spectacle.

The range of painful punitive measures extended from a combination of shame and pain in the pillory, where an uncomfortable position was combined with public harassment and ridicule. Public whipping was a common punishment, practiced even by ecclesiastical courts.[67] On the scale of severity, whipping (which presumably left little permanent marking) was followed by penalties of permanent mutilation and defamation: ear cropping, branding, and various other mutilations. In these cases the publicity was double: the maiming was first performed in public and was thenceforth inscribed in a person's body and public identity till death. Though the law considered these penalties defamatory—a matter of shame, not pain—one cannot ignore the fact that this ill fame was carved upon the culprit's body in a painful manner.

Execution was at the top of the scale of severity. There were different types of execution, depending upon local law, the culprit's status, and his crime. As a rule, throughout Europe thieves were hanged, murderers beheaded, and traitors executed in slow, painful stages that took their bodies apart.[68] The exact practices varied from country to country, with German executions being the most drawn out and painful. Given the chroniclers' relish for great drama, we naturally possess records of the most solemn executions.[69] Most famous late medieval executions were described, not as occasions for mass entertainment, but as dignified educational events, conducted according to a strict, solemn ritual. A great deal of thought, inventiveness, and expenditure went into staging these events. Such executions were preceded by carefully traced processions along symbolically charged routes (e.g., passing by specific churches or crime scenes), sometimes interrupted at significant points by educational sermons, declarations of guilt, and petitions for prayers for the culprit. In political executions, affiliations and guilt were mirrored in heraldic symbolism and specifically colored clothes.[70] Outside Germany there is little evidence of preexecution torture before the sixteenth century. What appears in German illuminations is usually pinching with hot pincers, but those illuminations usually accompany general texts like the *Sachsenspiegel* or later the *Constitutio Carolina*, and there is no evidence that they mirror actual practice.[71] Executions were meant to be rituals of pain in the sense of penitence, not of infliction.

However, one must remember that for every famous, carefully staged, and widely attended execution there were numerous cases of plain punitive hangings. There is no evidence that run-of-the-mill criminals merited a solemn procession. Nevertheless, they did receive public attention after their death, if not before. The place of execution in most cities was public, often outside the walls, and visible to all incomers. Wherever there was a gibbet, it was found upon a hill not far from one of the city gates. François Villon's description of the dead hanging in the wind until their bodies disintegrated has remained the most pathetic reminder of late medieval and early modern executions. While Villon was speaking of Paris, his description fitted most European cities of the time. Thus, even the nameless petty criminal who left no record either in the sketchy trial protocols or the more selective chronicles of the period left a cautionary grisly vision and smell for the living.

The publicity of painful punishments stands in stark contrast to the closely linked practice of judicial torture, which, as we shall see, was invariably performed in the most secret of places.[72] Clearly, European public authorities (urban or territorial) had no inhibitions about inflicting pain in public. To the contrary, the spectacle of pain was salutary for the viewers as well as the sufferer. The difference between the two practices lay in the degree of culpability. A suspect tortured for the sake of a confession was not a proven criminal; hence, there was no virtue in the pain and no benefit in exhibiting it to the public. However, the penalties of *iustitia* were all public for good reason: as well as retribution, they clearly advocated the virtues of pain not only for the personal body but also for the body social.

The body social, however, was rather selective when it came to the choice of members destined for amputation. Noblemen could find themselves on a rather-ornate gallows for treasonable activity. The poor might find themselves hanged, or drawn and hanged, for offenses that wealthier criminals could compensate for with discreetly paid fines or private settlements. For the most part, European crime records show that letters of grace could be obtained for murder much more easily than for theft, and that obtaining such a remission hinged more upon "honest" status than upon the crime.[73]

Public physical penalties were thus part and parcel of life in medieval cities. They may well have been part of rural life, but villages had their malefactors hanged on a convenient tree by an itinerant hangman and left too few records of punishment. Cities maintained, as part of their standard expenses, a permanent gibbet and at least one full-time, salaried hangman, whose job it was also to flog those sentenced to public whipping. Cities also had the symbolic space in which to conduct lengthy processions as educational spectacles. But whether it was an adulterer in York, whipped three times around the Cathedral church, or a Parisian thief hanged on Montfaucon, the punitive infliction of pain was invariably public, for it was useful for spectators even more than for the culprit. However, after death the public spectacle vanished almost entirely, to remain only in the mouths of the witnesses to underworld punitive pain: the preachers who spoke of purgatory and hell.

In the Afterlife

A famous exemplum, told by several writers of sermons and exempla collections, recounts the tale of a man who suffered from a bitter illness. When complaining, he was granted a vision in which he was offered the choice between a lifetime of pain and two hours in purgatory. The man first opted for the latter choice, but after one minute in purgatory he recanted, choosing a lifetime of pain instead.[74]

This is one of the rare cases in which preachers enthused over the pains of purgatory; as a rule, they were more prone to tell in detail what happened in hell. Hell, however, had no use whatsoever. It was eternal punishment, and none of those entering its gates could profit from the pain. Its only use was as a deterrent to the living. The difference between purgation, medical or moral, and absolute punishment was essential. According to most authors, purgatory was meant mainly for two categories of people: first, those who had repented and confessed but had not been able to achieve their penance before death overtook them and, second, all those whose sins were venial rather than capital (e.g., those who had clung too fondly to life: wife, children, or possessions).[75] In general, it was the place for all those who had shown some penitence and remorse during their lives.

Notwithstanding Jacques Le Goff's insistence upon the birth of purgatory in the twelfth century, earlier thinkers had acknowledged its existence.
Augustine of Hippo, Caesarius of Arles (468/470–542), and all the visionaries who had toured hell and heaven knew all about purgatory.[76] They knew
that it was a place of fire, and, almost to a man, they asserted that the pains
of purgatory were no different from those of hell except that they had a set
term. Thus, the fires of purgatory had a use: like the crucible, they purified
souls, readying them for paradise through pain, whereas the fires of hell
simply burned on endlessly.

All the same, purgatory earned little attention in comparison with hell.
Most authors contented themselves with repeating that purgatory was no
different from hell, barring the hope that prevailed in it. When Stephen of
Bourbon treated the pains of purgatory, he simply referred his readers back
to the chapter on hell, barefacedly borrowing Augustine's list of penalties
of living criminals for those of purgatory.[77] Thomas of Chobham transposed the comment on the direness of purgatorial flames to his section on
hell, commenting that hell was even worse than purgatory. The pains of
purgatory were subsumed under the heading of hell, and before reaching
the topic of purgatory these authors had already exhausted their tales of
suffering.[78]

Nevertheless, when preachers spoke of purgatory, they usually sounded
a different message. In his sermons Jacobus de Voragine insisted that purgatory was distinct from hell, a *forum mixtum*, for there was not only punishment in purgatory but punitive justice that granted a minimal measure
of glory to the place.[79] In the Holy Monday sermon, Jacobus used the cup
of unmixed wine in Christ's hands to expatiate upon three interpretations:
unmixed wine signifies heaven, mixed wine signifies purgatory, and the
cup of dregs signifies hell. Purgatory is where "after the addition of pain,
one receives glory." It is a mixed forum, where justice is done and, because
of the certainty of a future in heaven, hope exists.[80] Two centuries later,
the Franciscan preacher Roberto Caracciolo (1425–95) insisted too upon the
separate character of purgatory.[81]

Visionaries also paid close attention to purgatory. Although it was usually sandwiched between the tour of hell and that of heaven, it did earn
one entire and distinct vision: the *Purgatory of Saint Patrick*, written in
twelfth-century England, was a best-seller translated into several vernacular
languages. The twelfth-century poet Marie de France produced the Anglo-
Norman version.[82] The description, however, supports the theological terse
position: as far as pain and punishment went, purgatory was no different
from hell. The only one to make a clear distinction in her vision was Santa

Francesca Romana, who noted that, whereas the fires of hell burned black, the fires of purgatory shed light.[83]

Interestingly enough, most preachers did not harp upon the virtues of pain; they spoke of alleviating the pain of others. Rather than being warned of their dreadful postmortem future, people were told what their loved ones were suffering now. They were urged to contribute subventions for the dead, to pray, to aid their departed friends toward salvation. It was an act of supreme charity, for the suffering of souls in purgatory (while not eternal) was still worse than anything on earth.[84] Sermons included the *clamores* of suffering souls, begging for help and liberation like all prisoners.

Jacques de Vitry, John Gobi, and Stephen of Bourbon told many stories of sufferers appearing in dreams to the living, begging for help.[85] Nevertheless, exhortations did not stop at enlisting subventions. It was also possible to secure early release for suffering souls through individual penitence. Several holy women, including Christina Mirabilis and Catherine of Siena, had done so; however, simple believers could also practice penitence for the sufferers.[86] In these exhortations the pain of purgatory was not the focus; rather, the emphasis was upon how to shorten others' time there by dint of praying, securing indulgences, and making subventions.

While the fires of purgatory shrank in the medieval imagination in comparison with those of hell, they helped stress further the usefulness of pain. Pain could provide salvation, even beyond the grave. One could buy off purgatorial time not only with subventions but, more so, by taking upon one's self the punishment due to another. Catherine of Siena rescued her father in this way, and several other holy women performed similar feats. While no preacher advised his flock to attempt this themselves, the practice existed among those who felt themselves to have sufficiently mastered pain so as to use it.

Healing through Pain

Illness, misfortune, penitence, and punishment could bring salvation precisely because they were painful. In contrast, nobody extolled the virtues of pain as a healing force. To the contrary, all physicians and surgeons were in accord as to the need, in some cases, to sedate the pain prior to performing a procedure. No medical authority praised pain as a health-giver, but all of them recommended procedures that were unquestionably painful. Physicians and surgeons did not choose these procedures over putatively painless ones because of the merits of pain, but because they saw no other alternative. Moreover, they did not overtly consider the possibility of avoiding certain procedures because they were painful. For instance, one would take care not to bleed an overly weak patient, for fear of killing her, but avoiding cauterization because it was painful and frightening was inconceivable.[87] Unless the pain resulting from treatment was severe enough to kill, there was no medical reason to avoid causing pain in the process of healing. Pain attendant upon a procedure was not a category healers considered as an argument for avoiding it. Only in *consilia* did physicians distinguish between tolerable and intolerable pain, and the distinction concerned only pain as part of the disease, not the treatment. Of painful treatments healers have nothing to say.

I have been unable to find any procedure or medication that was recommended *because* it was painful. The point may seem moot to us. However, given the context of the late medieval preoccupation with pain and occasional praises of pain in nonmedical texts, this attitude is by no means obvious. The ancient linkage of *dolor* with illness and the later one with punishment (*poena*) indicate that, beneath all the cultural constructs that praised and sought pain, the original human shrinking from pain remained unaltered. When all was said and done, the healer's job was to rid the patient (directly or indirectly) of the pain. Surcease might not have been the primary goal of physicians, who often considered pain an ancillary phenomenon, but in the end the recommended cure was meant to also bring freedom from pain.

It is important to remember that the great majority of the suffering sick agreed with this point of view. People turned to saints, physicians, or simple healers to have their pain eased, not increased. No matter how vociferous the literature in praise of pain is, it cannot silence the evidence for the basic human search for painlessness.

Conclusion

This chapter began with the multifarious uses of pain for the betterment of humanity: it armed people against temptation and helped them recant; it kept social order and maintained justice; it accompanied common medical and surgical practices without healers questioning it.

How does one explain the uniformly utilitarian attitudes of professionals in different fields toward pain? Given the basic human recoiling from pain and the search for painlessness, this attitude raises questions. Why did professionals consider pain so useful? It might be argued, on a superficial level, that authoritative spokespeople of various disciplines did no more than make the best of a bad business. After all, they had no means of ridding humanity of pain, so they might as well make a virtue out of necessity. I would argue the opposite, however. Finding ways to ease pain was not considered the problem. The main reason that healers did not search for such means was that there was no reason to do so. One would not wish to annul such a useful force.[88]

Having disposed of the facile answer, I would suggest that the merits of pain were so much a part of Western culture in other fields of thought and action that when it came gauging the role of pain in a moral and utilitarian manner, the answer was obvious, if somewhat tautologous. Aside from a purely medical point of view, pain was useful because it was good, no matter how one felt.

CHAPTER TWO

"Twisting the Mind"

Torture and Truth-Finding

Torturing suspects in order to gain a confession is, according to legal historians, a phenomenon typical of European Continental legal systems from the thirteenth to the eighteenth century.[1] According to John Langbein, with the abolition of ordeals in 1215, European legal systems had no way of finding the truth other than through confession. The rules of evidence demanded by the ensuing development of the Roman-canonical system were so rigid that only a confession could meet all demands.[2] This thesis is perfectly valid, provided one assumes that all early medieval trials were resolved by ordeals and similar ritual methods. Despite the colorful nature of ordeals, which have captured a great deal of historical attention,[3] research into early medieval legal practice has shown that the great majority of cases were settled by compromise, testimony, and circumstantial evidence rather than ordeals, duels, or oaths.[4] True, ordeals were used in cases where there was no evidence, but their abolition, and the establishment of new rules of evidence, did not automatically entail the use of torture. As the case of England shows, one could rely upon juries for the truth. The literature of ordeals and torture contains very little description of pain. All the same, both procedures, especially torture, were unquestionably agonizing. In this case, we must dig below the dry descriptions of procedure to elicit through imagination and empathy what the *patientes* felt when tortured. The suffering is implicit in the texts, although they practically never mention it explicitly.

In this chapter, I will make two arguments. First, it is my hypothesis, though I cannot prove it, that torture in secular courts never really vanished in medieval Europe between the disintegration of the Roman Empire and the thirteenth century. Second, that one cannot explain the practice within a purely legal context. I intend to contextualize the practice of torturing suspects as a means of truth-finding within ideas of pain and truth prevalent from the thirteenth century onward. Furthermore, I will distinguish between the theological and legal ideas of confession and analyze the influence of one system upon the other. In both cases, the purpose was to reach the truth via confession. Finally, I will describe to the best of my ability the different methods of torture and their development over time.

Trying to prove truth by one means or another is fairly common to all human societies. The practices that were familiar to medieval thinkers distinguished various types of truth. Side by side with Aristotelian logic, truth was sought in astrological configurations and bibliomancy.[5] A third way of arriving at the truth was by divine revelation. When it came to verifying the truth in law, the standards were necessarily different, for logic could not prove ownership of a house or the identity of a murderer. Legal truth required facts, and fact-finding was subject to rules that were different from those of logic. Nevertheless, no search for a truth is context free. The very method of search defines the nature of what the searcher considers "truth." If truth is the transcendent meaning of life or the sum of angles within a triangle, one cannot expect a charter to supply it. If truth is the boundary line between two fields, one can indeed expect a charter to prove it, though in certain cultural contexts divine intervention could do so as well.[6] At the same time, divine intervention does not prove the sum of angles within a triangle: human reasoning does. Different truths, then, require different methods of proof.

Legal fact-finding, as we have ascertained, can rely upon a number of methods, and pain need not necessarily be one of them. Indeed, though late medieval jurists relied heavily upon Roman law as justification, most of Roman law did not assume that fact-finding involved torture. When the Roman jurist Ulpian (170–223) wrote about torture, it was in the context of extracting evidence of adultery—always a difficult accusation to prove—from household slaves. Only slaves and suspected traitors could be tortured in classical Roman law, a limitation that essentially made torture fairly useless as a tool of criminal investigation. Whatever was done in practice—if it diverged from the written texts—left no traces, and medieval jurists knew only the written texts. Most of the sixth-century *Corpus iuris civilis* section upon torture (*Digest* 48.18) is based upon Ulpian, and thus irrelevant to medieval reality.

From Roman Law to the Twelfth Century

The Roman Law of Torture

The honor of shaping the theoretical underpinnings of the practice of medieval torture falls to Roman law, enshrined in the *Corpus iuris civilis* of

Justinian (482/83–565).[7] While torture practices changed throughout time, the theory changed very little.[8] The *Digest* provided Ulpian's original definition of judicial torture, or *quaestio*, as it is called already in antiquity: "By torture we mean the infliction of anguish and agony on the body to elicit the truth."[9] This definition, with numerous minor variants, was to reappear in practically all late medieval torture treatises. The *Digest* also stated that torture was a last, not first, resort in a criminal investigation—when all the facts were in, and only a slave's corroboration was lacking. Furthermore, the law demanded that torture should avoid causing permanent physical damage, "so that the slave will be whole, either to [achieve] innocence or to face the death sentence."[10] Minors under the age of fourteen were exempt unless the case was one of treason. The argument was usually that the harshness of torture might well kill a young boy, and certainly make him lie.[11] Finally, in a group of suspects, the *Digest* suggested that it was best to begin with the most fearful or the youngest.[12]

Between Ulpian's time and the codification of Roman law four centuries later, the scope of torture grew gradually wider. By the compilation of the *Codex Theodosianus* (438), even high-class people could be tortured if suspected of witchcraft, while lower-class ones could be tortured upon almost any criminal suspicion.[13] Though Justinian's later codification mitigated some of the severity of the Theodosian code and narrowed the scope of torture, a great deal of the fourth-century legislation did remain in practice.

All these bits and pieces, and several more interspersed in other sections of the entire *Corpus iuris civilis*,[14] were incorporated into the scholastic law of torture a millennium or more later. As early as the second century there ran the thread of uncomfortable knowledge that some (or most) people would say anything their questioner wanted to hear in order to free themselves from torture. Ulpian claimed that it was *res fragilis et periculosa*, "a chancy and risky business." People confessed to whatever the judges wanted, if only to avoid pain, regardless of the truth. Further, he elaborated: "There are a number of people who, by their endurance (*patientia*) or toughness under torture (*duritia tormentorum*) are so contemptuous of it that the truth can in no way be squeezed out of them. Others have so little endurance (*inpatientia*) that they would rather tell any kind of lie than suffer torture; so it happens that they confess in various ways, incriminating not only themselves but others also."[15] At the same time, the *Digest* also incorporated an edict of Emperor Augustus that posited almost the opposite: "I do not think that interrogations under torture ought to be requested in every case and person; but when capital or more serious crimes cannot be explored and investigated in any other way than by the torturing of slaves, then

I think that those [interrogations] are the most effective means of seeking out the truth and I hold that they should be conducted."[16] The ambivalent attitude toward the efficacy of torture was to continue throughout the Middle Ages.

When it comes down to medieval practice, there was little in the Roman law of torture that could serve jurists. In medieval times neither the types of people who could be tortured nor the reasons for their torture nor the methods had much to do with ancient Roman law. It was useful as academic camouflage, but no more. When thirteenth-century jurists were faced with a practice of venerable age and no acknowledged intellectual ancestry, they happily adopted the *Digest*.

Ordeal as Truth-Finding

The closest we can come to torture in the early Middle Ages as a mode of eliciting the truth from a body in pain is through ordeals. Recently, Patrick Geary has claimed that "judicial violence" had existed in the Carolingian Empire. This violence, however, is predominantly punitive, not investigative.[17] The ordeal procedure, undoubtedly painful, was clearly unknown before the fifth century, when it is first mentioned in histories and Germanic laws. Until a few decades ago, legal historians could still claim that ordeals, duels, and oaths were the standard modes of proof in early medieval courts.[18] But even when modern scholars argued that ordeals functioned well within the social dynamics of small communities (thus achieving the epithet "rational"),[19] they still believed that these methods were arbitrary and their outcomes preconceived and prejudiced. The results of ordeals were ambiguous, requiring manipulation and communal interpretation. Respectable community members could even avoid an ordeal by producing champions or serfs to take their places or a sufficient number of oath-helpers (respectable people to support their oath), an option denied to lesser members or to strangers. In sum, historians considered the procedures primitive and superstitious, whereas the new torture-based methods were modern and scientific.

Primitive and modern, superstitious and scientific, are malapropistic epithets for the two methods. Early medieval court decisions mentioned written documentation and eyewitness testimony as standard modes of proof.[20] The use of supernatural means for ascertaining the truth was reserved for those cases where no other proof was available. Oaths, judicial duels, and ordeals were the exception rather than the rule.[21] What evidence there is for the use of "irrational" proofs usually comes not from court records, nonexistent before 1215 (the usual date for declaring ordeals obsolete)[22] but from chronicles, letters, or records of ecclesiastical councils. In fact, most of the evidence for ordeals (other than the liturgy, which is prescriptive) is anecdotal and dramatic: a legendary queen (Iseut or Cunigunde) proving her chastity through the ordeal of hot iron or a Catholic defeating an Arian in an argument by pulling a ring out of a boiling cauldron unharmed.[23] There is no indication that ordeals were used as a matter of course when there were other possible avenues of verification. In contrast, inquisitional torture was part and parcel of the daily activity of European courts in later centuries and was recorded as such in protocols. The much-vaunted dramatic shift from ordeal to torture never took place. The transition that did take place, slowly and fragmentarily, was the transition from a flexible system of multiple types of proof that privileged litigants to a strict system that accepted only the most stringent standards of direct proof, thus privileging personal confession over testimony and circumstantial evidence. The latter system also privileged the authorities over the litigants.

Even when it came to ordeals—ostensibly the most painful of the pre-inquisitorial methods—very few texts contained an admission that holding a red-hot iron or plunging one's arm into boiling water was actually exquisitely painful.[24] Certainly, none of the legislation or the liturgy does. The reality of pain in ordeals surfaced only in exempla and in miracles. Miraculously, an innocent undergoing an ordeal felt no pain. Equally miraculously, confessed and repentant sinners remained unscathed by the red-hot iron, but if they relapsed, they were burned even by the cold iron and screamed with pain. A heretic who had failed his ordeal, recanted, and confessed prior to execution had his wound and pain miraculously disappear.[25] These exempla were repeated long after ordeals had become a rarity. But they were based upon one genuine experience: undergoing an ordeal was at the very least frightening, probably very painful, and possibly lethal. If, as Edward Peters says, torture was a kind of ordeal because surviving it somehow proved innocence,[26] then the ordeal was a kind of torture too. Though in stories the innocent remained unscathed, the real omnipresence of pain in ordeals argued that all those put to the ordeal were a priori guilty.

The Blurring of Ordeal into Quaestio

Two traits were traditionally presumed to characterize the new system: the inquisitorial procedure and the Roman-canonical standards of proof.[27] The inquisitorial procedure meant that all criminal cases were initiated, prosecuted, and punished by public authority rather than by private, injured parties.[28] The new standards of proof meant a narrow definition of what constituted acceptable proof. By the thirteenth century, confession had become the "queen of proofs," better than any other form of evidence.

The legalistic view was usually tied to papal legislation. "It is a commonplace among legal historians to observe that the abolition of ordeals led to the adoption of torture as an investigative device," observed Richard Fraher.[29] Bluntly put, since the courts had lost their method of ascertaining the truth with the banning of clerical participation in ordeals in 1215, they needed a substitute tool. Stephan Kuttner has offered an alternative explanation: torture was an imitation of Roman practice, tied to the revival of legal studies in the twelfth century.[30] In contrast, both Raoul Van Caeneghem and Edward Peters have insisted that the inclusion of torture in judicial practice did not result from Roman law studies, nor was it a purely judicial phenomenon: "It was not the revived study and application of Roman law in the twelfth century, nor a leaving off of earlier barbarian practices alone that caused these changes, but a complex combination of changes in society and political authority that influenced the new legal procedure in several different ways."[31] Judicial practice, not the ivory tower, was responsible for the increasing use of torture.

Reality, however, refused to fit neatly even into this juridical transition. Torture appears in sources before the abolition of ordeals and the latter survived after its abolition. As Jacques Chiffoleau has shown, there were ordeals recorded all over Europe in various places after the Lateran Council of 1215, to say nothing of duels, which persisted well into the modern era.[32] Some of the earliest instances of torture mentioned in the sources testify to a confusion between the two practices. As early as the late ninth century, Pope Stephen V (886–89), writing to Archbishop Ludbert of Mainz, forbade the clergy from subjecting to an ordeal parents suspected of accidentally suffocating their children during sleep. While such prohibitions were fairly common in the following centuries, what is most striking about Stephen's letter is his own confusion. Apparently, the pope was unfamiliar with proof by ordeal; he thought that the procedure he had disallowed was investigative torture, meant to extract a confession: "for the holy canons do not permit extorting a confession from someone through the test of hot iron or boiling water."[33] The test of the hot iron or boiling water was supposed autonomously to prove guilt or innocence by the state of the damaged limb (following the burn or immersion) a few days later. No confession was necessary, and none asked for. What the pope knew was that confessions were extorted by the application of physical pain, and he assumed that this was done by means of the heat of iron or water. In other words, the manipulation of pain blurred the lines of demarcation between the two practices. Some

juridical authorities could still see little difference between torture and ordeal as late as the twelfth century. The *Tübingen Lawbook*, a learned legal
text presumably composed in southern France during the 1160s or 1170s
and influenced by Bolognese learning, sounds remarkably like Pope Stephen:
"The testimony of men of respectable lives, who cannot be corrupted by
favor, friendship, or money, shall be accepted upon their oath. However,
men of low standing [*vilissimi*] and those who are easily corrupted shall not
be believed according to their oath but shall be subjected to torture, *that
is, the judgment of fire or boiling water*" (my italics).[34] The first legislative
text to mention torture, the *Liber iuris civilis urbis Veronae* (comp. 1228),
spoke of torture as coexisting with the duel and the ordeal. The *podestà* was
enjoined by these statutes to search out the truth in controversial matters
either by means of a duel or another ordeal or by means of torture.[35] Roughly
at the same time, Emperor Frederick II's *Liber Augustalis* (1231) spoke of
torture and ordeals (especially judicial duels) as two alternatives available
for interrogating people of dubious reputation, whose standing did not allow
them to clear themselves with an oath.

From the strictly utilitarian point of view, both practices eventually
achieved the same result. They provided knowledge or truth at the price of
bodily pain. They were both applied as a last resort, when no other evidence
could be found. And they were both applied only to people whose credibility was doubtful, and who therefore could not clear themselves by oath. In
other words, they were relevant only for *vilissimi homines*, either suspects
or people of no credibility or community standing. People rightly feared
both procedures and did their best to avoid them.[36] It made little difference
that ordeals and torture used different methods to elicit the truth and that
the source of truth differed depending on which system was used. Even the
names were similar: in canonical discourse, ordeals were *purgatio vulgaris*,
while torture (or oath, in the case of a clergyman) was *purgatio canonica*.[37]
Purgation—a cleansing, a means of violently expelling the truth from a person (either from his body or through his words) at the cost of pain—was
essentially the same.

There were also instances of judicial torture openly and licitly applied
without any confusion as far back as the eleventh century. Hildebert of
Lavardin (1056–1133) mentioned secular torture in one of his letters, object-
ing to clergymen's involvement in such a practice.[38] There is also evidence
from the diocese of Laon indicating that torture was informally used during
the early twelfth century, between 1113 and 1117. It is entirely possible
that bishops before Hildebert had also known about secular torture and not
intervened, or even had initiated it.

Together with Paul Hyams, I believe that the gradual disappearance of ordeals was due to "merely the cumulative effect of many individual acts that arose from actual cases."[39] Given Pope Stephen V's confusion, it is possible that interrogatory torture, legal or otherwise, had never vanished from practice. Like the love that has no name, the pain of torture may have remained nameless but present until the Roman vocabulary, revived in Bologna, crept into judicial usage, thereby giving the procedure a respectable (though ahistorical) ancestry and a score of names.

Whatever the reasons for the gradual discontinuation of ordeals, the growing use of judicial torture was bound up with a number of twelfth- and thirteenth-century trends. It had to do with centralization of justice, with its professionalization, and with the growth of scholastic culture. But most of all, I argue, it had to do with the contemporary climate and culture of pain. In a world that eulogized and enshrined suffering, infliction of pain upon blameless people could not be considered wrong. As we shall see, the pain of martyrs and of criminal suspects had some parallels in late medieval language.[40]

The Ecclesiastical Shift

Judicial torture may well have survived in Western practice from Roman times to the eleventh century, when it surfaces in written sources. Since ordeals were practiced only rarely at the time, it is very likely that those classes of suspects subject to torture under Roman law would remain so in later centuries. We have no sources to prove this assumption, but the earliest mention of torture makes it clear that it was customarily used in secular courts. Hildebert of Lavardin, bishop of Le Mans, knew of torture in secular criminal courts. Hildebert's letter is a rebuke to a priest who, as a theft victim, had had a suspect tortured. The bishop's reaction was sharp: "Subjecting suspects[41] to torture or extracting the truth by means of torture lies within the discipline of the [secular] court, not the church. . . . You are not an executioner but a sacrificer."[42] It is better for a priest, said Hildebert, to let his lost money go rather than subject another to certain pain and danger because of dubious suspicions.

Neque enim carnifex es, sed sacrifex. A priest is one who celebrates a sacrifice, not one who executes. In this sentence, Hildebert squarely identified torture with capital punishment. He was leaning heavily on late antique Christian discourse. From the time Christianity had become legal, Christian thinkers and communities had had to face the unpalatable fact that their own coreligionists were now no longer acting as martyrs and victims of the law but as its enforcers and executioners.[43] Augustine had faced the problem more than once. In *The City of God* he concluded that Christians must serve as judges, even if it meant condemning suspects to torture.[44] But in another letter, quoted by Hildebert, Augustine was extremely disapproving of clergymen who used pressure and even ecclesiastical sanctions to recover stolen property: "Since we are reluctant to give up what we know was both wrongly abstracted and can be returned, we accuse, we blame, we denounce them secretly and publicly. . . . Sometimes, if there is nothing more important, we even deprive them of the sacrament of the altar."[45] Hildebert quoted these sentences, concluding that, although Christian laymen could send suspects of uncertain culpability to the certain sufferings of torture because the judge's office must be done, the clergy had no such privilege. Clerics must resign themselves to loss rather than resort to torture and sanctions against suspects. Very much like early Christians, early-twelfth-century clerics were not to appeal to secular authorities, who used torture.

Hildebert's letter has been cited as proof that torture was in use in secular practice much earlier than expected, at least in the diocese of Le Mans.[46] The bishop of Le Mans, however, was hardly voicing a unanimously held clerical position in his letter of reproof. Hildebert's colleagues in the episcopate had no inhibitions about torturing suspected heretics long before the legal rules of inquisitorial practice were established by Pope Innocent III.[47] Corroborating evidence of secular practice, though not of ecclesiastical disapproval, comes from the diocese of Laon, indicating that torture was used during the early twelfth century. A thief who had stolen the church's treasury was identified thanks to an ordeal by cold water, and then he was "tortured from morning to evening, ten times hanged [i.e., on the strappado] and ten times taken down, until the judge saw him falter, and swore that if he allowed him to hang any longer he would not be brought down alive."[48] The torture was not aimed at getting a confession, for guilt had already been proven by ordeal, but to find out where the thief had hidden the treasure. In this case, to regain church property, Bartholomew, the bishop of Laon, had absolutely no inhibitions about ordering a secular judge to use torture.

There is one point about which the bishop of Le Mans and the bishop of Laon seem to have agreed: there was nothing wrong in extorting confessions through torture, as long as the church spilled no blood. Hildebert may have been more squeamish than Bartholomew, but neither of them disapproved of torturing laypeople in principle. Furthermore, there was not a shred of doubt as to the veracity of the extorted confession.

Within the span of one generation after Hildebert and Bartholomew, canon law came openly to accept torture. Gratian (fl. 1140–50) strongly disapproved of bishops who tried to extract confessions from suspected priests by means of torture, but if a bishop stood accused of an infamous crime, and the accusers were not credible, the truth had to be elicited by torture:

> Those who are suspect in their Catholic faith or of enmity should not be allowed to accuse bishops. Nor those who confess [testify to] crimes at other people's will. For so carefully should the truth be made manifest that it cannot have a voice *in those who have discarded their own will* [my italics]. Here the God-fearing torturer must extract [the truth] by means of various tortures from its hiding place, so that while they are subjected to corporal pain, what has happened should be faithfully and truly ascertained.[49]

One could not accept an accusation against a bishop unless the accuser proffered it spontaneously and would repeat it *under torture* as the truth. The paradox of torture and free will is patent in this case: witnesses who were coerced into testifying at others people's will were not trustworthy, since they had discarded their own will; therefore, truth could not use them as a voice. Was truth then consonant with one's free will? Only, it appears, as long as that will was subject to torture. Being unreliable, such accusers (even those who came forward of their own free will) had to be tortured so that they revealed the truth—not at their own will, of course, but at the god-fearing executioner's will. Truth, it appears, stood revealed when the accuser relinquished his will to the appropriate authorities. Torture was the means for extracting the truth even *against* the accuser's will.[50] Neither Hildebert nor Gratian ever doubted the efficacy of torture in extracting confessions and neither did they doubt the veracity of these confessions. In this matter, canon law was to alter its attitude in later centuries: Gregory IX's decretals only threatened reluctant witnesses with excommunication. His decretals, however, concerned clergymen involved in illicit marriages, so the omission of torture is not surprising.[51]

Early ecclesiastical ideas about torture may be better documented than secular ones, but the practice is not in doubt. Torture in secular courts existed long before it was wrapped in academic discourse. Once the learned secular tradition began in the thirteenth century, not a single jurist referred back to the question of veracity. At the same time, they did point to the many dangers of torture as a reason for avoiding it whenever possible. The attitude toward torture had been inverted: whereas earlier it was a secular procedure, execrated by churchmen, it now became the prerogative of religious procedures. With the beginning of the systematic hunt for heretics in

the thirteenth century and the establishment of inquisitions for this purpose, any pretence of distance between church and torture vanished.[52] "[I]t
was standard canonistic doctrine that all ecclesiastical judges were able to
employ it [torture], especially the torture of vacillating witnesses or those
of 'vile condition.'"[53]

What stood at the basis of late medieval practices of torture was—among
other things—a strong belief that causing pain was salutary and that it
brought out the truth. The twelfth century was the time when confessions
began to become private rather than public,[54] when confession was first tied
not only to the guilt of deeds but to a genuine inner penitence as essential
for absolution, when all salvation or damnation became centered in the
human will. Ordeals had nothing to do with one's will. Like a laboratory
test, they could work on any body submitted, be it the suspected person or a
proxy. In contrast, torture was a contest of wills between judge and suspect,
and the suspect did stand a slim chance of emerging victorious. The privacy
of confession and the privacy of torture, as opposed to the publicity of the
ordeal, were both part of a changing, more inward-looking worldview.

While canon lawyers were debating the uses of torture, theologians and
preachers started forging a totally new argument. It neither favored nor
condemned judicial torture in earthly matters but instead drew a fascinat-
ing new parallel between confessional practices of law and religion. While
modern French can distinguish between the judicial *aveu* and the religious
confession, and modern English between admission (of guilt) and confession
(of sin), late medieval Latin definitely, and probably deliberately, transferred
the religious term to the juridical framework, using the same word in both
contexts: *confessio*. The use of the same term in two different fields, both
dealing with guilt and its acknowledgment, was originally meant to promote
religious confession but ended up granting judicial torture an unsought-
for legitimation.

There is little question about who borrowed from whom. Though continuously evolving, the theology of religious confession of sinners had coalesced by the mid–twelfth century.[55] At that time, secular juridical theories
were vague to the point of nonexistence. It is hard to find much in the works
of the early glossators of Roman law that would deal with this point, and
most customary-law texts were not written until a century later, by which
time Italian jurists were producing an entirely original corpus of criminal
law dealing with torture.[56] By then, theologians had already produced a considerable body of literature to draw upon.

The difference between the two types of confession was noted when
preachers began making comparisons between them: "In this world's court

of justice, he who confesses his misdeed is immediately condemned; but in God's court, it is the opposite: he who admits his guilt is completely liberated."[57] These words were written long after torture had become a standard means of fact-finding in courts and obviously indicate the need of clerics to distance themselves from the awful implications of a secular confession. Religious confession saves, secular confession damns, and believers should be made aware that safety, rather than danger, lay in religious confession. They should not be confused by the deliberate judicial adoption of religious terminology.

There was, however, a certain similarity in the dynamics of the two types of confession. Viewing the development of each case, they often seem like mirror images (although, like Alice's looking-glass image, from the other side things are not quite the same). The process begins with a misdeed. The church labeled it a sin; the law, a crime. Often the two categories overlapped, as in cases of adultery or bigamy. Both systems made clear distinctions between degrees of misdeeds according to their gravity or their degree of publicity—there was a point when a personal misdeed, become public, turned into scandal—and both assumed that the punishment would accord with the degree of guilt.

Guilt was indeed the next step. Both systems had determined that certain acts carried automatic guilt with them. This was an impersonal, objective fact. Feelings of guilt and contrition were something very different. However, a deed was labeled sinful or criminal through legislation or custom and, once so labeled, automatically carried with it guilt and punishment. The awareness of this guilt was personal and subjective. In the case of sin, it was necessary that the sinners be aware of what they had done. Contemporary writings are full of complaints about the lack of such an awareness, from Gerald of Wales's story of the cleric forced to convince a group of Welshmen that murder was a misdeed to the thirteenth-century clerical condemnation of group confessions to an imaginary standard list of misdeeds the "sinners" had never actually committed.[58] Since believers could not be expected to know what was or was not sinful by themselves, the church began, as of 1215, to require an annual confession, in which the priest was to lead the way for the sinner. Handbooks insisted that the dialogue between sinner and confessor lead the former first to the awareness that his acts had constituted a sin.

In the secular mirror image, however, internal awareness of objective guilt was not the issue. The person who needed to become aware of the crime was the judge, whose job it was to investigate and prosecute crimes. As we have seen, the judge could be informed in a number of ways. If the crime were public and notorious, it would come to his ears in any case. If not, the injured party could bring an accusation, taking upon himself the onus of proof and prosecution. Alternatively, if the injured party did not feel capable of sustaining the charge by himself, he could resort to denunciation, which essentially meant bringing the facts of the case to the attention of the authorities and letting them deal with the prosecution. In any case, this was the point at which the two systems parted company: pastoral Christianity concentrated upon bringing inner awareness; secular justice, upon public knowledge. Either way was to lead to certain actions by the knowledgeable party.

The next stage is the one most authors consider the beginning of the process. Abelard named it one of the three constitutive elements of confession: *contritio in corde,* the feeling of internal, subjective guilt. Twelfth-century theology claimed that shame occurred only later, when contrition had led to confession. Shame could not be sustained alone within the self; it depended upon the existence of an external condemning viewer and upon the willing articulation of guilt. Theologians did argue whether genuine contrition could wipe away sin, Abelard insisting that it was so, while Peter Lombard later claiming that an actual confession had to follow. All theologians, however, insisted that free voluntary remorse was an essential element in the process of self-purification. Another question, which took precedence, was the causal relationship between contrition and confession. With a self-aware, educated culprit, presumably contrition would precede confession and lead up to it. Given an ignorant sinner, however, contrition might have appeared only during the confession, after the confessor had awakened the sinner's conscience and awareness. Unquestionably, though, while confession could be forced and ordained, contrition was entirely a matter of one's free will. No one could coerce it. Witness Abelard's merciless analysis of his own self and his sins: he had known all along, none better, that his relationship with Heloïse, before and after the marriage, was sinful but felt no remorse, no contrition, until after it was ended.[59]

By contrast, in law the stages were much clearer. The stage following the magistrate's learning of the crime was the stage of investigation, interrogation, and torture. Like the religious confessional dialogue, this was the stage of truth-finding. The investigation would include the collection of *indicia,* or indirect pointers to guilt, and the interrogation of witnesses—building up a body of evidence. Interrogation, meant to elicit a confession, was to set a seal upon this evidence. Should it be unsatisfactory, the judge could resort to torture in order to elicit the required confession. Unlike the consistent theological framework, the juridical one was paradoxical. Freedom of will played different roles: ill will displayed by a homicide suspect toward the victim was an *indicium*. At the same time, a spontaneous confession without any torture could not "prejudice" the suspect. It was not sufficiently credible without torture and coercion of the will. It was acceptable only if, after confessing under torture, the suspect "freely" persevered in court. Though no jurist said so, the basic assumption behind such procedures was that spontaneous, uncoerced contrition was an impossibility in the realm of the law. It was only after torture that people could be expected to tell the truth *of their own free will*. The order of things was clear: first interrogation, then contrition and confession.

The act of confession (*confessio in ore*)—admitting one's guilt before a priest—was, despite the preachers' vehement need to deny it, not too different in the two spheres under comparison. Two central elements played a role in both: privacy and shame. By the twelfth century, private confession of individual people facing the priest had become common. Though the physical structure of the confessional was post-Tridentine, the contents of confession became private, secret, and hallowed four centuries earlier. Twelfth-century theologians argued whether a priest was indispensable; the usual conclusion, which Peter Lombard sustained, was that only in the absence of a priest could one confess to a layman. They also agreed that, when confessing, one ought to cleanse one's soul totally and confess all one's sins, not only the most recent ones. Most importantly, the very act of confession was essential. As Peter Lombard and the Victorines insisted, contrition was not enough to cleanse the soul.[60]

What was there in the act of oral confession that was so powerful? After all, the knowledge of guilt came with contrition. The act of sharing one's sins with another person was shaming, and the shame (*verecundia, erubescentia*) was already a punishment that began the process of cleansing the sinner's soul. The greater the shame, the greater the merit in confessing. The element of shame had always been part of confession and penitence, especially within the context of the Carolingian *penitentia publica*, which was undertaken for having committed a public, scandalous crime. The Carolingian ritual was special; though theoretically a once-in-a-lifetime event, which left penitents in a quasi-ecclesiastical status, unable, for example, to hold public office, it had been known to be repeated. Its shameful and infamatory character, however, was not in doubt. Mayke De Jong has shown that the ritual was connected with secular rites of shame and penitence, such as the *harmiscara* (publicly carrying a saddle on one's back for a prescribed distance).[61]

Twelfth-century confession carried a new kind of shame. It had no public consequences; the penitent needed not leave public or secular life nor be publicly branded as a sinner. Nobody but the priest knew the nature of this shame, but even that sufficed. It was the shame of actually acknowledging in words, quite literally getting out of one's mouth, like vomit, the damning words. If confession could be private, so could shame. It had nothing to do with being disgraced in the eyes of society, but in one's own eyes, and in the priest's eyes. Skillful preachers made two very important pastoral points: first, that a partial confession was invalid and, second, that fear of shame was no reason to avoid confession. To the contrary: only by bearing the shame of confession could one cleanse oneself.[62]

As far as most theologians from the twelfth century on were concerned, once confession was done, the sinner was cleansed. Twelfth-century and later theology tended to discount penance, claiming that contrition and confession remitted sins. And yet, the element of *satisfactio in opere*, or making amends, did survive from the older procedures, as concrete proof of genuine, heartfelt contrition. It was not a punishment, such as the church imposed upon heretics, but rather a visible expression of an interior and private process.

The satisfaction provided by criminals was of a different order. Once torture was over, the rest of the criminal procedure took place in a blaze of publicity: not only the public perseverance but also the punitive ritual that followed. Accounts of public executions stress the long procession preceding the actual putting to death, during which the culprits were to proclaimed their guilt vocally, begging the audience to pray for their soon-to-depart souls.[63] During the fourteenth and fifteenth centuries condemned criminals in France, Italy, and the Holy Roman Empire gained the right to priestly confession and absolution just before their execution, though there was nothing private about the foot of the gallows. Preachers fighting for the right of the condemned to receive the Eucharist claimed that the criminals deserved it because they had confessed and expressed contrition, just like any other communicant.[64] In this, they were not claiming that the confession in court counted as a sacrament or was proof of contrition. Contrition was there in the declarations along the processional route to the gallows and in the second, foot-of-the-gallows confession. Criminals were thus subsumed into the general *corpus Christianorum* by virtue of sacramental confession.

Did this mean that the effects of criminal confession were identical to those of the sacramental confession of sinners? Not quite. It did not erase their crime, for which they paid with their lives or their bodily integrity. While common sinners were reintegrated back into the community after confession, contrition, and satisfaction, criminals essentially remained outside it. If physically branded, the marks remained on them lifelong. If executed, they did not merit burial in holy ground but remained to disintegrate on the gallows.

Not unnaturally, dead criminals were quit of all further obligations, their souls presumably cleansed enough to get them into purgatory rather than hell. Sinners had to comply with one more requirement: perseverance. In religious terms, perseverance was as private as confession and equally dependant upon contrition and free will. No confession and contrition bore any validity if the sinner relapsed. Perseverance in this context meant a mode of acting, not a public verbal act of acknowledgment of guilt.

The net result of this quasi similarity was a system of truth-finding by torture and pain masquerading as a system of truth-finding by question and answer, of coercion masquerading as free will. Torture, or *quaestio*, could have flourished only in a world where guilt was invariably extracted by questioning and confession, where inner knowledge and awareness of guilt were the basic requirements for ultimate satisfaction. Nor is it surprising that torture survived so very long in European judicial systems. It looked remarkably similar to a very respectable, and physically painless, procedure.

Juridic Theory

More than half a century ago, when Walter Ullmann wrote about medieval and early modern torture, he argued that the system had so many safeguards built into it that it was, in the end, far less brutal than twentieth-century illegal, and widely practiced, torture.[65] His argument relied entirely upon the theoretical literature, which indeed sets up very stringent (albeit contradictory) rules for the use of torture. But too often one finds the wry comment that this restraint was more honored in the breach than in observance. In reality, jurists admitted quite often that things were not necessarily done by the book.[66] There is not enough judicial material to substantiate any thesis concerning widespread abuse of torture, but there is no doubt that such abuse existed. Most authors adduced this fact as the reason for producing yet another torture manual.

Confessional practices were a partial cause for the rise of legitimate torture. Torture had never been really illegitimate, only disreputable. We have already mentioned above the growth of scholastic Roman law studies and the professionalization of legal expertise as further supporting elements. In addition to the spurious respectability of a pseudoreligious practice, torture achieved the further dignity of becoming a fitting subject of scholarly writing. Beginning with Albertus Gandinus (d. 1310), speaking and writing about torture became a jurisprudential convention, just as much part of the successful jurist's list of publications as a collection of *consilia*.

In reviewing this literature, one must bear in mind that torture was definitely part of the law of evidence, not of penal law. Causing pain might reveal the truth, as one might today consider that laboratory experiments do.[67] Whether pain did or did not penalize or harm the possible source of certainty was not really relevant. Many of the treatises on the matter of torture and questioning were written by practicing judges rather than university professors.[68] Although torture was used in France and Germany, the practice there failed to generate the sort of intellectual literature that it did in Italy.[69] Relying mostly upon Italian writings (with a smattering of French and Flemish material), it is possible to try and elicit the views of practicing jurists—judges, advocates, university professors—on the subject.

Surprisingly, these views were not unanimously supportive of pain infliction. In those parts of Europe where a litigant could employ a lawyer, lawyers fought to have their clients exempted from torture. In the first place, they could demand an accusatory, rather than an inquisitorial, procedure. In an accusatory procedure, the onus of proof rested upon the plaintiff rather than upon the defendant, a situation that made the judge's decision all the more difficult.

As torture treatises are an exotic form of scholastic writing, long relegated to the ash heap of history, it might be well to describe them. The task is made easier by the authors' tendency to copy each other and by the existence of an original, anonymous *Tractatus de tormentis*. It has appeared under the names of most leading Italian jurists from the late thirteenth century onward.[70] As Albertus Gandinus was the most famous and one the earliest copyists of the treatise, it is as well to summarize his version as the basis for a conflation of torture treatises.[71] The treatise begins, in the best scholastic manner, with a list of questions. What is torture (*quaestio*); who may be tortured; how should torture be conducted; in what order should people be tortured and for what causes; what are the conditions necessary for ordering torture; and what are the effects of torture?[72]

Also at the beginning of the treatise is an exhortation against cruel judges, *immodice sevientibus*, who rush to torture. Similar invectives appear in practically all the treatises. Gandinus's teacher Guido de Suzara (fl. 1260–90) spoke of *assessores autem honores avidi*, who manipulated procedure in order to get quick confessions, and Gandinus's 1378 editor, Ludovico Bolognini, added the comment that his own contemporaries were equally rash and cruel.[73] By the fifteenth century, Franciscus Brunus (fl. 1493) spoke against *perversi* judges who invented new forms of torture for their own pleasure, openly asserting that they were criminals (*male-ficiunt*).[74] Following the general warning, Gandinus provided the standard definition of torture, taken from the *Digest*.[75] This is the only place in the treatise where the word "pain" is mentioned at all. The following article, which grew longer in subsequent treatises, dealt with those vulnerable to and those exempt from torture. Unlike his Roman predecessors, Gandinus allowed the torture of witnesses only if they vacillated in their testimony. The young (under fourteen) and the aged were exempt, though Gandinus was at a loss to define the age of decrepitude. Magistrates and their families, military commanders, and nobility in general were exempt, unless the case involved *lèse-majesté*. Other authors exempted the clergy as well.

Torture, said Gandinus, should be applied moderately, carefully tailored to the physical fortitude of each suspect, so that "he should be delivered unharmed either to innocence or to death"—another useful Roman maxim.[76] If several people were to be tortured in one case, there was a careful order established by which a son ought to be tortured before the father, but in his presence, and a woman before a man, for she was likelier to break down faster.[77] Torture was applicable in both civil and criminal cases but only in severe cases, and very rarely in civil ones. Before it was applied, however, there had to exist some evidence in the form of *indicia*. Precisely what pointed toward guilt, but did not establish it, varied from author to author. Gandinus warned, once more, that each judge should carefully consider whether he has enough evidence to send a suspect to the dungeon, for the consequences were irreversible and "many perish when tortured."[78] At this point, agreed all jurists, the weight of responsibility rested upon the judge's shoulders alone.

When it came to sending someone to torture, the social standing and public fame of the person were central. The *Tractatus de tormentis* listed the following reasons for sending someone to torture: previous enmity between suspect and victim, the suspect's bad reputation (*fama*) and low social status, body language (stability of voice and body, pallor or blushing), family networks, past record, disposition, circumstances, and so on. A homicide suspect, echoed Bartolus of Sassoferrato (1313–57) more than a century later, could even be condemned without witnesses (but not without a confession!) if he was known to have been the victim's enemy, was commonly believed to be guilty, and was a man whose character was consonant with such deeds; a suspect's master or someone who had received a suspect in his house following the murder could also be condemned without witnesses. It is important to note, though, that Bartolus required all of these *indicia* together, rather than any one of them, as proof sufficient for conviction.[79]

All the criteria were subjective and amenable to bias. Gandinus's treatise repeated the usual statement that it all depended upon the judge's decision, a further reinforcement of the subjectivity of presumed guilt. In any case, the *indicia* had to be sufficient and credible, whatever that meant in practice. Testimony was half a proof and hence served as an *indicium*. It was therefore incumbent upon the judge to seek out all the witnesses, whether to testify as to character and biography or to facts. At the same time, the judge had to make sure that the witnesses (especially character witnesses) were swayed by neither amity nor enmity with respect to the suspect.

Interestingly, a voluntary confession without so much as fear of torture was not invariably considered either incriminating or even an *indicium*. In fact, in the wake of the Roman precedent concerning slaves, an uncoerced confession was often unacceptable. Having surveyed ancient and modern contradictory opinions concerning the weight of unextorted confessions, Gandinus firmly accepted voluntary confession as sufficient for final sentencing without torture. Not all his followers agreed. The rationale for doubting free confession was that it was a unique event. Extorted confessions were not valid unless repeated in court without pressure, and that, asserted Gandinus, was *communis opinio doctorum*. The confession under torture, then, was declared twice over, once in the dungeon and once in open court. According to Franciscus Brunus, by the fifteenth century judges were hastening to send suspects to torture without any *indicia* at all, with the consequence that they achieved quick confessions. While invalid in law, such malpractice did help to advance judicial careers.[80]

All authorities followed Gandinus in stating that if a suspect did not confess following torture, he could not be submitted to further torture without any new *indicia* coming to light. Nevertheless, too many ambitious judges ignored this restriction. But even honest judges were enjoined not to accept silence as proof of innocence. The defiant suspect must continue to be tortured until the end of the prescribed torture session and then kept in jail until further evidence should surface. A semidefiant suspect, who confessed under torture but retracted the confession later in court, could not be condemned, but his first confession was held as partial proof (*semiplena probatio*) and hence as a further *indicium* to justify another session with the torturer.

Despite these generalizations, in Albertus Gandinus's time people of dignity could request and receive a postponement of the torture and use the time to prove their innocence. This, said Gandinus, is because, if innocence was proven after torture, "never can one recover the damage to one's limbs through the appeal."[81] Furthermore, noted the knowledgeable judge, it often happened (presumably in political cases) that suspects who were tortured, confessed, and sentenced to death were then pardoned by the ruler. As we shall see, such people did take vengeance upon their torturers at the first opportunity. In general, the intervention of rulers in legal proceedings was a nuisance that all judges faced. Sometimes the *podestà* (*princeps, potestas*) sent people to torture with no evidence whatsoever. Needless to say, the offense against the dignity of justice automatically voided the validity of any confession extracted without prior evidence. Nevertheless, at the end of his treatise Gandinus devoted a long section to the role of rulers as prosecutors of crime and hence as initiators of torture proceedings. As a strong supporter of the inquisitorial method of justice, Gandinus was all in favor of government initiative (unless it was motivated by private hatred) in criminal matters.

One of the most central aspects was the fear that the threat of torture induced, for a confession extracted by threats remained invalid. Curiously, while actual physical coercion did not invalidate a confession as long as the confession was repeated in court "freely," fear was pronounced a stumbling block to confession. Just as people varied in their reactions to pain, so did they react differently to threats. Some people were constant (steadfast); others were *meticulosi*, fearful. What constituted an extremely frightening threat to one barely affected another. Already Bernard of Parma (d. 1213), writing in the twelfth century, noted that "the fear that affects the constant often depends also upon the courage or cowardice of the sufferer, since what is insignificant to the courageous will be found to be violent in the fearful."[82] It was therefore necessary to define exactly the sort of fear that would induce the constant man, a figment of jurisprudential imagination, to confess. The term *vir constans* goes back to Roman law, and according to the *Codex*, it was fear of death or torture that would break the constant man. The *Digest* gave examples of threats of death, flogging, and servitude that affected even constant men: "not just fear, but fear of a great evil."[83] Ulpian had stated that a threat of torture was indeed such a fear, not a *levis territio* but a genuinely frightening intimidation. By the twelfth century Sicard of Cremona (ca. 1155–1215) instanced the situation in which a knife was held to one's throat as a parallel.[84]

The purely juridical question was colored in the thirteenth century by scholastic debates concerning free will and coercion. A genuine confession had to be made freely and willingly; otherwise, it was invalid, insisted canon law. Could the will be coerced? In purely scholastic circles, the answer was usually negative, with some qualifications. Thomas Aquinas implied that constancy negated coercion by claiming that the constant man could

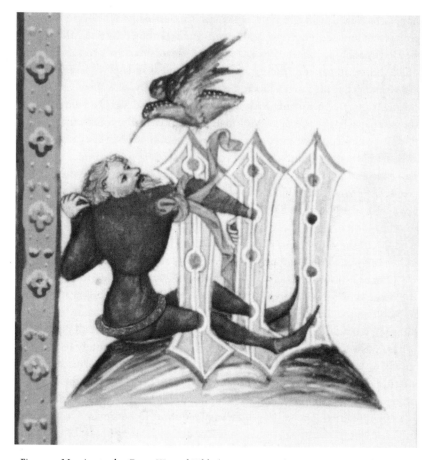

Figure 1. Man in stocks. From Wenzel Bible (ca. 1389–1400), Austrian National Library, Vienna, Cod. 2760, fol. 18r, margin miniature, right side.

always choose the lesser evil (i.e., torture) as opposed to the greater (i.e., lies). In other words, a constant man would prefer torture to a false confession, and therefore fear had no hold upon him.[85] Jurists, dealing with practical experience, were more skeptical. Already Azo (fl. 1190–1220) had noted that, although theoretically torture could not break the will, he had known instances when it had.[86] The problem for the judicial system was that cases were known in which confessions had been extorted by torture.

The assertion that the will of a constant man could not be affected by threats and fear or even of torture was a dangerous yardstick for judges. If a constant man succumbed to threats of torture and confessed, the confession was invalid because it had been extorted under fear. Hence, to begin with, one had to define the precise stage of the proceedings at which a slight fright turned into genuine fear of torture, affecting even the constant man. After all, the judge could hardly resort to Roman examples, threatening suspects with murder or enslavement or laying a knife to their throats. At this point, legal opinions varied. Albertus Gandinus drew a line between the courtroom and the dungeon. Fear counted as torture only if the suspect was actually conducted to the dungeon and shown the instruments, but threats in court did not count, for "light frightening with torture outside the place of torture is imaginary [facta illusoria est]." His followers as a rule agreed with this distinction, for, as we shall see, the symbolic spaces of courtroom and dungeon were two carefully separated realms. Baldus de Ubaldis (1327—1400) asserted that manacles already induced genuine fear. Bonifacius de Vitalinis (d. 1388) began by claiming that any confession made at the place of torture, tied to the instrument, was invalid. But since he continued by defining torture not only as the actual act "but also if he is undressed and put out in the cold, or if he is denied food, or exposed to smoke,[87] or had cold water poured over him in cold weather, or into his nose, or was subjected to the leg-screw, as is very often done," he greatly extended the scope of legitimate fear. Franciscus Brunus followed Gandinus in defining the point where light fear turned into legitimate fear as being tied up at the place of torture.[88] Other judges also ventured to consider cold, hunger, and jail as fear inducers amounting to torture.[89]

The opinion of jurists was reversed one generation after Brunus. Paulus Grillandus (fl. 1525) asserted that tying a man to the rope "so that nothing lacks but raising him" did not count as torture, "for indeed the body is not tortured, nor does he feel pain; it is more a mental fear."[90] It is consonant with the general growing severity of the late fifteenth and sixteenth centuries that fear of pain was no longer considered a torture that would make a constant man lie. In reality, Grillandus's position completely emptied the restraint of fear of any meaning. Grillandus defined five levels of torture, but the lowest level needed the clearest definition, for if threats counted as torture, any confession under threats required repetition in court. Conversely, if threats were frightening enough to make a constant man confess, they could disqualify the entire trial. There is, on the one hand, an embarrassment of circumlocutions about the theory of torture and, on the other hand, an embarrassment of silence about the actual practice. In a world that praised, indeed glorified, the acceptance and tolerance of pain, the problem of recalcitrant suspects who refused to confess was fraught with religious and philosophical pitfalls. Truth without pain hardly existed within the realm of criminal law.

A system that claimed to uncover inner truth and bring it into the daylight but that was predicated upon coercion, negation of free will, and pain was bound to be self-contradictory. To understand the medieval ambivalence concerning torture, it is important to understand the way it worked. The entire procedure presents one contradiction after another. No person was to be tortured unless there was proof that a crime had been committed and unless there were sufficient *indicia* pointing to the suspect's culpability.[91] Suspects, in theory, were sent to torture only under an interlocutory (intermediate) sentence. This sentence declared that there were good *indicia* for suspecting that there was more involved than what the suspect had hitherto been willing to reveal, listed those indicators, and interrupted the trial until a new confession was forthcoming. *Indicia*, declared the jurist Baldus de Ubaldis, must be clearer than light, sure, and credible.[92] The line between proof sufficient for torture and proof sufficient for condemnation was extremely unclear. Theoretically, at the end of the procedure a suspect could be found innocent and released without punishment, but in reality recalcitrant and obdurate suspects who refused to confess were often found merely stubborn or resilient. Those who did confess when in pain were forced to repeat the confession in public "of their own free will" after a suitable period for recovery.[93] The system had little to do with free will, truth, or credibility. If what the sources tell us beyond the theory is true, then only one thing really deterred judges from sending people to the dungeon: the fear of being sued if the suspect died under torture.

Practice: Methods

When dealing with practice, one must remember that no city or kingdom in Europe followed explicit Roman law. Every judicial authority had its own statutes, which judges and rulers were bound to follow. Many of the complaints concerning abuses probably stem from local particularities that a specific doctor of law decided to exclude from the *ius commune*.[94] However, since the generalizations of jurists provide a useful basis for analysis, the following description of torture practices is based largely upon torture treatises.

Of all legal dealings with pain, torture is the topic that elicited most of the literature. The first thing to strike anyone investigating the subject is the contrast between the vast amount of theoretical material available on judicial torture and the dearth of real accounts or actual descriptions. But the writing about torture is convoluted and ambivalent. Unlike corporal punishments, which were described in great detail, tortures were all the more terrifying because presumably nobody really knew what happened in the dungeon. The deliberate infliction of pain was hedged by a great many rules and controls, at least in theory, but the silence surrounding the real events and sensations prevents all possibility of writing in depth about the pain of torture.

Medieval torture sessions were shrouded in secrecy. In blatant contrast to the public confession in court, the preceding torture and primary confession were avowedly secret, and secrecy pointed to infamy. The place of torture, *locus torturae*, was secret and private—so private that the judge must make sure that every word of the suspect was written down, "otherwise he will not be believed." Conversely, the courtroom, where the suspect must repeat his or her confession freely, was public and honorable, *locus publicus et honestus*.[95] Openness was equated with *honestas*, the term usually applied to people whose status was above reproach or suspicion. *Personae honestae* were usually people whose oath was accepted without the need for torture, the opposite of the *vilissimi*, whose very status made them liable to torture when implicated in some crime. When referring to a witness's testimony extorted under torture, a secret confession sufficed: "Admittedly it is safer and less suspicious if witnesses are brought to confession and persevere [in it], as said above; all the same, it is valid if the document is written down by a notary in front of the judge in secret and without witnesses . . . thus it is done by general custom, which has the power of law."[96]

Western culture was not squeamish about the public infliction of pain, but torture, carrying the burden of shame and semilicit practice, had to be private. It was an unconvincing secrecy: even the lightest of tortures damaged a man's dignity and innocence, asserted another expert.[97] Such a statement reveals that the fact of torture, with its damaging and dishonorable implications, was not likely to remain secret in reality. All the same, the act of torture was carried out in such a way that none of those implicated in it would be seen to perform it.

It is not until the sixteenth century that questioning under torture during trials before the Inquisition was recorded in detail.[98] Sixteenth-century protocols were meant to include everything that happened in the dungeons, including screams and pleas for mercy, but the earlier ones say nothing of what actually happened. Both ecclesiastical and secular trials merely stated the indirect incriminating evidence leading to torture, sometimes the type of torture, and the fact that before confessing in court the suspect was allowed respite, warmth, and drink. The confession record always included the statement that the confession was produced without coercion or torture.

Who was to be present in the dungeon, other than suspect and executioners? The judge, says Gandinus, must be there to witness the first confession. This presence raised once more the question of the judge's responsibility in cases of irreversible laming or death. The judge must bear the punishment for his deeds only if he acted out of private malice; as long as he did no more than his duty, he was not held culpable.

Local variations abounded not only in procedure but also in the means of torture. In trying to dig through layers of verbiage to the original infliction of pain, one must also examine the various instruments of torture. In fourteenth-century France methods ranged from stretching victims over a racklike trestle to pouring great quantities of water into their mouths. Since most torture treatises were written in Italy, they speak of the strappado (also called the "rope," *funis*) or the *stanghetta*.[99] Franciscus Brunus is almost unique in listing a variety of methods, specifying which were "safe" (i.e., that would not kill or permanently maim a suspect) and which were "dangerous":

> Some force water down the nose, and some also insert a stone to block the drinker's mouth. This type of torture, I have heard, is dangerous, for the suspect may suffocate. Some put small dice [*taxillum*], commonly called *losso pazzo*, between the toes. Some put a mouse on the abdomen or in the umbilicus, and on it they put a cat to keep it in, so that it cannot come out. Some torture with a goat's tongue thus: they wash the feet of the tortured with saltwater, and tying him down on the rack [*scannum*], make the goat lick his soles, which it will willingly do because it loves salt; and I hear that this is a very hard torture, and totally safe. Some torture by putting rods between the fingers and tying the hands with a cord. Some use a rope, with the hands tied behind the back. This type of torture is the most common. And one of the judges has such an instrument, which we can see everywhere, and it is approved by custom and law . . . but in this one must use great care and moderation; otherwise, there are many dangers. Others tie only one hand to the rope and let dangle this way above the ground. I have also heard that they give the prisoner much salty meat to eat and refuse him drink. Others wash his feet and smear them with pork fat and, tied to the rack, put the soles of his feet next to the fire and leave him thus.[100]

This horrific list comes from the pen of the man who sternly warned against inventing new and sadistic methods of torture. Brunus was inventing nothing, merely listing all the methods he knew. In actual fact, it seems that the most common method was probably the strappado.

Brunus's list indicates again the fear that a suspect might die during torture. Suspects were—at least theoretically—meant to emerge from torture not only alive but physically unscathed. Judges and jurists were constantly in search of a "safe" method of torture, one that would make people confess without endangering them. Thus, Hippolytus Marsili happily described in a letter the latest ingenious method: deprivation of sleep. "You do not allow the suspect ever to sleep or rest, so that he will confess all after two nights and one day at the latest, if you promise him rest. . . . you must bear in mind this type of torture, for it is supremely effective and does not damage the body, so that no judge would ever be put on trial for it."[101]

All of these methods could be applied at different degrees of severity or for different lengths of time. In the early sixteenth century Paulus Grillandus defined five different levels of torture, each including the use of the strappado.[102] The first degree, which Grillandus considered no torture at all, was fright. In general, Grillandus argued that fear was an excellent tool, not to be thrown away as a disqualifier of confessions. After all, real torture had to be carefully and discriminatingly administered, for not all were robust enough to withstand it, but fear could be instilled in young and old alike. The second degree was when the suspect was lifted a short distance above the ground, held there for a short time (as long as it takes to say a Pater Noster, a somewhat longer Ave Maria, or an even longer Miserere, depending upon the suspect's fortitude), and then lowered back gently, without breaking or dislocating any bones. This Grillandus called *levis tortura*, recommended for cases when the evidence was in fact too flimsy for torture. Performing a wonderful scholastic sleight-of-hand, Grillandus asserted that light torture was not really torture either, just as a light fever was not a "real" illness sufficient to excuse a sick man from appearing in court.[103] Hence, the procedure just described did not conform to the definition of a torment causing pain to both mind and body. This level of torture, noted Grillandus, also had great advantages: since it was not properly torture, if it failed to elicit a confession, one could still call for a second—and more severe—torture session on the basis of the same *indicia*, with no further evidence. Furthermore, it could be applied to people who had immunity, such as noblemen and the clergy. All the same, Grillandus cautioned that, if the tortured person felt any pain at all, or if his good reputation was damaged, this level did constitute torture. Personally, he never applied it unless he had sufficient evidence for genuine torture.[104] Furthermore, any confession made under light torture required confirmation in court.

The third level, undoubtedly torture, was when a suspect remained hanging for a time longer than it took to recite one Miserere, albeit still without having the ropes tightened or being suddenly dropped. This torture, recommended Grillandus, ought to be used in cases of ample evidence but of a crime that was not heinous, such as a modest theft or a nonlethal wound. The fourth degree included keeping the suspect hanging for an hour or so, with added sudden pulling on the ropes. This degree was to be applied only when, in addition to solid evidence, the suspect also had a robust constitution and was accused of a grave crime—a major theft, sacrilege, forgery, or murder. The last, and most severe, degree, added to the hanging suspect heavy weights on his feet: "And this is the most savage of tortures. Jurists who wrote of this said that then the suspect's body is torn to pieces, limbs and bones are broken apart from the body. This is said to be a worse punishment [poena] than the severing of both hands."[105] Even Grillandus was horrified at this torture, saying that it was almost never used, and only in the case of the most terrible crime—treason, heresy, assassination of a cardinal, and so on. The results were undoubtedly tantamount to an extremely painful execution. Only here did Grillandus forget the rigid juridical distinction between torture and punishment, calling such a torture poena. Torture had to entail the greatest and most savage infliction of pain before jurists were prepared to admit that it was indeed punitive.

The judge was to decide the type and degree of torture and the length of each session.[106] Bartolus of Sassoferrato (1314–57), probably the greatest jurist of the fourteenth century, had nearly had a young and healthy suspect die under torture when still a young judge. The experience marked him for life.[107] Baldus de Ubaldis told in a (probably putative) consilium the nightmare of each and every judge: a suspect who had died under torture. Baldus was posing the question whether, under certain circumstances, the judge should be prosecuted. The suspect had been accused of counterfeiting, which was by definition a crime of lèse-majesté. Thus, he definitely qualified for the inquisitorial procedure and the possibility of torture. Under questioning, the man had prevaricated. Furthermore, according to credible witnesses (fide dignorum virorum) he was of evil reputation. Prevarication and reputation were both separately considered indicia, and together they provided sufficient proof for legally submitting the man to torture. Thus far, the judge had displayed no lethal overenthusiasm. The torture, however, was harsh: the man was lifted on the strappado; when he refused to confess, he was lifted again and suddenly dropped this time. The procedure was repeated for a third time. The judge did not believe the suspect would die of the torture, "even though he could not tolerate the pain in the said third torture," and even though the executioners warned him of the man's state. They did give the man some water to revive him, but he died later on. Should the judge be penalized? Predictably, Baldus concluded that, though the judge had exceeded the measure of torture, he was innocent of any intention to kill and thus should not be prosecuted.[108]

Baldus omitted in his opinion one crucial factor: the suspect's physical condition prior to torture. If a previously robust man died under torture, said Bartolus of Sassoferrato, the judge was not responsible as long as he had not exceeded the usual degree of torture. However, if he had sent a weak man to torture, the judge must answer for his deeds.[109] Brunus too stated unequivocally that a judge who had let his suspect die from torture must be executed by decapitation.[110]

The judge's responsibility was probably theoretical in most cases. All jurists complained of continuous abuses. People who had immunity were nevertheless tortured, and through technical manipulation of a single "discontinued" and "resumed" session, recalcitrant suspects were subjected to a second session of torture without any further evidence being submitted against them. In some cases, even witnesses were tortured, contrary to the laws enunciated in most treatises. Finally, often suspects without a shred of evidence against them were still sent to torture.[111] The practice of torture lent itself excellently to abuse.

Practice: Cases

Though jurists avoided to the best of their ability the discussion of pain in torture, the subject inevitably arose within the context of individual cases. Judges were faced, on a daily basis, with the decision of whether or not there was sufficient evidence to warrant torturing a suspect, and to what degree. The line between theory and practice was fine indeed, at least in Italy. In the following, I survey a number of cases for which we have some individual evidence. Not all are real; two at least are found in judicial *consilia*, which means that they might or might not have been real. Nevertheless, they are the best we have.

The common denominator in all of these cases is the social standing of the victims. As all the cases concern illegitimate torture and a lawsuit either to prevent or redress it, only people of position and wealth could have left records of such suits. Common thieves and criminals in an inquisitorial procedure were not usually allowed defense lawyers, nor could they afford them. One encounters lawyers involved in cases of torture only on the rare occasion when an overzealous judge made the mistake of ordering the torture of a respectable citizen.

Such was the case of Giovanni Giovannini. In October 1294 in Bologna, the commune prosecuted one Galvano, formerly *capitano di popolo* of the commune. Among other accusations of official malfeasance was the denunciation by Giovanni Giovannini, who accused the ex-magistrate of having had him illegally tortured. The illegality lay both in the nature of Giovannini's case and in his status: the case had not come under the statute of torture, and the suspect had had a privileged immunity from torture. For this act, Galvano was fined one hundred Bolognese pounds. It is worth noting that both sides employed lawyers (*procuratores vel curatores*).[112] Clearly, Galvano was not being sued for causing pain. He was being accused of having done so illegally. Giovannini's lawyer was obviously familiar not only with the local statute *de tondolo et tormento* (concerning torture)[113] but also with the general jurisprudence concerning who might and might not be tortured, and under what circumstances. Giovannini was not a plaintiff in an accusatory procedure but a denouncer who brought his evidence before the authorities and initiated an inquisitorial, public procedure. He brought the facts before the syndics of the commune, who then prosecuted and tried Galvano for a series of misdeeds. There was no question of compensation for an injured party, only of a fine paid to the public treasury. All the same, Giovannini had gone to the trouble and expense of hiring a lawyer, who had presented the syndics with a *libellus* containing all the facts of the illegal torture. He did all this knowing full well that he would receive no compensation for his injury. Whether Giovannini wanted revenge for his injured status and honor or for his physical pain remains unknown, but it is highly probable that both factors played a role in his decision to take revenge through the courts. Not a word was said about the trauma of torture.

Our next case also concerns illegal torture of a man of standing and is unique in its descriptiveness. In 1320, in the Avignonese papal chancery with two cardinals present, Bartolomeo Uberti Canholati gave a deposition concerning the judicial torture that had been inflicted upon him. The illegal torture was perpetrated at the orders of Matteo Visconti, *signore* of Milan (1250–1322). Bartolomeo, a Milanese cleric, had apparently had a reputation as a magician. When Matteo Visconti, leader of the Italian Ghibellines, wished to get rid of the "Guelph pope" John XXII (1249–1334), he had Bartolomeo summoned to his presence and gave him a silver statuette of a man for the purposes of maleficent sympathetic magic. The statuette was hollow and bore various mysterious symbols, and the magician was expected to subfumigate it (i.e., fumigate its lower parts) with *napellus* poison[114] while performing whatever magic was necessary to kill the pope. Bartolomeo, a cleric of nebulous standing, refused repeated orders and requests to perform the deed, even excusing himself from going to Verona to find another magician on the grounds of ill health.

All this had happened in February 1320. Sometime between this meeting and September of the same year, Bartolomeo went to Avignon, ostensibly to undo a curse laid upon the pope's nephew. On his return he was set upon by the lord Scotus (one of Visconti's men), and—despite his clerical status—imprisoned for forty-two days in shackles and leg-irons in total darkness. Furthermore, he was severely tortured to make him confess that he had gone to Avignon to tell the pope about the statuette and the spell. Though Bartolomeo had suffered only one torture session, which left him broken (*confractum*),[115] this one session was enough to have killed a less-resilient man. Bartolomeo was put to the strappado; his hands were tied behind his back, and he was raised in the air for quite a while and then, "terribly and suddenly," dropped almost to the ground. This degree of torture matches the highest degree that Grillandus mentioned. The procedure was repeated seven times. Nevertheless, the suspect remained constant in his refusal to confess, and when subsequently Galeazzo I Visconti (Matteo's heir, 1277–1328) suggested again that he perform the fatal magic (or, alternatively, bring in Dante Alighieri to do the job), he still refused. He managed to escape Milan with the magical figurine only after promising Galeazzo that he would indeed do the deed.[116]

Unfortunately, we have no further evidence in the matter. The tone is dry, precise, unemotional. The notary who took down the deposition did not mention pain even once. The only emotional note in the account comes from the repeated use of the term *martirium* [*sic*] to describe the torture and the single use of the phrase *martirium seu tormentum*.[117] Though legal treatises on torture borrowed freely from the martyrological vocabulary, they were careful to avoid the hallowed term. The feelings of outrage and pain and the desperate, stubborn adherence to the one version of events that could save him emerge in this one word from behind the dry account.

The use of martyrological terminology in this case does raise some questions. Why did Bartolomeo file this declaration in the papal chancery? Clearly, there was no chance of claiming redress from Milan. Most likely, papal authorities suspected that Bartolomeo had indeed broken down under torture and was involved in a plot to murder the pope—hence the need for a self-clearing declaration. Bartolomeo's claim that he had steadfastly refused to change his explanation for his sojourn in Avignon echoes the refusal of martyrs to change their declaration of Christianity. Just like the ancient martyrs, he claimed that he had not allowed the pain to change his statement.[118]

In sharp contrast to the hapless Bartolomeo, Tanin de Porte of Vienne was saved from torture by the efforts of a good lawyer. The fifteenth-century jurist Gui Pape (d. 1477) wrote a *consilium* to prevent his torture. Tanin de Porte had been accused of perjury by the fiscal procurator of the commune of Vienne. De Porte, a merchant and a citizen of Vienne, had appealed to the *parlement* of the Dauphiné (where Pape was a counselor) against the commune. Pape's primary defense argument did not concern guilt or innocence. Rather, he claimed that, in criminal matters, in the absence of a private denunciation (obviously lacking in this case) public authorities could initiate an inquisition only if the judge could establish a previous evil reputation, "not only once, but many times, so that it creates a public scandal, such that cannot be tolerated without danger [to the public]."[119] Pape's argument rested on no lesser an authority than Guillaume Durant's *Speculum iudiciale* (first published in 1271) and on the opinion of Angelo de Perigli (d. 1453), who had taught Roman law in Perugia. As Tanin de Porte was a man of good reputation and had proven that much to the Viennois judge, the inquisition carried out in his case was null and void. The premise behind this argument was that torture was meant only for the dishonorable and the manifestly criminal, and "honest" people should not be subjected to it. As we have seen, this premise had had a long history.

The judges who ordered torture also sentenced criminals to death or whipping. While causing pain as punishment was unlikely to place the sentencing judge on the dock for cruelty or abuse of power, here too a legal misstep could cause him some trouble. The canonist Panormitanus (1386–1445) told in his *consilia* of an urban *capitano di popolo* (commune unspecified) who, in an inquisitorial procedure, had condemned a certain Domenico in absentia to either a fine or loss of a limb. As it turned out, Domenico had been contumacious (i.e., absent from court) because, at the time, he was in jail and had had no knowledge of the ongoing trial, to say nothing of proper summons. Though we do not know the nature of the crime, Panormitanus himself strongly disapproved both of the sloppy procedure, conducted in the absence of the condemned man, and of the sentence. In general, he asserted, no man is lord of his own limbs, and mutilation was not a punishment he could approve of.[120] Once more, the main concern was with malpractice and shoddy procedure, not with gratuitous pain.

The first three cases cited here were real, while the last one might have been purely theoretical. But they all reflect an almost total disregard of bodily pain as a factor that ought to have deterred the judicial system. None of the advocates condemning torture did so in principle. Saying openly that systems of government (ecclesiastical as well as secular) relied upon what horrified and repelled all human beings was not possible, so technicalities were summoned to prevent the torture. Despite the specific objections in certain cases, there seems to have been a consensus that torture as a truth-finding method was legitimate. This legitimacy lasted over half a millennium in Europe. Daniel Baraz claims that jurists espoused humanity as opposed to cruelty, but it is rare to find any mention of such an attitude in torture tractates.[121]

The clearest evidence of malpractice in the system comes from the sixteenth-century witch-hunt. Since trial protocols rarely record concrete infringements of the rules, the best source to shed light upon the darkness of the dungeon is the one inquisitor who had absolutely no inhibitions about declaring his practices. When Heinrich Kramer—Dominican inquisitor and preacher, not a jurist—published the *Malleus maleficarum* in 1487, he was not trying to vaunt his erudition. His argument was that witchcraft was such a very dangerous crime that all judicial safeguards should be bypassed. Thus, he provided all the ammunition necessary for any judge wishing to bend the rules. Interestingly, the danger of witches was not sufficient, in his eyes, to warrant the creation of a new procedure; he merely found ways of legally subverting the system. Jurists, not surprisingly, avoided citing him. Kramer broke all the rules by dispensing with references to earlier authorities, arguing time and again that experience, not jurisprudence, was the best teacher. Though his writing echoes previous inquisitional manuals, scholastic theories, and theological knowledge, he rarely used quotations, unlike contemporary jurists.[122]

The third part of the *Malleus* is devoted to procedure.[123] Kramer advocated the inquisitorial mode over the accusatorial because it gave the judge more power (3.1). Beginning with the witnesses, all rules were thrown overboard. Everybody's testimony was acceptable: the word of excommunicates, accomplices, criminals, serfs, and infamous people was valid against suspected witches. Even open, mortal enemies of the suspect could testify (3.12). The suspect could neither see nor question the witnesses, could not even know their identity, but their testimony sufficed to send the suspect to torture. Reluctant witnesses were to be compelled to testify and questioned several times (3.2–6).[124] During the trial, none of the maneuvers a skilled advocate might use—postponements, appeals, exceptions, a flood of witnesses—were to be accepted in the urgency to stamp out heresy. In fact, the judge could debar any advocate who was considered litigious, accepting only those he found honest and cooperative. If the advocate demanded to see the charges, he could receive only an anonymous list (3.11). Since the devil invariably operated in secret, standards of proof became extremely elastic and minimal.[125] If even then sufficient evidence were lacking, one could always sentence the suspect to many years in prison, hoping new evidence would turn up. In any case, suspected witches were to be kept in prison until the entire procedure was over.

Kramer dedicated two long questions (3.15–16) to torture. The first, surprisingly, deals with a perfectly standard interlocutory sentence. If, once told of upcoming torture, the suspect confessed (and this, said Kramer, often happened, because the devil abandoned her then), she should still be moderately tortured, preferably without spilling blood (3.15).[126] If she did not, she was taken to torture; after one lifting on the strappado, the judge was allowed to fallaciously promise her her life if she confessed. If she persisted, she was to be shown the other instruments. If neither promises nor terror opened her month, "then for a second or third day her questioning must continue, but not be repeated, for one cannot repeat [torture] without new *indicia*" (3.15).[127] The formal continuation, rather than renewal, of torture, was the way to avoid the most basic of safeguards, the prohibition against renewed torture without new evidence.

The rest of the section on torture deals exclusively with witches, on the assumption that they had special supernatural powers to protect them from pain. As long as they had those powers, they would not confess, so they had to be entirely stripped of them. The stripping began with clothes, continued with removal of all bodily hair (to find hidden charms), and ended with abrasion of the skin of the entire body, for the charm might have been embedded under the skin. All this was not torture, merely a way to ensure torture worked. Run-of-the-mill torture treatises also assumed that suspects might use charms but contented themselves with the stripping of clothes and a search of the hair, for they dealt with run-of-the-mill criminals, not with witches. What is remarkable about this section is not so much the overt contempt for legality but the absolute rejection of any acceptable standard of proof. How was one to know if the suspect was really a witch? The judge was to exhort her to weep in memory of Christ's tears. Witches, however, were unable to weep, so if the suspect wept, she was not a witch. But witches too knew this, and they very craftily shammed tears. So crafty were they that a judge faced with tears ought not to believe the evidence of his eyes. The suspect was still a witch. Similarly, if no charm was found anywhere on the witch, it did not mean that the suspect was innocent; all it meant was that one must continue searching in the secret places of the body.[128]

Kramer's knowledge of legal procedure was sketchy at best, and he filled the gaps by relying upon his experience. For historians, Kramer may very well be the hand that draws back the curtain, the one voice that tells what went on behind closed doors in criminal trials if the judge happened to be arbitrary. How far anybody might have followed his abominable ideas in practice we cannot know. What does remain is the incredible discrepancy between the caution professional jurists advocated and the arbitrary coercion Kramer supported. After all, judges were liable to prosecution if a suspect died under torture. Kramer was not.

Conclusion

The times and places that saw the menacing flowering of torture were the same times and places that saw a number of other phenomena, all growing in the same context. The burgeoning of governmental punitive authorities was contemporary with the search for truth and the glorification of bodily pain. Though juridical discourse was carefully unemotional and seemingly devoid of intertextual references to other discourses of pain, the embeddedness of torture within late medieval cultural contexts is evident. The interconnectedness of truth and pain, the need to bring the secret, tortured confession into the light of public gaze in the courtroom, the insistence upon evidence—all these were part and parcel of contemporary culture. Similarly, the connection of pain with social shame and honor and the ever-present (but never mentioned) parallel with ancient martyrdom, which valorized pain, gave a cultural context to late medieval torture that could well explain the fact that not a single voice condemned the actual practice, only its abuses. This contextualized pain disintegrated in the sixteenth century. We have seen the decline of safeguards and the growth in severity in the theory and practice of torture. Nevertheless, those were the symptoms, not the phenomenon. The sixteenth century saw the politicization of torture, which was probably one of the reasons for the increase in its savagery.

The infamous strappado is still in use. It has been described as one of the most painful sensations a human being has ever undergone, a total disintegration of the self: "Frail in the face of violence, yelling out in pain, awaiting no help, capable of no resistance, the tortured person is only a body, and nothing else beside that," says Jean Améry, speaking of his own atrocious strappado experience. Nor does the pain end with the session: "Twenty-two years later I am still dangling over the ground by dislocated arms, panting, and accusing myself."[129] Given that human sensations cannot have changed much over a few centuries, it is fair to assume that medieval people reacted similarly. The procedures Franciscus Brunus listed as torture must have been efficient in one sense: most of those subjected to such tortures undoubtedly confessed. It is also likely that many of them did not survive the experience.

CHAPTER THREE

Alleviating Pain

The face of pain, seen from the perspective of medicine, was clearly different from the one seen through religion or law. Despite the universal acceptance in the Middle Ages that pain was an integral part of life and that there was much to praise in feeling it, throughout the period pain alleviation was written about and practiced extensively, with sporadic attempts at totally eradicating pain. Many of the efforts to alleviate pain, consisting primarily of herbal concoctions applied in the form of unguents or plasters to the body, would not be classified today as scientific. However, such methods should not be dismissed as merely popular remedies by any means. The tradition of pain relief through medication runs from Dioscorides (first century) and Galen (second century) to the later Middle Ages with remarkable consistency and continuity, appearing in learned medical writings just as frequently as in antidotaries and receptaries.

Theories and Definitions of Pain

Late medieval medical thought was the basis of much scholastic discourse about pain in other disciplines as well. Late medieval physicians were heirs to two separate traditions: the international medical culture and the growing scholastic discipline. They had inherited the wealth of Greek, Latin, Byzantine, and Arabic medicine but their thoughts and experiences were shaped in the scholastic matrix. This meant that certain rules of thought and proof had to apply in their writing. Thus, citing an earlier authority was proof—as good as, if not better than, clinical experience. Furthermore, their approach to any phenomenon (be it gallstones or geological petrified formations) was to categorize it. If one dealt with pain, one had to define it, place it within a specific framework, corporeal or animate, and break it down by type. Once one knew what sort of phenomenon it was, one could understand it.[1] Finally, one needed to pose questions concerning all those points and prove all claims by argument.

Systematic European thinking about pain began with Galenic medicine.[2] While ancient Greek medicine considered pain a diagnostic device and a useful prognostic tool, there was no theoretical framework for it. Hippocratic medicine was concerned with pain, but not enough to warrant definitions and clear-cut categories.[3] Galen, the most famous physician of his time, part heir to the Hippocratic tradition, part innovator, and a prolific author of medical texts, did cite causes for pain but did not offer a clear interpretation or taxonomy.[4] He did, however, provide the basic definition of pain. In his most detailed work on pain, *Of the Affected Parts* (*De interioribus*), Galen included what sounds like a well-worn (albeit unknown to us beforehand) definition of pain: "I remember often saying that the two types of pain are the sudden change of temperament and the rupture of continuity."[5] Galen inserted this statement casually, indicating that by his time this was already a truism beyond argument. Galen had probably not formulated it, nor did he devote much thought to it. In modern parlance, Galen's definition meant that pain could come from either inside or outside the body. The temperament—*krasis* in Greek, *temperamentum* in classical Latin, and *complexio* in late medieval Latin—was the balance of the four humors (blood, phlegm, choler, and black bile) in the body and their relationship to all other elements within it. All organs have an intrinsically labile complexion. When change—from hot to cold, for example—occurs, the organ resists the contrary force, and thus pain appears out of a resistance to change of the natural condition. The second element—the body's continuity—was the fabric of the body, as one saw and felt it. Any breach of the body's integrity—a break, a wound, or any other local dissolution of tissues and vessels—disturbed the smooth uniformity of skin, limbs, organs, or bones. Such an external trauma, interrupting the wholeness of the body, also caused pain.

Throughout Arab, Latin, and vernacular medieval medicine, all subsequent generations were destined to repeat this statement as an article of faith. The Galenic tradition was adopted by most of the antique medical world and subsequently introduced into Persian, Jewish, and Arab medicine. Centuries later, with some alterations, it was incorporated into the great medical compendium of Abu Ali al-Husain ibn Abdallah ibn Sina (Avicenna). Gerard of Cremona's (1114–87) Latin translation of the *Canon of Medicine* became a classic of Western universities during the late twelfth and early thirteenth centuries. Its effect was significant.[6]

Avicenna began his treatment of pain with the assertion that pain was *res non naturalis*. It was thus one of the six nonnaturals (i.e., external forces) affecting the body.[7] This, said Avicenna, was why he had placed the discussion of pain and its categories in the first book of his *Canon*, which was supposed to deal with universal, theoretical problems.[8] Avicenna was the first to include pain among the nonnatural forces. The only explanation for this innovation is that presumably Avicenna subsumed pain under the passions of the soul, commonly understood as emotions rather than sensations. Whatever his reason, the Latin Avicenna granted pain a place hitherto unknown in Western medicine. By placing human pain in relation to nature and as a nonnatural, Avicenna elevated what had been a somewhat-unpopular diagnostic tool to the rank of a primary affective force with a theory of its own. In a state of perfect balance and health, people ought not to feel pain. The idea that the natural, pristine state of humanity was free from pain and that pain meant a deviation from the natural state had survived separately in Western medicine and theology in a muted form. Following the dissemination of Avicenna's writings, it revived, entrenched in the Christian context of prelapsarian Adam.[9]

For Avicenna, following Galen, pain was primarily the result of a drastic change somewhere in the human body. Alteration immediately caused a protesting reaction of the organism, which resisted change and tried to preserve the status quo: "Pain is a sensation produced by something contrary to the course of nature, and this sensation is set up by one or two circumstances: a very sudden change of complexion—or the pathologically unbalanced complexion[10]—and a rupture of continuity."[11]

Before the arrival of Arabic medicine, Western medicine mostly confined itself to attempting pain relief, without inquiring too far into the causes, effects, and nature of pain. With Avicenna and Galen in hand, Western physicians began addressing pain as a subject of scholastic study. Most medical authors, and some theologians, cited the standard definition of pain with slight alterations. Taddeo Alderotti (1223–95) in Bologna, Arnau de Villanova (1238–1311) and Bernard de Gordon (ca. 1258–1320) in Montpellier, and a score of other medical writers repeated the definition.[12]

The definition of a thing provides it with its individuality and character, as Guy de Chauliac (d. 1368), papal surgeon, stressed.[13] Having defined pain, one could discuss it as an independent phenomenon and treat it accordingly. While there seems to have been unanimity concerning the causes of pain, physicians differed when it came to its locus. Many, among them Arnau de Villanova, followed Aristotle, placing it within the sense of touch (and thus within the sensitive soul).[14] Others, among them Taddeo Alderotti, adhered to Galen's theory in arguing that pain was perceived through the sensitive nerves and the spirit.[15]

None of these learned arguments, however, could help in the alleviation of pain or in its healing. When it came to actual practices, late medieval medicine tended to rely far more upon a tried-and-true tradition of herbal pharmacology (with some animal elements as well) than upon scholastic definitions. The place where the voices of university professors join those of surgeons and healers is in the practice of alleviation. "The notion that nothing in nature was without power underlies much of medieval pharmaceutical practice, and accounts in part for the enormous variety of substances medieval people employed in their medicines," notes Faye Getz in the introduction to her edition of the Middle English translation of the works of Gilbertus Anglicus.[16] When it comes to the composition of medicines, her comments are relevant for painkilling recipes and incantations throughout Europe. While variants exist all over, substances considered to be painkillers seem to have been a common tradition. In principle, every substance could be hot, cold, moist, or dry. Consequently, if a patient suffered from a cold, moist headache, he required a medicine composed of hot, dry substances. This principle stands at the base of all recipes, medical and popular alike.

Alleviation as Healing Practice

The most common historiographical assumption concerning pain treatment by healers in the Middle Ages used to be that they paid no attention at all to their patients' sufferings and never lifted a finger to alleviate pain. This attitude was assumed to have been born not out of indifference but from incapacity.[17] The dark ages of ignorance apparently lacked all means of pain sedation, and the best physicians could do was to avoid harming their patients by "ignorant" treatment.[18]

On the whole, the historiography of pain skipped over medieval history. What little work that did appear usually relied not upon medical but upon the more accessible theological sources, where praise of pain and suffering abounded.[19] Augustine's writings were taken as sufficient evidence for a millennium of medical learning and practice. The greater availability of theological than medical writing fostered a tendentious selection of evidence that stressed the significance of pain for Christian religiosity and supported the premise that pain was either ignored or deliberately exacerbated throughout the Middle Ages.[20] This view was reinforced by the well-entrenched construct of "the medieval man."[21] This curious figure, the brainchild of historians, was primitive enough to lack sensory delicacy and was thus immune to pain. That is why he was able to tolerate all the pain nature and other people inflicted upon him. In contrast to modern man, who was sensitive to pain but restrained by culture, medieval man (and it was invariably a man) stood closer to the imaginary Neanderthal man than to modernity. Nineteenth-century history of medicine supported this construct, which Daniel de Moulin ably demolished only in the 1970s.[22] De Moulin marshaled all the evidence he could find to show that human beings six or ten centuries ago were as sensitive to pain as modern humans and that any attempt to argue neurological changes over such a short evolutionary term was nonsense. De Moulin's examples ranged widely from medical to lay writings, but like his opponents, he relied upon stray examples. His best argument for a fairly stable pain threshold for the past few thousand years is the constant harping on pain in nonmedical literature; had it not frightened and repelled people, there would have been no point in threatening them with corporal punishments or with hell, where pain was the major retribution.

Was medieval medicine callous toward pain? By no means. When they did refer to pain, many medieval medical writings insisted that pain must be sedated, often even before the causal illness was treated. The same is true, and even more so, for the writing of surgeons. I will treat the means of analgesia, or easing pain, and anesthesia (the removal of all sensation) in the following sections, but we must begin with the decision to treat pain. The evidence for such treatment is contradictory and too thin to draw firm conclusions. Some physicians and some types of medical literature almost invariably included pain management, others omitted it, and there does not seem to be a clear-cut development from indifference to sensitivity (or vice versa), from lack of understanding to a coherent theory of treatment. Still, one would be hard put to find a healer who did not recommend any palliative care at all.[23]

The clear distinction between learned and popular medicine appears in the prescribed order of treatment. While more popular collections concentrated upon curing the immediate pain, the first thing to be done about any disease, including pain, according to scholastic medicine, was to make the patient adopt a healthy regimen of life, with proper diet, rest, and baths. This general prescription goes back to antiquity, reappearing in twelfth-century Salerno and recurring thereafter in general textbooks and *consilia*. The main principle of the regimen was moderation in all things: not too much wine, but also not too much exercise and not too much sleep. Drugs or other forms of medical intervention only came into use when a healthy lifestyle failed to heal disease. Nevertheless, in England John of Mirfield (1362–1407) distinguished between *experimenta*, or expedients that rid the patient of painful symptoms, and proper cures, which take time. In his view, most patients did not have the patience to wait for a disease to run its course but demanded prompt alleviation.[24] This yielding to patient pressure for prompt relief is specifically English. None of the Continental authors recommended pain relief for no other reason than the patient's comfort. Nevertheless, John of Mirfield's trenchant statement concerning the dangers of pain and the importance of alleviation can be found echoed all over Europe:

> In all procedures of medicine, when pain is present we ought first to alleviate the pain. Of this Galen says: "Strong pain has a character which supersedes any other factor." And again, "Painful parts, also, or parts having pain: The pain is itself the cause of attracting the worst of the humors. . . . When pain occurs in a wound, therefore, or some other evil distemper, then we ought not to strive for the consolidation of the wound; but first we ought to alleviate the pain and remove the distemper which was there; then we should cleanse away the sanies, then generate flesh, and last achieve a scar."[25]

To understand this almost-universal attitude, one must return to medical perceptions of the nature of pain. As Avicenna had said, pain could be one of three things: the sign and manifestation of an illness (like the pain that follows fever), the cause of another sickness (for pain causes humor to concentrate in one spot, producing a swelling, a syncope, or a spasm), or an independent disease (as in the case of headaches or earaches). If pain was only a signal, one needed to interpret it and cure the disease behind it. But if it was an illness, or worse, a motive cause for a further illness, it was imperative to treat it before it caused further harm or even death.[26] Even if pain did not bring about anything as dramatic as Avicenna feared, it still weakened the patient and interfered with the normal functions of the organs, making breathing difficult. Therefore, said Constantine the African (ca. 1020–87, quoting Galen), one must hasten to perform a phlebotomy to cure the pain, lest the patient be further weakened by waiting and end up too weak (*ne virtus deficiat*) to withstand the bloodletting.[27] Surgeons William de Saliceto (1210–77) and Guy de Chauliac warned that in cases of nerve wounds the pain was severe enough to cause a possibly lethal spasm and therefore had to be treated before anything else was done; Bernard de Gordon repeated the same urgency several times, claiming that pain could cause fever.[28] Michele Savonarola (ca. 1385–1466) counted sedation as the second of the intelligent physician's Ten Commandments.[29] In sum, medical lore assumed that pain could cause fever, spasms, and even death and hence ought to be treated independently and immediately.

In Paris, where Avicenna was better accepted than in Montpellier, Jean de Saint-Amand published his *Concordantiae* sometime in the last decades of the thirteenth century.[30] The book is an alphabetized collection of short sentences from Galen's works and Avicenna's *Canon*, sorted by topic. The animadversions concerning pain faithfully appear under *dolor*, giving any searcher a pithy summary of classical opinions on the subject of sedation and its utmost importance. Physicians in Italy, Montpellier, and Spain also supported this attitude, counseling sedation before all else.[31] Pain should be sedated before any curative action was taken. This abundance of statements in favor of analgesia might not argue great efficacy, but it does prove, beyond doubt, that pain was a serious concern for healers of all sorts. Beyond the need to please the (paying) patient, many practitioners argued that pain was harmful and that sedation was an essential part of the cure.

Methods of Soothing Pain

There was no clear distinction in the Middle Ages between popular and learned medical recipes. The borderline between what we would consider folklore and what we would consider "proper" medicine was extremely porous. Herbs, incantations, animal excrement, and human-female milk all permeated this border. Much as surgeons and physicians might decry the practices of "old women" healers and *empirici*, the ingredients of analgesic prescriptions were fairly similar. Receptaries and antidotaries appeared during the early Middle Ages, and even respectable late medieval physicians did not scruple to include entire collections of prescriptions in their *opera*.

Thus, there is little difference between "low" and "high" analgesia. For one thing, almost all analgesics were external rather than meant for ingestion. They were to be used mostly in salves and plasters and sometimes for inhalation or fumigation. All unguents and plasters included some sort of fat: Guy de Chauliac recommended using the fat of chickens, ducks, or geese. Alternatively, one could use oil (preferably rose or violet oil) or linseed. Jacques Despars (1380?–1458) recommended rosewater and rose oil for hot pains and lily oil for cold ones.[32] Other standard additives (probably for their binding qualities) were egg yolk and egg white. Next, there was an array of plants used for different kinds of aches and pains: mallow, chard, oregano, lettuce, purslane, cucumber. The plants that could put someone to sleep or cause death—poppy, henbane, hemlock, crocus, mandrake—were in a different category of stupefacients. They were not, properly speaking, sedatives of pain, since they put the person, rather than the pain, to sleep.[33] As a rule, they were very sparingly used, for obvious reasons. Opium, due to its high price, appears only in the writings of surgeons and physicians, but even these avoided it if at all possible.[34]

In practice, recipes tended to mix the categories of analgesics and anesthetics. Thus, Mondino de'Liuzzi (ca. 1270–1326) recommended an embrocation composed of cold elements (lettuce, dill, poppy, henbane, and mandrake root) compounded with warm ones (oregano, melilot, chamomile, rose, and laurel). The principle here was to mitigate the cold effects of the first group of herbs. In cases of severe pain, one was to use purely stupefacient medicines: henbane juice, water lily, powdered mandrake root, opium, crocus.[35] Like all other recipes, painkiller recipes were vague. Quantities appear in medical, but not popular, recipes. The embrocation cited above contains ten ingredients, but the recipe mentioned quantities only for the roses and the mandrake root. The stronger recipe, meant for a salve, contains no quantities whatsoever other than "some" opium. Nor does it specify which part of the crocus or the water lily to use, and how. This vagueness, though, was by no means an indication of carelessness. The prevalent belief that one learned more about compounding medication by practice and imitation than from theoretical handbooks, further strengthened by the idea that proportions and quantities were entirely individual and specifically tailored to each patient, made exact measurements irrelevant.[36] Moreover, given the lack of a universal system of weights and measures, whatever quantities were listed might have been incomprehensible.[37] Usually, narcotic recipes prescribed quantities of the dangerous substances, for every antidotary insisted upon the dangers of an overdose.

Animal excrement and urine were also standard ingredients for painkillers. Guy de Chauliac and John Arderne recommended using pigeon excrement in an analgesic plaster; Jehan Sauvage de Picquigny prescribed gargling with the urine of a white dog for a throat infection. The first was the pope's surgeon, the second a surgeon in Newark, and the third a clerk and author of a dubious receptary.[38] Occasionally, one comes across exotic medicines that required the blood of a virgin (preferably noble) or, more often, a woman's milk.[39] Modes of preparation were also similar. Mashing, soaking, boiling, distilling, or infusing plants and mixing with a binder to make a poultice, with animal fat for an ointment, or with wine for drinking differed little from one recipe to another.[40] Poultices and embrocations for soothing pain could also be hot or cold. Surgeons from the learned tradition preferred hot poultices, but there are many prescriptions for cold ones as well, if the pain was classified as hot.[41]

Finally, our information about charms and amulets is not limited to the so-called popular literature. Guy de Chauliac might have despised them, but English authors cheerfully included charms in their treatises.[42] Some collections included invocations to St. Apollonia against toothache (her martyrdom had consisted of having her teeth drawn), inserted after a series of sedatives composed of herbal medicines.[43] Other charm cures contained an entire narrative:

> Item, carry this note. Peter sat on a rock, and the Lord said to him, "Peter, what is the matter with you?" Peter answered, "My teeth hurt." The Lord said to him, "Peter, remember by this sign: father and son and holy ghost." Whoever carries this note will not suffer toothache.[44]

The most remarkable incantation is one recommended by Gilbertus Anglicus. It is a narrative incantation in which three pious brothers meet Christ, who queries their destination. They answer that they are going to the Mount of Olives to gather herbs for healing blows and wounds (the incantation is for head wounds). Christ supplies their need by telling them to call upon him and then take sheep's wool steeped in olive oil and put it on the wound, saying, "As Longeus the Jew pierced the side of our Lord Jesus Christ, *who did not bleed nor was corrupted nor suffered pain nor decay*, let not this wound occur which now I chant, in the name of the Father and the Son and the Holy Ghost, Amen."[45] Gilbertus Anglicus was a cleric who also practiced medicine.[46] Nevertheless, the total nonorthodoxy of claiming that the posthumous wound on Christ's side neither bled nor caused pain did not seem to trouble him at all. Incantations were passed on from receptary to receptary, with little difference between the learned and the popular.

The practice of collecting recipes in antidotaries, probably composed in monasteries, goes back to the High Middle Ages.[47] Almost every recipe in these collections is recommended for several purposes, among them pain relief. Thus, the ninth-century Bamberg antidotary recommends an antidote "that is given all year long to those suffering from gout." The compound is supposed to help gout, all pains of joints, headache, stomachache, pain in the eyes, dysentery, calluses, and pain in the liver, spleen, and kidneys. Boiled, thickened, and used as an ointment, it loosens stiff joints. There is also a recipe for a fortifying potion that is useful for pain anywhere in the body.[48] Seemingly, the word *dolor* in the Bamberg antidotary is synonymous with "illness," but it is remarkable how many of the prescriptions are supposed to be analgesic in one form or another. The Bamberg antidotary contains 78 recipes. Of these, fewer than two-thirds (46) state the uses of the recipe. Slightly fewer than one-half of the recipes with a stated purpose (21) include analgesia among their effects. Such a frequent mention of pain argues for a pain-conscious pharmacopeia; efficacious or not, one of the main purposes of the drugs was to free people from pains in various organs.

The *Antidotarium Nicolai*, the most famous and most copied medieval pharmacopeia, was probably written in Salerno between 1160 and 1220.[49] It is a composite of the old Salernitan antidotary tradition and new Arab knowledge and has a much richer pharmacopeia than the older antidotaries for physicians. However, the multipurpose character of prescriptions remained unaltered. The Agrippa salve, for example, helps cure dropsy, tumors in any part of the body, and restless nerves. It is also a diuretic, relaxes the abdomen, and cures cold pains of the kidneys.[50]

The word *dolor* is far less common in the *Antidotarium Nicolai* than in the Bamberg antidotary. This does not necessarily mean callous indifference on the part of Salernitan physicians, but that the vocabulary had grown more diversified. *Dolor* was no longer a synonym for "illness." The prescriptions have a much richer language for describing diseases, and many diagnoses that earlier would have been simply "headache" now refer to a specific type of headache—*hemicranea, foda*, and so on. A prescription meant specifically for a migraine does not need to add that it eases the pain of the head. In contrast, toothache and earache still had no name but the generic one.[51] In other cases, medication for sedating the pain inherent in certain diseases was separated from the medication meant to cure the illness: thus, a prescription (one of several) for treating kidney, gall, or bladder stones was meant primarily to pulverize the stone, not to ease the pain.[52] In older antidotaries, where *dolor* was often synonymous with "illness," both migraines and kidney stones might have been labeled "pain." In contrast, the later ones clearly distinguish between the disease and the ensuing pain.

An appropriate pharmacopeia had developed together with a new variety and richness of diagnoses. It is possible to see in this shift the beginnings of stress upon the cure of a disease rather than care for its symptoms. Despite the linguistic development, the presence of sedatives still looms large. The *Antidotarium Nicolai* includes 142 prescriptions, of which 41 have primarily sedative qualities; several soothe more than one organ, so that sedation appears 63 times in the text. Headaches top the list of aches and pains (14 prescriptions), followed by pains of the stomach (8), intestines (7), teeth (6), kidneys (5), and breasts (4). Most prescriptions are of the stupefacient variety, including opium or poppy, henbane, and mandrake.[53]

By the early thirteenth century, a new collection of Arab pharmacology had reached the West. The *Grabadin* of Pseudo-Mesue (Yūh'annā Ibn Māsawaih, 777–857) was a highly valued and important source that included many hitherto-unknown prescriptions.[54] Many of the new recipes were incorporated into late medieval receptaries. To what extent those new medicines were applicable, even feasible in the West, remains questionable.[55]

Anonymous receptaries proliferated in the later Middle Ages.[56] Many of them were vernacular, and most of them mixed medication with incantations and means of medical divination. Thus, one will commonly find in those receptaries means of discovering the sex of an unborn child, the state of a woman's virginity, and the prognosis for a severely ill patient in danger of death.[57] Like the early medieval antidotaries, late medieval receptaries rarely distinguished between pain and illness. Consequently, *dolor* looms large in them.

Was this "popular" type of medical literature divorced from academic writing on pain? Unquestionably, physicians had a wide vocabulary for different types of pain, but when it came to plasters, inhalations, and other pharmaceutical recipes, they had recourse to the same ingredients. The one clear difference is that benedictions and charms to be pronounced upon medication prior to administering it appear in recipe collections but not in the writings of professional surgeons and physicians.[58] The great distinction, however, between the popular and the learned lies in the form: receptaries have no clear internal order, while scholastic pharmacology created order from chaos, ending up with the same medications but presented in a better-organized way.

The late medieval proliferation of academic and semiacademic medical textbooks had a formative effect upon the structure of composition. Salernitan twelfth-century works usually followed the head-to-foot model of surveying the entire body, top to bottom, whether dealing with anatomy or pharmacology. The same system was kept later in anatomical works: once the author began the description of the body, he followed the same order (rather than organizing by bones, nerves, skin, etc.). Pharmacological works, like the *Antidotarium Nicolai*, had no specific internal order at all, barring a vague tendency to follow the alphabet. Once Arab science and university discipline grew, the structure of medical works became clearer. A specific text on a specific problem might not deal with medication, but general works, following Avicenna's pattern, included an *antidotarium* as their last chapter, often partially culled from the *Antidotarium Nicolai*.[59] Painkillers did not deserve a full section. Within the pharmacological section of a general work, however, scholastic medicine applied its own order.

The prime example of reorganization of the pharmacopeia according to scholastic principles comes from the prime representative of the rational surgery.[60] Guy de Chauliac's antidotary does not resemble the traditional one. First, it includes other means of healing in addition to drugs. Second, the drugs are not organized alphabetically or haphazardly but according to their function. Thus, Guy begins with bloodletting in all its forms: phlebotomy, cupping, and leeches. From there he moves to purgatives, cauterization, and the preparation and manner of application of antidotes. Chapter 5 begins a series of three chapters that list medications according to what the surgeon would use them to treat: apostemes (i.e., abscesses), flesh wounds, and fractures. For each situation the surgeon distinguishes the types of medication according to their use: thus, the chapter on apostemes lists repercussives, attractives, resolutives, softeners, maturatives, cleansers, and sedatives. The order follows roughly the envisioned progress of the illness. When the aposteme first appears, there are medicines aimed at arresting inflammation. These are followed by drugs that attract noxious matter (be it an infection, an embedded arrow, or snake poison) from noble, internal organs to the vulgar, surface ones, so that it can be easily extracted. If the subcutaneous infection still exists, the resolutives help rid the wound of any remaining infection; the softening drugs make the wound amenable to treatment; if there was no choice but to mature and lance the aposteme, the maturatives were used; cleansing drugs rid the wound of the remaining pus; and sedatives eased the discomfort. The following chapters are also arranged in a functional way for the surgeon who requires a different drug at different stages of treatment. All in all, Guy de Chauliac's pharmacy is a far cry from the old antidotary or from haphazard receptaries.

Guy de Chauliac did not invent his antidotary *ex nihilo*. He was heir to a learned surgical tradition going back to the first half of the thirteenth century.[61] Along with a rational organization of material, he included phlebotomy and cauterization, methods that previously had not belonged in an antidotary. These two procedures were indeed a surgeon's stock-in-trade, and we do know that many surgeons from all strata of the profession practiced them. With what success they did so is open to question. All receptaries contain numerous recipes for stanching hemorrhages.[62] One does wonder whether all these cases were of bleeding wounds or whether occasionally a barber's botched phlebotomy may have had to be stanched.[63] Given that phlebotomies were used not only for immediate cures but also as part of a regular health regime, the possibility does seem realistic.

In contrast to surgeons, physicians, who did not battle pain on a daily basis, were the more likely to try and plumb the origins of pain before sedating it. Unlike surgeons, they were not faced with the extreme suffering of surgery without anesthetics and in fact were often not faced with the patient at all, only with his or her urine in a uroscopy flask. One might well expect them to have been more callous to pain than their less erudite brothers and sisters. If they were, however, it is hard to tell, for physicians left behind several types of writing, each displaying a different degree of concern: most great medical compendia treat pain theoretically, manuals of practice are one degree closer to the patient, and *consilia* evince most care for pain alleviation.

Applying an embrocation or a salve to the ill body was not the central practice of scholastic medicine. If illness and pain resulted from an imbalance of humors, the best way to rectify the imbalance was by expelling from the body the superfluous humor. The same could be said for pains caused by corrupt matter or humors. The main practice argued for getting rid of the bad so that the good could recover its natural place. This could entail evacuation of the digestive system by means of emetics or laxatives or the lancing of inflamed spots, but mostly, it meant phlebotomy.

Arnau de Villanova devoted considerable space to pain in his commentaries on Galen's work, but only on its diagnostic uses. In some cases, he insisted, sedating the pain without dealing with the real problem would only endanger the patient. Once sedated, the warning signal was gone, but the illness had yet to be cured. For example, in the case of a hot aposteme, nothing but evacuation would help.[64] His other elaborate analysis of pain, within a treatise on phlebotomy, also has more to say about the theory of pain than about pain management.[65] More interesting is the Parisian physician and author Jacques Despars, who wrote a massive commentary on Avicenna's *Canon*. In his commentary on book 1 (which contains Avicenna's treatise on pain), Despars paid no attention to Avicenna's work on pain. However, he did comment on one specific chapter, "the effects of pain on the body."[66] Whereas Avicenna stressed most emphatically the destructive character of pain, Despars took precisely the opposite attitude. He cited the case of Adam de Baudribosc, president of the Chambre de comptes, who took to drink as a soporific rather than adhering to a strict dietary regimen that would have allowed the ulcer in his bladder to get better, and ended up dying of it.[67] The implication is fairly obvious: Despars did not think sedation was of prime importance in this case; perhaps he even disapproved of his patient's demands for ease. In this case, pain was a symptom, and like Arnau de Villanova, Despars believed in treating the disease, not its symptom. These statements stand in clear contradiction to the practice of always trying to ameliorate patients' pain, but they appear only in medical writings meant specifically for professionals.

Professors of medicine were usually also practitioners of the art, so one cannot distinguish between clinicians and academics. Manuals of practice, though, usually do show more preoccupation with pain than theoretical treatises. Mondino de Liuzzi began his *Pratica de accidentibus* by insisting that pain must first be eased in every sickness.[68] Furthermore, Mondino prescribed his own recipe for a painkiller for each pain, testifying to his own ability to distinguish the different types of pain. As his treatise is concerned only with noble (i.e., mostly inner) organs, beginning with the head, and these were invariably the most sensitive to pain, his concern is understandable. Going farther, he insisted that "the primary cure of pain is the cure that seeks the reason that is proper to the sensation, and therefore such a cure is through those [medications] that remove all sensation or block it, and those are universally stupefactive and narcotic, and these we use only when the pain is strongest, so that it destroys the strength."[69] In short, Mondino advocated anesthesia rather than analgesia in cases of great pain. Cristoforo Barzizza's (ca. 1390–1445) *Introductorium practicae medicinae* contains numerous chapters that address pain as illness (of ears, head, teeth, spleen, etc.) and in every one he prescribed sedation. Like Mondino, Barzizza distinguished different types of pain.[70] One can clearly see the difference between theory and practice of sedation here. While sweeping statements concerning the need for sedation appear everywhere, in practice healers first examined the case at hand before deciding whether to sedate or not.

A single voice stubbornly insisted also in literature addressed to the laity that the physician first diagnose the illness hiding behind the pain and cure it, incidentally also ridding the patient of the pain. In his *consilia* Arnau de Villanova remained steadfast to the opinion expressed in his commentaries. In a *consilium* dealing with quartan fever, he sternly warned his putative correspondent not to believe quacks (*dolosi*) who promised to lower fever by using cold stupefacients (such as opium or mandrake) without recourse to phlebotomy or evacuation. Making the pain go away without ridding the body of superfluous matter would cure nothing.[71] Arnau's opinion was destined to become standard wisdom two centuries later, when prompt sedation became a "popular error."[72]

Whether physicians also practiced what they preached is impossible to determine. The literature of *consilia* is problematic in this sense, since it is impossible to know which cases are real and which imaginary, and it is doubtful that physicians wrote only about their real cases.[73] Furthermore, *consilia* almost never include a clinical follow-up after the patient had complied with the doctor's advice. Clearly, too, a *consilium* for a real case, in which a patient had paid for treatment, would include discussion of how pain was managed, while theoretical texts would pay less attention to pain. Still, if a physician described his putative treatment of pain during the care of an illness, the fact that he troubled to do so is significant.

Faithful to the idea that headache is a disease, Bartolomeo Montagnana (fl. 1422–60) described how he sedated *dolor gravativus capitis a materia frigida et humida* in one case but in another insisted that one must cure the plethora of cold and humid humors causing the headache by purgation and diet.[74] Sedative measures and recipes were prescribed in cases of hemorrhoids, gallstones, kidney and bladder stones, cancers, headaches, earaches, and toothaches. Unlike Mondino, Montagnana restricted the use of opium to toothache and recommended for stones simply warm and dry analgesics to counteract the cold and humid matter causing the illness.[75] Cases of gout also earned sedation; Arnau de Villanova and Taddeo Alderotti gave several prescriptions, many of them including opium. Painkillers were prescribed when the pain was the illness (as in headaches and toothaches) and when its violence caused fear that it would sap the patient's strength before recovery. "For pain, in its extremity, sometimes makes us break all rules," noted Michele Savonarola. Baverio Maghinardo de Bonetti (1405/6–1480) recommended analgesia not only for kidney stones but also in terminal cases. He had diagnosed a woman with terminal cancer of the womb and recommended painkillers, "so that life may be lengthened and the pain made more tolerable."[76] It is always possible to find a *consilium* that neglects to mention sedation for certain illnesses, but the general picture is one of common practical resort to sedation in painful illnesses. Practice manuals and *consilia* were expected to deal with clinical, rather than theoretical, problems, and so sedation in various forms seems to have been standard practice.

Nevertheless, most *consilia*, regardless of the diagnosis they arrived at, begin by prescribing a general regimen of health: exercise, moderate intake of food and drink, rest, and regular purgation.[77] Purgation included laxatives, diuretics, and emetics.[78] Purgation might also occasionally stop pain if the humor being purged caused the pain. Indeed, a thorough cleansing of what Guy de Chauliac terms *cacochimia* (a superfluity of bad humors) was useful for many purposes, among them alleviation of pain. Still, purgatives were powerful medicine, not to be given to the young or the old. The underlying perception was indeed the one voiced by Arnau de Villanova: pain is more often a symptom of another illness, not an illness in itself. In most cases, therefore, the serious physician would first heal the patient of the illness rather than sedate the pain. Presumably, the pain would disappear once the illness was gone.

Childbirth Sedation?

Medical literature, especially books of practice and *consilia*, passed over in silence those cases in which alleviation of pain was not an option. The texts speak of action, not a deliberate withholding of action. Nevertheless, there are some rare descriptions of pain situations in which no palliative is recommended, and it is incumbent upon us to query those cases. The clearest case of pain unquestionably present, yet unalleviated, is childbirth.

Almost every obstetric textbook contained recipes for hastening birth or easing postpartum pains, but almost none suggest any mode of relief during labor. The best-known medieval gynecology manual, Trotula's *Of the Diseases of Women*, is silent on the subject. Trotula and others suggested violent sneezing as a mode of hastening contractions, and several texts recommended a variety of oils for anointing the vaginal tract.[79] These measures were meant to hasten and ease the birth, so that both mother and child would survive. The option of making the delivery less painful for the parturient is mentioned nowhere in these tracts.

The reason did not lie in any medical or masculine callousness. Nor, surprisingly enough, did medieval physicians adduce the curse upon Eve as a reason. It seems that the scholarly medical tradition considered uterine contractions and the resultant pain as one and the same. Consequently, easing the pain would slow the contractions and endanger the entire birth. Thus, Michele Savonarola inveighed against the female custom of walking around during labor precisely on the grounds that it eased the pain: "Furthermore, the constant movement of the parturient woman to and fro, not wishing to suffer the pain, adds much to the difficulty of the delivery; the delivery chair, or *catedra*, adds much to the ease of the birth, because staying upon it and not moving away from it, the pains continue and become stronger."[80]

This perception may have deterred physicians from prescribing painkillers to parturient women, but less academic healers did not share it. An anonymous, pseudo–Arnau de Villanova book of practice proves a most interesting link between the different levels of writing. The author began by borrowing Trotula's recipe for soothing water, in which mallow, fenugreek, and linseed had been cooked. He also recommended several sedative oils and subsequently pepper to make the woman sneeze hard with mouth and nose covered and thus hasten the birth. The significant difference between Trotula's twelfth-century text and the fourteenth-century one is that Trotula indicated those recipes for a *difficult* birth, while pseudo–Arnau de Villanova recommended them for a *painful* one.[81] Subsequently, the anony-

mous author tells of a *vetula* (wisewoman) who recommended an incantation that included the Pater Noster and some gibberish. Having cited the
entire incantation, he ends with a comprehensive condemnation: "all this
I condemn, and I think that all the true faithful should flee such diabolic
medicines."[82]

Pseudo–Arnau de Villanova may have cited an incantation only to condemn it out of hand, but the incantation forms part of a considerable corpus
of prayers and incantations for parturient women, practically all of them
intended to ensure a painless delivery. Many of them, the *peperit* charms, cite
the births of Samuel, John the Baptist, the Virgin, and Christ as successful
(albeit not necessarily easy) precedents.[83] Similarly, exempla speak of miraculously painless births granted by the Virgin and St. Margaret of Antioch.[84]
There is no way of knowing whether women had a hand in composing those
prayers and charms. It does seem plausible, however, that whoever did
compose them knew enough of childbirth not to ignore the element of pain
in the search for a safe and quick delivery. The incantation cited by pseudo–
Arnau de Villanova might have come from the pen of a wisewoman, but it
might far more plausibly have come from the pen of a cleric who had heard
and seen midwives at work and women in labor.

In sum, medical texts treated childbirth extensively but avoided the
subject of labor pains. All the references to a difficult delivery do not necessarily mean a painful one but rather a protracted and dangerous one. At the
same time, the literature of charms saw no reason not to provide for painlessness, and many charms and prayers do voice the parturient's wish for a
pain-free delivery. Occasionally, but very rarely, those same charms seeped
into medical literature.[85]

Exposure to Pain

Besides sedating the pain of illness, healers caused much pain through treatment. They did not do so to satisfy the demands of theologians who praised
pain; it was simply that some healing practices were inherently painful.
Most painful procedures were handled by surgeons, those notorious semi-
butchers of medical invective. In the later Middle Ages university-trained
surgeons often shared the opinions of physicians rather than those of plain
village barbers and itinerant tooth-pullers.[86] Such surgeons left their writings,
studded with learned quotations, for posterity, and in those writings they
advocated several practices that could heal but that caused pain. Learned
surgeons spoke with two tongues about pain: on the one hand, it was necessary to sedate pain before attempting a cure,[87] and severe pain could be

dangerous. On the other hand, when describing surgical procedures, they often ignored completely the problem of pain. For instance, the removal of an arrowhead, doubtlessly a painful operation, deserved a purely technical instruction with no mention of sedation.[88] Indeed, it is probable that pain alleviation was applied far more often in cases of illness or wounds than during surgery.

Some painful procedures gained sufficient academic esteem to merit their description in medical and surgical literature. As we shall see, most of them had a great deal to do with extracting from the human organism those noxious elements that caused imbalance and illness. When it came to maintaining and restoring health, it was necessary to restore the balance of humors by actively drawing out the excess of whichever humor was causing the imbalance. The restoration of balance was not necessarily invasive or painful; fumigations and sweat-baths were often recommended.[89] Other means were more drastic, and surgeons were exhorted to make sure the patients could tolerate them. Expulsion of matter could take place through either end of the digestive tract, by use of emetics, laxatives, clysters (enemas), and diuretics. These were often used to evacuate noxious "unnatural" matter promptly from the system.[90] Many medical *consilia* advised drastic artificial evacuation as a regular part of a health regimen and in cases of illness, even if it was uncomfortable. For example, the manifold problems of several of Montagnana's putative patients stemmed from a cold and humid complexion, which caused many problems in all parts of the body.[91] Such a complexion invariably generated *materia*, unwanted phlegm or an excess of black bile, which required evacuation. In most cases, clysters and purgatives could expel the unwanted matter, but when the problem was not simply ill health but a specific disease that generated undesirable matter, physicians often advised phlebotomy. Phlebotomy was undoubtedly the best way to evacuate unwanted natural matter, for blood in the veins contained all four humors at once, and the proper bloodletting from the correct vein at the right time could solve many problems. Furthermore, unlike the use of leeches or the administration of purgatives, it was amenable to the surgeon's control: he could always stanch the flow of blood if necessary, so that the patient was not excessively weakened. "Since phlebotomy is the most common of all [methods of bloodletting] and a great help, one must begin with it. Phlebotomy is the incision of a vein which evacuates blood and humors that flow with it."[92] Not a single text mentions that phlebotomy is also painful. On the contrary, it was often considered an analgesic procedure.

The practice of bloodletting is of venerable antiquity, going back to Hippocratic medicine. Barbers often performed it, much to the irritation of university-trained surgeons and physicians, who insisted that the procedure required more than the skill to use a knife. One had to know which vein to open for which disease and under which astrological configuration. Technical treatises listed a whole panoply of diseases for which bloodletting was useful, especially in febrile conditions: hectic, quotidian, tertian, and quartan fevers. The principle was double, of derivation and revulsion: either the surgeon could let blood out of the vein nearest to the locus of the illness (e.g., the cervical vein for headaches), thus ridding the body of unwanted matter, or one could do the opposite—bleed a vein on the other side, thus forcing new blood into the ill organ.[93]

Phlebotomy was considered a cure for numerous illnesses. Already Constantine the African had recommended it as a general painkiller.[94] Bleeding the frontal vein was good for a headache in the back of the head, but not for other headaches. It was, however, efficacious against melancholy and madness. Headaches with fever, resulting from too much hot humor, required the bleeding of the *vena capitalis*. Petrus Hispanus (d. 1277) recommended phlebotomy of the frontal vein for migraines; for pains in the chest and lungs, one had to bleed the circular vein that ran through the arms. The cephalic vein, which ran through the entire body, was good for all pains but dangerous to bleed. Phlebotomy was also good for toothache, dizziness, and pain in the eyes.[95] It was also recommended for gout, kidney stones, melancholy, and pleurisy.[96] Since external injuries attracted matter and corrupt humors, they could cause inflammation and additional pain unless the matter was drained away, and so phlebotomy was recommended also in cases of external trauma. It accorded with other practices of extrusion, such as lancing hemorrhoids or other subcutaneous infections. Getting the vitiating matter out was the main medical imperative, and phlebotomy was the best way to do it. It seems to have been the treatment of choice for many physicians, though patients may not have shared their enthusiasm. In the sixteenth century, Laurent Joubert (1529–83) had to hotly argue the virtues of phlebotomy to the recalcitrant, erring populace, who feared the procedure and the pain:

> I am astonished by some, who will more willingly take twenty different drugs than endure one bloodletting that is necessary, given its great ease and simplicity. For one can control perfectly the amount we wish to let flow; it can be stopped at will and be repeated later so as not to weaken the patient too much in a single application. This is not the case with drugs, for often they cause more voiding than is desired and cannot be stopped when we want. These are considerable drawbacks, not to

mention the nausea, the upset stomach, and the severe intestinal cramps
they usually bring about.[97]

Those who argued that they had seen people die after phlebotomy were
arguing for a nonexistent causal relationship, said Joubert. People also died
after eating or sleeping. True, some practitioners were overly hasty with
dangerous treatments, but phlebotomy was safe, even as a preventive measure. Not all physicians, however, agreed that phlebotomy was invariably
safe and desirable. Arnau de Villanova, though he often recommended the
procedure, did warn that a sharp pain was a clear contraindication for phlebotomy. Antonio Cermisone, in the wake of a long medical tradition, forbade it in cases of weak, young, or elderly patients, and Michele Savonarola
insisted that it was not to be applied to gout patients.[98]

Joubert was stating the common medical point of view. What he failed
to mention was what emerged from the texts as well: first, that the incision hurt, and second, that bloodletting weakened people considerably.
Still, long after the principle of blood circulation was established in the seventeenth century, physicians still insisted that regular phlebotomies were
essential for good health and that emergency phlebotomies were excellent
cures for many illnesses.

The conviction that healing consisted of removal of noxious elements
was not limited to medicine. Similar ideas percolated through other disciplines of soul and body. Confessors urged penitents to "vomit out" their
sins.[99] Similarly, the metaphors of corrosion as necessary cleansing moved
from the disciplines of the body to those of the soul. Clearly, in this case,
medical practice was the source of theological metaphors. As my discussion
of William of Auvergne has shown, the use of corrosive substances to erode
putrid flesh and infections was a common metaphor for spiritual discipline.

An equally painful method of curing was cauterization of the open blood
vessels with a hot iron. Guy de Chauliac considered both cauterization and
the application of corrosive substances as use of fire, either real fire that
heated the iron or potential fire that appeared only when the corrosive medication—sulfur, caustic soda, or quicklime—was applied. He recommended
the use of cautery because it was quicker ("quickly done and the impression
also passes quickly"), less painful, and more localized than corrosive substances, "unless it is the case that the patient because of his cowardice does
not dare to accept fire, or in the case in which we wish to cauterize for the
sake of evacuation and derivation [i.e., as in lancing an infection]; then the
caustic [ruptorium], because of the pain and big burn that it leaves behind,
weakening the place, provokes a greater flux."[100] Corrosives, as older sources

had warned, were also far more dangerous than cautery.[101] They also took a long time to work, causing much pain and fever, and their effect could not be completely controlled. Both methods, said Chauliac, were less common in his time than in antiquity, largely because, as Henri de Mondeville had complained, they were practiced by laymen and ignorant practitioners (*ydiotas et operantes inperite*), with predictable results.[102] Nevertheless, they were viewed as belonging to the same category as purgation and phlebotomy, only in an extreme degree. Cauterization was even recommended as a painkiller in cases of extreme pain.[103]

A good example of the virtues of evacuation by any means appears in the writings of Arnau de Villanova. If a thorough evacuation of the digestive system did not precede a phlebotomy, the direst results could be expected. Any attempt to cure an aposteme without evacuation would only result in its changing into a scirrhus.[104] Even hemorrhoids had to be opened, and the blood let out, by medication, phlebotomy, or lancing. If they were not opened, it would be dangerous to lance them, since they contained a plethora of blood and could cause too much bleeding. Opening the great veins of both legs would divert the blood from the hemorrhoids elsewhere.[105]

It is therefore not surprising that cautery was recommended for as wide a variety of problems as phlebotomy; in addition to stanching bleeding and lancing apostemes and other abscesses, cautery was recommended for eradicating small cancers,[106] a cold complexion, gout, wounds, headaches, and strong pains.[107] Perhaps the most telling comment about cauterization comes from the fourteenth-century English Franciscan philosopher John Duns Scotus, who denied the need for any external factor for the mind to sense pain: the mind alone could comprehend pain and the need for pain.[108] For this, he instanced the cauterization iron—painful but indispensable. John was probably a patient as well as a philosopher, and the very thought of cautery was sufficient to create the sensation of pain in his body.

Cauterization was also in integral part of surgery. Guy de Chauliac attributed to Avicenna the pouring of boiling oil upon the stump of a sixth finger to stop the bleeding.[109] As for himself, Chauliac advocated tying a ligature around the corrupt member until it simply fell off, "because it is more honorable for the physician if it falls off than if it is amputated. Whenever there is amputation, there remain in the patient anger and the idea that it could have been saved."[110] The rationale for allowing a gangrenous limb to die and fall off rather than amputating it had nothing to do with the patient's pain, only with his or her anger. Nevertheless, in every case of amputation, cauterization was the fastest and surest method of sealing the wound.

Cautery extracted nothing from the human body. To the contrary, it sealed the incisions made by surgeons from which too many humors might flow. At the same time, it was conceived very much as part of the same methodology that employed clysters and phlebotomy. It was part of the economy of painful removal for the sake of health.

Medieval surgery was a procedure of taking out (kidney or bladder stones) or taking off. It was employed to remove projectiles, tumors, lesions, and putrid limbs. When a wounded part of the body refused to heal and became gangrenous, it was necessary to amputate, lest the corruption spread to the entire body. This metaphor, the ultimate justification for executions, was first coined by John of Salisbury in his *Policraticus*,[111] which likened the body politic to the human body. Thereafter, it became common also in treatises of penal law and religious works advocating the extirpation of heresy.[112] One gangrenous part could contaminate the whole, and it was incumbent upon the ruler to sever that part.

All surgery, including amputation, was performed without any anesthesia until the nineteenth century. Anesthesia, as distinct from analgesia, was difficult to achieve. The literature is rife with warnings about the dangers of an overdose of opium and other stupefacients that could just as easily kill the patient as anesthetize the pain of surgery.[113] Guy de Chauliac was willing to allow their use only when all other painkillers had failed and the patient was in danger of dying from the pain. Even then, he said, one must use them only in suppositories, for this method was safer than ingestion. Others, he said, actually gave people opium to drink, which was even more dangerous.[114] Clearly, Guy did not consider the pain of surgery as mortal. There were methods of surgery that made amputation, at least, less painful, and he preferred to avoid stupefacients altogether. Ambroise Paré, who in the sixteenth century also followed the tradition of learned surgery, also recommended sharp knives and quick surgery rather than anesthesia.[115]

What, though, was a healer to do in situations of extreme pain? Worse, what was a surgeon to do to stop a patient from thrashing around while being cut up? According to premodern sources, up to the nineteenth century the options were tying the patient up, getting her drunk, and performing the surgery as quickly and as efficiently as possible. Nevertheless, medieval surgery acknowledged the possibility of using stupefacients in modest quantities.[116] The possibility of total anesthesia does crop up in various sources, but in no clear prescription.

The earliest medieval source mentioning an anesthetic drink, either opium or a mixture of mandrake and wine, is Isidore of Seville (ca. 560–636),

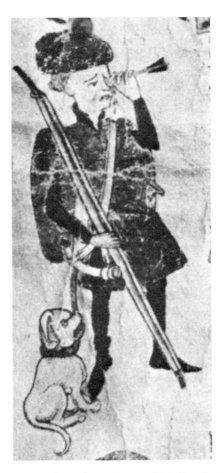

Figure 2. Arrow in eye. From John Arderne, *De arte phisicali et de cirurgia (1412)*, trans. D'Arcy Power, Research Studies in Medical History of the Wellcome Historical Medical Museum 1 (London, 1922), pl. III, right side, fig. 3.

quoting classical sources.[117] All Isidore said was that the drugs make men sleep; he made no mention of surgery and pain insensitivity. During the ninth century three monastic manuscripts describe the soporific sponge, which is meant to render candidates for surgery completely insensitive. One is the Bamberg antidotary, another one comes from Monte Cassino, and the third, presently in Copenhagen, is probably also from southern Italy.[118] While those manuscripts form a very small group, they are a departure from the previous tradition. The prescription they describe is not meant as a painkiller but as a desensitizer in surgery. Furthermore, the mode of inges- tion is not by drinking but via inhalation of fumes stored in a sponge.

The original ingredients of the sponge were opium (specifically opium from Thebes), mandrake juice, hemlock (*Conium maculatum*), and henbane, all well crushed together and mixed with water. This mixture was to be soaked into a fresh sea-sponge, which could then be allowed to dry and remoistened when needed. The surgeon was to place the wet sponge under the patient's nose; for awakening, he was to use a sponge soaked in warm vinegar. It is obvious from the early recipes that great care was taken in the dosage and the avoidance of ingestion. All the early recipes specified quantities (though these varied with local variations of weights and measures). Anesthetic sponges appeared in several twelfth- and thirteenth-century sources. The *Antidotarium Nicolai* has a recipe with several ingredients added to earlier ones.[119] Other authors came up with different prescriptions, including one from England, for the use of opium and henbane ointments in surgery.[120] Best known is the recipe of Theodorico Borgognoni, bishop of Cervia (1205–98), which is a variation upon the *Antidotarium* recipe. Borgognoni, educated in Bologna, attributed his recipe to his father, Hugo of Lucca (d. ca. 1252). This recipe is the last detailed sponge prescription.[121] Although Borgognoni himself did not claim to have applied it, he did assert that his father had used it when performing surgery.

In fact, there is no evidence of any surgeon having used such a sponge. The only surgeon to mention the method specifically—and disapprovingly—was Guy de Chauliac. He knew Theodorico Borgognoni had mentioned it, and he knew the ingredients, but he had neither the quantities nor a mode of preparation.[122] In Guy's opinion, the anesthetic was far too dangerous to use.

The centering of the anesthetic tradition in medical writings of university-trained surgeons raises the question of actual practice.[123] Paintings of late medieval surgical procedures show patients restrained with ropes, a clear indication that anesthesia, if applied, was ineffective.[124] Indeed, Michael R. McVaugh, in his study of the rational surgery in the Middle Ages, dismisses the soporific sponge as no more than a literary tradition.[125] I agree that the evidence for the existence of soporific sponges remains unproven.

While the sponge may not have existed, anesthesia in the form of a drink remains a very stubborn tradition, at least in the British Isles. There is a twelfth-century literary tradition concerning a drink named Letargion. Jocelyn of Furness noted in the *vita* of St. Kentigern, patron saint of Glasgow: "many have taken the drink of oblivion which physicians call 'Letargion' in order to sleep, and have endured incisions in their limbs, and sometimes burning and abrasions in their vital parts, and felt it not at all. After being awakened they did not know of the physician's actions."[126] While the evidence is extremely weak, it does specifically mention anesthesia in surgery. Two centuries later, one finds John Arderne speaking of an anesthetic ointment, made up of ingredients similar to those of the sponge (adding fat or beeswax as binding), "with which if any man be anoynted he schal now suffre kuttyntg in any place of the body without felyng or akyng."[127] A milder concoction, containing minor quantities of hemlock, poppy, henbane, and lettuce mixed with a gallon of wine, appears in several English manuscripts under the name of dwale, "A drynke that men callen dwale to make a man to slepe whyle men kerven him."[128] There does seem to have been a persistent tradition in English medicine that such a thing as anesthesia during surgery was possible.

The horrors of surgery without anesthesia are present more in popular drawings than in medical literature. Pictures of people tied down, held down by stalwart assistants,[129] and thrashing and screaming with contorted faces were common, especially in early modern prints.[130] There is no question that surgery under those circumstances was difficult for the surgeon but gravely traumatic for the patient.

Surgery, therefore, remained extremely painful until the nineteenth century, and the learned traditions of both physicians and surgeons did not support the idea of anesthesia. Was this attitude mere callousness? Hardly, for healers invariably distinguished between different types of pain. Pain resulting from illness, or pain signifying illness, required alleviation. Pain that was part of the healing process required restraint and fortitude on the part of the patients. The healer was correct in inflicting it.

Conclusion

Late medieval medicine was not focused upon achieving painlessness. Its central aim was balance and health, with freedom from pain inevitably ensuing. At the same time, the means of alleviation were also limited. The lack of evolution in receptary literature—the repetition of the same ancient ingredients and methods—indicates that healers had devised no new methods for dealing with pain. Nevertheless, medieval medicine most certainly did not ignore pain. In certain situations, such as surgery, cauterization, and childbirth, pain was considered inevitable, even natural. But whenever pain was diagnosed as the result of an internal imbalance or an external injury, healers considered pain treatment as an essential part of healing. They were fully aware of the dangers of severe pain and did not consider its soothing an irrelevance.

While this attitude is a far cry from the modern one of allowing free access to analgesia, the two are not really comparable. The medieval attitudes described above are those of healers, not of sufferers. It is entirely possible that medieval sufferers wished just as ardently for relief as their modern counterparts but could not fulfill their wish. Physicians, then and now, have other considerations as well, some of them (such as fear of an overdose) still relevant today. Medieval healers were forced to accept the constant pain of their patients but never reached the point of making a virtue out of necessity. They did recommend, and probably used, all the means at their disposal when they considered the situation warranted it. What does differ drastically from present medical pain management is the range of pain situations that doctors believed merited relief. The distinction between past and present does not lie necessarily in the severity of pain but in its warrantability and manageability. There was almost nothing that could be done for the pain of surgery and childbirth, both of great severity, and indeed medieval texts rarely speak of managing those sufferings. Paradoxically, a light headache was more likely to be treated, and effectively, than the pains of a cancerous tumor.

How does the medical attitude compare with the theological and legal ones? Whereas theology and law focused on the uses of pain and not its evils, medieval medical culture did not embrace pain because Christ and the martyrs had suffered. It considered human pain an evil, but not one that could be banished with human resources.

CHAPTER FOUR

The Script of Pain Behavior

G iven the valorization of pain in theology and law, and the care for it evinced in healing, one would expect people in pain in the Middle Ages to broadcast their pains vociferously, both to gain merit in heaven and to receive help on earth. But "people in pain" are not, and never were, a homologous group. Mark Zborowski's pioneering work identifying different norms for different ethnic groups in different situations has given rise to much debate but has also brought to the forefront the subjectivity and variety of pain expressions.[1] Given that pain itself, albeit an almost-universal experience, is unshareable and intransmissible, the need for sufferers and those who surround them to understand and evaluate the experience is invariably urgent. Furthermore, those who recorded pain took the trouble to record the appropriate (or deliberately inappropriate) behavior of other sufferers. Indeed, throughout Western history, men of science attributed more or less sensitivity to pain to different social and ethnic groups at different times, partially on the basis of misunderstood behavioral codes. Conversely, the modern anthropological discourse on pain in a social context is very much aware of the sufferer's own attempts to couch her message in a comprehensible form. This form may be body language, spoken language, sounds, or any other means of communication that might be interpreted as pain by whoever is nearby. Modern pain research (both medical and anthropological), therefore, does not generalize about different levels of sensitivity but attempts to get sufferers to couch their sensations in a commonly understandable narrative as a form of transmission and sharing, an Esperanto of pain.

Medieval sufferers and their caregivers were no less anxious than their modern counterparts to establish a comprehensible connection between individual sensation and the surrounding world. Since pain is a multivalent sign, the behavior of sufferers is subject to varying interpretations. Was the screaming nun bound in ecstatic union with the crucified Christ, or was she suffering from kidney stones? Was the stern-faced king sitting still because he was listening, because he was angry, or because he was trying to conceal his headache? The answers to such questions lie in the eye of the beholder/ narrator. Clearly, norms of behavior dictated not only the actions of people in pain but also how those actions were interpreted in subsequent recording. But even within the same time and place, different norms applied to different people: norms acceptable for women were unacceptable for men, and vice versa. Social standing and space also dictated different modes of behavior.

What we have is almost invariably the normative model, not the actual description. Medieval descriptions are permeated with the purposes of their composition, and none of these purposes accord with present-day cultural anthropology. The authoress of a king's biography or a saint's *vita* would make sure that the protagonist of her work acted in the text precisely as he ought to. The chronicler describing a villain's downfall and death was bound to tell it just as it ought to have happened. And the more outstanding the hero, the more normative the actions would be. The norms of people outside the limelight were perhaps different, certainly less rigid.

"Lesser" humans had a greater variety of norms, and their behavior when in pain occasionally merited description rather than prescription. If all types of behavior are placed somewhere between absolute restraint and absolute expressivity (neither of which exist in reality), what would emerge is that concealment of pain was present throughout the later Middle Ages at one and the same time as the "extroverted" model of overt pain expression. It is possible to hypothesize that both models have coexisted throughout history and that only the sphere of prescription has changed from time to time. Thus, the sort of vocalization that was permissible to or demanded of parturient women in the twelfth century might have been shameful for a male knight at the time but proper for a contemporary abbot with mystical inclinations. The frenzy of pain that thirteenth- and fourteenth-century holy women showed was admired by some as saintly and condemned by others as improper, even insane or demoniac, while self-control evinced by sixteenth-century women in labor could earn them a stiff condemnation.[2] Always bearing in mind that expressivity does not mean lack of culture or control but is merely another cultural norm, it is possible to visualize these models as two partially overlapping spheres. At either extreme stand the absolute demands for restraint or expressivity. In the middle there is a gray area that allows a wider range of behavior. As time goes by, the intermediate area either grows or shrinks, and the spheres overlap to a greater or lesser extent.

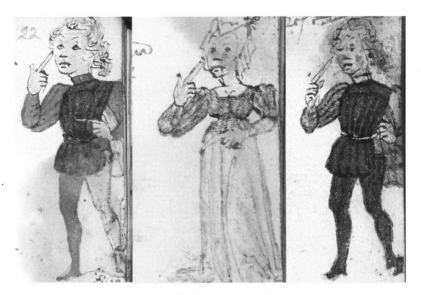

Figure 3. Eye disease. Edinburgh University Library, MS 314, fol. 22 (fifteenth century). With permission of Edinburgh University Library.

These models of behavior may have little to do with theories of pain, for theoretical assumptions about pain convey very little information about human behavior. The assumptions usually speak of the sensation as though it were an objective entity with an independent existence, a known quality amenable to analysis regardless of how it is conveyed to others. Thus, medical *consilia* state simply that the patient was suffering from percussive pain in his abdomen. They do not say how they had reached this conclusion, whether by asking, probing, or observing behavior. Furthermore, theories—with the exception of medical observations—often tend to regard pain as a uniform experience. Historians must perforce content themselves with second- and thirdhand information and so must read the description of expressions as generically proscribed scripts.

Means of Communication and Silence: Letters

One way to track the changes in normative expressivity of pain is to follow a specific genre across the centuries. Autobiography is the ideal genre for this purpose since it is the most consciously self-descriptive. Unfortunately, autobiographical writing appears only rarely before the sixteenth century, and when it does, it is usually written by public figures.

Letters, however, have survived from antiquity onward. Furthermore, the rules governing epistolary communication are clearly stated in manuals and epistolaries. Granted, in this field, too, the figures who do mention pain in their letters—and whose letters have survived—are usually well-known personages. All the same, there is a difference between an author describing the behavior of a holy man in public view and the same author describing himself in a letter on an ostensibly one-to-one basis. Even official letters of popes occasionally allow the personal element some room, and this fact is indicative of the mores of the period.

To follow the rules governing expressions of bodily infirmity and pain in letters, one must follow the *longue durée*. At least until the thirteenth century, when practical literacy became a lay and vernacular characteristic, one can trace how the rules of *ars dictaminis* adapted to the different mores of different eras.[3] The late antique letters of Augustine, for example, evince a code of decorum completely alien to modern-day manners: "According to the spirit, as it pleases God and the strength that he deigns to grant, we are all right; nevertheless, according to the body, I am in bed. I can neither walk nor stand nor sit for the pain and swelling of the fissures and hemorrhoids."[4] This is the opening sentence of one of Augustine's letters. As a personal statement of suffering, it is certainly eloquent, though somewhat startling to modern sensibilities since Augustine was writing an impersonal letter concerning the succession of the archbishopric of Numidia. He may personally have known his correspondent, Brother Profuturus, but opening a letter on church politics with the details of his anal pains, severe though they might have been, argued a code of vocalization that did not valorize heroic silence. It was neither querulous nor in bad taste to complain of one's hemorrhoids.

The tradition of describing one's pains in public letters was still present a century after Augustine, when Pope Symmachus (498–514) excused a belated answer by referring to physical pain.[5] At the end of the sixth century, Pope Gregory I made quite a habit of using his gout pains as an excuse. The prolific Gregory also expatiated on the pain in detail:

> It is a long time now that I cannot get out of bed. Sometimes the pain of gout tortures me, and sometimes it runs throughout my body like fire. And often both the fire and the pain contend with each other in me, so that I am left breathless. I have no wish to add more than I have said of the illness. But briefly I shall say that the infection of noxious humors so depletes me that it is punishment for me to live, and I look forward to death, which, I believe, is the only remedy to my sufferings.[6]

This text can be mined for two types of significance. For one thing, it provides a rare account of personal pain by an articulate hypochondriac. At the same time, it gives us a glimpse of the norms operating in sixth-century Rome. For a high-ranking Roman of the time, it was quite suitable to adduce pain as an excuse for a delayed answer. Gregory even considered such complaints to be part of his public persona. Physical pain seems to have permeated social interaction much as complaints of lovesickness did in the late eighteenth century. The fact that it surfaces quite often in such a strictly constructed genre as letter writing is indicative of the normative place of such complaints in late antiquity. Coming from Gregory the Great, who wrote so widely on the benefits of physical pain for the human soul and about the sufferings of souls in hell, it shows the disjunction between theories and actual sensations. Gregory could freely expatiate on the uses of pain as long as his own infirmities were not involved. When he was suffering from gout or a kidney stone, the tenor of his words changed dramatically. Gregory reacted to his pain in public papal letters very much as any ill person would: he wanted the pain to go away. It would be another millennium before Montaigne felt impelled to write in such a vein about his kidney stones in his essays.[7] For Montaigne, though, physical complaints were part of his candid self-investigation and self-exposure, not something to be addressed in formal writing to a fellow *parlementaire* in Bordeaux, for example. Gregory addressed his pain to his interlocutors and to all subsequent readers of his letters, for letters were not private scripts.

One can find similar expressions of illness and pain occasionally in Carolingian letters. Einhard, summoned by the empress to court, excused himself (and asked a friend to intercede for him, too) on the grounds of severe spleen and kidney pains which made it impossible for him to ride.[8] In his letter to an anonymous friend he expatiated further upon his suffering:

As both the excessive diarrhea and the kidney pain alternated in me, there was not one day since I left Aix-la-Chapelle that I did not suffer from one or the other illness. Both and other problems stem from last year's illness—that is, the continuous weakness in my right thigh and the intolerable pain in the spleen. Affected by these passions, I live in great sadness and lacking all joy.[9]

Gerbert of Aurillac (d. 1003), later Pope Sylvester II, had no compunction about addressing his predecessor, Pope John XV, in similar terms.[10] Illness and pain, while not a necessary part of epistolary communication, seems never to have been a censored subject.

The rigid rules of *ars dictaminis*, formed mainly during the twelfth century, concentrated upon letter structure rather than licit or illicit topics. Physical pain became more emotional in the text of letters. When Hildegard of Bingen's will was crossed, she could take to her bed with violent migraines and write about them as eloquently as any man to the abbots or archbishops who had rejected her liturgy.[11] Significantly, when letters told of personal pains, they were written by those who had considered the theoretical implications of pain. St. Anselm of Bec and Canterbury, known for his deep emotional involvement with his monks and his groundbreaking theological interpretation of the Passion,[12] felt the pains of his monks and his own body to be apt matters for correspondence. In one letter, he complained to Abbot Gilbert of Saint-Etienne in Caen:

> In this space of time I was afflicted in France with many bodily aches and pains; above all a sudden fever broke out within me, and it dared to attack your servant twice, terrifying me immensely and violently menacing me until I was afraid of never seeing you or our other monks of Bec again. . . . Therefore, I have not yet been able to rid myself of these three ill effects; loss of appetite, insomnia, and the accompanying weakness that tends to follow upon going-on-all-fours [*terra vestigia*].[13]

Again, the detailed description was the introduction to an apology for nonappearance. While still the abbot of Bec, he was equally concerned about a young monk, a nephew of Archbishop Lanfranc, who had developed severe headaches:

> divine chastisement has daily afflicted him in a fatherly manner for many months with such a headache that his enjoyable company has sometimes been cut off from the whole community and his intention has been completely turned away from reading or any serious meditation . . . his temples always seem to be throbbing, his brow feels heavy, especially when he is lying down. The greater any light and noise are, the more they bother him.[14]

Perhaps the impression of a growing stress upon pain in correspondence is the result of the increased number of letters we have from the twelfth century. Of course, not every letter began with a detailed list of aches and pains, and it is impossible to imagine some correspondents ever being so forthcoming, even when retelling the story of their calamities and persecutions. Neither Abelard nor Heloïse, though bitterly bewailing their fates, ever mentioned physical pain, not even that which Abelard must have suffered during his castration.

From the thirteenth century onward, there are a great many letters describing pain, but most of them were written by mystics describing their experiences and are a totally different genre. Catherine of Siena's letters are full of pain, blood, and fire, but they are in fact visionary minitreatises of emotive religiosity, not records of illness. Her writing was not governed by the constraints of rhetorical models. There was no question of complaining about her aches and pain, for she rejoiced in them. Unfortunately, this is true also for much of the secular correspondence of the later Middle Ages. A merchant writing to an associate or a wife to her husband also had no reason to follow epistolary models. Whether he did or did not write about his latest headache indicated nothing about what was or was not appropriate to write about. Correspondence had become functional rather than literary, and hence the norms no longer applied. Literary letters, such as those of Francesco Petrarca (1304–74), were as carefully crafted as Cicero's or Abelard's and just as much of a model for future generations. Yet Petrarch, who wrote extensively about pain, produced no detailed descriptions of his illnesses in his entire copious correspondence.[15] Pain had been well and truly elided from scholarly formal letter writing and was not to return before the sixteenth century.

The evidence from formal correspondence is disappointing. At the time when mystics began ardently meditating upon Christ's Passion and experiencing stigmata and other painful phenomena in empathy with Christ, formal letters ceased dwelling upon personal infirmities. At the time when scholastics debated all the minutiae of Christ's particular sufferings and preachers enumerated the nine pains of hell, letters—or, rather, the letters we possess—avoided the subject. Possibly, with the evolution of a new style of vernacular in Italy, ideas of rhetorical decorum came to exclude uncomfortable personal sensations. Seemingly, the genres in which it was suitable to discuss pain changed. Lives of saints, martyrologies, miracles, and theology might well describe pain, but in formal letter writing, it was no longer acceptable to describe one's illnesses, whether to excuse oneself for a belated reply or otherwise. Narratives of pain were simply channeled elsewhere.

Letter writing was one way to communicate pain, but it was reserved to the literate. Descriptions and prescriptions of conduct, while a less direct source, are a much richer one. While as rigorously constructed as any epistle, such descriptions tell us about the norms of a much wider group of people than the letters do.

Conduct: Emblematic Figures and Others

Other than martyrs, almost every narrative including protagonists followed specific rules of conduct: saints practiced asceticism, sinners either repented in a flood of tears or went to hell screaming and gesticulating, parturient mothers screamed and noblemen caught in embarrassing accidents kept a stiff upper lip. But the most rigid norms of behavior applied to emblematic figures. Since the richest biographical and autobiographical descriptions of physical pain come from the pens of mystics and their biographers, they form my model for emblematic behavior. These narratives are constructed as a journey towards union with a beloved God, whose main manifestation was through pain.

Saints in and out of Rapture

In the later Middle Ages it was standard for saints and visionaries to speak and write about their own illnesses with little emotion. A millennium separates them from the irritable Augustine's hemorrhoids, but more importantly, so does a conceptual chasm between two sets of relationships between self and body. Julian of Norwich nearly died before she received her first revelation, but all she said about the illness was that she had suffered a shortness of breath. Angela of Foligno apparently suffered the pains of ill health throughout her life, but this fact is mentioned in her biography only at her deathbed. Her biographer took care to note that she had suffered but that she manifested properly controlled pain behavior.[16]

But when experiencing rapture, the same people behaved in a completely different manner. Those who live close to the divine, constantly tossed willy-nilly by ineffable forces from joy to despair, from uncontrollable vocalization to equally uncontrollable silence, from pain to exaltation, are uncommon in any social milieu. We tend to think of them as fairly common during the later Middle Ages simply because at that time it was acceptable to broadcast such experiences and write about them. But their experiences and behavior were not presented as standards for others to follow. Such people were a law unto themselves. Those who gained some fame, local or widespread, became emblematic figures of the unusual and the miraculous. Different types of "unquiet souls," as Richard Kieckhefer termed them, followed different rules.[17] When they did express pain, their behavior was often described and adjudged in terms of its similarity to madness in the abandon of their movements and vocalization.

Vitae of saints, especially female saints, repeat the same motif incessantly. As a rule, public saints spoke little of their illnesses and suffering, as long as that suffering was neither self-induced nor religiously charged. The same principle sometimes also applied to self-inflicted pain. Heinrich Suso carved a cross on his own chest, telling of it only years later in his autobiographical writings. Catherine of Siena prayed to receive Christ's stigmata and was answered, but the stigmata were internal, and she could only feel the pain, not show it to others.[18] In the following, I will try to distill the codes governing the pain behavior of visionaries and the authors of their *vitae* from the lives and writings of five women and one man: Christina Mirabilis (1150–1224), Douceline of Digne (ca. 1215–74), Colette of Corbie (1381–1447), Margaretha Ebner (1291–1351), Elisabeth Stagel of Töss (ca. 1300–ca. 1360), and Rulman Merswin (1307–82). The choice is not accidental: each one of these people was reputed to have suffered physical pain to a severe degree; in each case, we have a description, either autobiographical or of an eyewitness. In each case, there is a different interpretation of the pains, contextualized according to status, gender, and circumstances. Furthermore, each sufferer and her behavior were paradigms of different dialogues with pain. Behind each individual case stand several similar figures.

The life of Christina Mirabilis has undergone a great deal of scholarly attention in the last few years.[19] After a youth spent herding sheep and communing quietly with God, she died and came back to life. Then, for several years, Christina's behavior resembled that of a demoniac or madwoman more than it did that of a holy woman; she was "the village lunatic," according to Barbara Newman. She threw herself into burning ovens and icy rivers, screaming with pain, practiced extravagant and visible asceticism, hung herself on the gibbet, and stretched herself upon a torture wheel. Though nothing showed on her body, she was constantly in pain, largely because of her determination to save souls from purgatory by suffering in their place. But the smell of human beings was unbearable, and the food given by unjust people tasted like the intestines of frogs and toads, and the death of any of the townspeople of Saint-Trond—if they went to purgatory—released a wave of projected suffering. Her behavior on all those occasions was extravagantly expressive. She shied at the smell of human bodies. She howled like a woman giving birth, she screamed and writhed with pain in public—in short, she was pain incarnate, visible, audible, olfactory, and tactile.[20]

This behavior was not part of an ecstatic vision but merely her reaction to the world. Christina's projections of pain were involuntary. Indeed, at first, her behavior led her to be classified as insane: "Her sisters and her friends were greatly embarrassed because of these things and the manner in which they were done, for men thought that she was possessed by demons. They made an agreement with a most wicked man who was very strong and they bribed him to follow and capture her and to bind her with iron chains."[21] Christina managed to escape several times, at the cost of several wounds, but was eventually caught and tied up, fed "like a dog" on bread and water. Her wounded buttocks and thigh festered, causing her great pain. God, taking pity upon her, did not ease her pains but produced miraculous oil from her breasts, so that all were awed and she was freed. It was only after her death, when Thomas of Cantimpré wrote her *vita*, explaining that her first death was a tour of the otherworld, that her behavior was accorded public sanction. The extravagances of a saint, especially a defunct one, could be acceptable.

Nobody could be as different from the illiterate herder of Saint-Trond as Douceline of Digne, in Provence. Aristocrat, abbess, sister to the local bishop, and strict ascetic and disciplinarian of her nuns, Douceline was indeed a different type of suffering saint.[22] Such was her devotion to the Crucifixion that any mention of anything connected with Christ's death promptly sent her into a state of ecstasy. Under these conditions, she occasionally levitated, but mostly she manifested a state of perfect impassibility: while her rapture lasted, people could inflict upon her whatever pain they chose; she felt nothing. When this happened in the middle of the Franciscan church of Marseilles, someone "tested" her by sticking an awl into her. Others inserted needles into her body. Later the count of Provence in person verified her raptures by having molten lead thrown on her feet, without any immediate effect. When she came out of her ecstasies, however, she felt her pains severely, "although she did not complain."[23] Despite her efforts to avoid public raptures (leading her to avoid attending public sermons and conventual masses), she could not prevent them and soon became a public spectacle. The countess of Provence added insult to injury by making her a court spectacle as well. Wishing to see the miraculous impassibility, she invited Douceline and a "good friar" to court, intending that his sermon would provoke the expected reaction. Douceline could not escape, and to avoid another public ecstasy she unsuccessfully tried to use self-inflicted pain to distract herself: "She had so tortured her hands during the sermon that they were covered in bruises."[24] For these marks, and for her total insensibility to pain during her raptures, Douceline gained much pain (after the rapture) and an equal measure of glory among the people of Provence.

Other holy women experienced impassibility during rapture. The canonization procedures of St. Francesca of Rome (d. 1440) note precisely the same phenomenon.[25] In fact, Francesca's confessor, Giovanni Mattiotti, resorted to precisely the same methods of pain infliction to verify impassibility. And just as in the case of Douceline, the pain was felt after the ecstasy had ended. As a trait of suffering saints, impassibility is fairly rare. The uniqueness of Douceline's case stems from the fact that her biographer was a woman, not a man.

When it comes to rules for manifesting pain, Colette of Corbie's case is undoubtedly the most complex and illuminating one.[26] Colette was a Poor Clare and abbess-at-large for reforming the order (already noted for its strictness). Pain and behavior while experiencing pain loom large in her *vitae*. Colette suffered from many illnesses and they all caused acute pain. She distinguished, however, between two types of illness: those illnesses she deemed natural were in her opinion to be treated by physicians, and she suffered the pain patiently. Other illnesses, however, she considered a gift from God meant to bring her closer to perfection. Those she refused to have treated or eased.[27] These were the worst pains, gripping her entire body so that she could never sleep and barely drew breath for an hour in eight days. The pains were so severe that her companions could hear her sinews creaking, blood flowed from her mouth, and she admitted that her head felt like a boiling pot. But she knew them for God's gift because they could be turned on and off at need. In general, Colette's body seems to have been constantly burning. "Often, moved by curiosity, I looked at the blessed Colette's face, and I noticed that her teeth looked as though they were burning from the force of her pains. Similarly, I noticed her feet, which had a scorched color."[28]

Colette was described by Pierre de Vaux, one of her biographers, as a martyr in all senses, a Christ figure:

> Sometimes she was tortured by fire, like St. Lawrence . . . and that martyrdom usually lasted for a whole night. Sometimes she was tortured like St. Vincent, sometimes she was crucified. Sometimes she was excoriated like St. Bartholomew, sometimes she froze, sometimes she boiled; and sometimes it seemed to her that her heart was breaking open. . . . Sometimes it seemed to her, and she felt it in her senses thus, that under her belly she had a blazing torch that burned her completely; at other times that she had burning coals at the roots of her eyes, consuming them; or that sharp irons pierced her whole body and all her limbs from end to end.[29]

All this meekness and toleration of pain vanished at once when she meditated upon the sufferings of Christ. Her empathy with Christ went as far
as total identification, so that she felt the nails stuck into her hands and
feet and the lance piercing her side. Her pains were worse than those of
any parturient woman. When feeling these pains, she displayed absolutely
no reticence. To the contrary, she displayed the power of tears. "She wept
abundant tears, most pious crying, desperate sighs," every Friday. So strong
was the pain that one Friday after mass the sisters were shocked to see her
face looking battered and disjointed.[30]

A third type of behavior followed the example of Douceline. While in
ecstasy, Colette was completely frozen and immobile, on one occasion remaining thus for three full days, manifesting no pain.[31] Nevertheless, her
biographer had no doubt that she suffered severely during the raptures.
Perrine de Baumes, her second biographer, claims that, though she could hear
Colette's bones and sinews coming apart during her ecstasy, the saint never
made a sound.[32] Nevertheless, once she awoke from her trance, she cried,
groaned, and complained. Her hands and feet were burning, and the sisters,
fearing for her life, washed them in cold water and called a physician. Colette's behavior was never seen as anything but normative, for her followers
saw her as a saint: the power to identify with Christ to the point of living
martyrdom and the power to temporarily transcend the senses while seeing
a vision were conceived as holy charisma. Nobody dared to test her impassibility by inflicting pain during her ecstasies. Colette and Douceline were
typical of many late medieval saints, who drew a clear distinction between
heavenly or self-inflicted suffering and materially caused pain. The first was
cause for an exuberant, demonstrative show of pain (once the rapture or vision was over), while the latter required strict silence. Douceline may have
lost control of her own self among the religious *voyeurs* of her time,[33] but
she remained careful to evince no suffering during her ecstasies, and this
behavior gained her popularity and respect.

Colette of Corbie was a much-respected living saint of heroic asceticism,
a reformer and visionary. It is highly unlikely that she had ever heard of an
obscure abbess who had lived in Marseilles a century and a half before her
time. Furthermore, should we consider the pain behavior of both saints the
products of their biographers' minds, Douceline's biography was written in
Provençal, while Colette's were written in the French of the north. The incontestable model for Colette was St. Clare and no other. And yet, the two
saints manifested many common characteristics of behavior in pain and
painlessness. Roughly phrased, one might say that respectable holy women

showed their power, as men did, by weeping copiously in empathy with Christ while meekly bearing human ills. Raptures demanded the code of impassivity. The saint was to remain immobile, stonelike, while in trance, devoid of all sensory input. Afterward she was to sense all that the trance had deprived her of, and more. Not all people, however, were granted such license. Beginning visionaries could well encounter wonder and hostility when they behaved according to the norms established for respected abbesses, as the case of Margaretha Ebner shows.

Margaretha Ebner was merely a German nun from a well-to-do urban family, not an abbess or a famous visionary. More importantly, our source is not a worshipful hagiography produced by a faithful disciple after the saint's success and death but her own record of her experiences, setting down her career (at her confessor's instigation) from her youth onward. She first suffered from illness and only later associated her pains with spiritual experience. According to her testimony (written when she was in her fifties), Ebner was twenty years old when God first revealed himself to her in 1312. At the time of the writing, she claimed she could not describe herself as she was before the experience, for she had had no self.[34] Her religious experiences during the following decades were closely intertwined with sensory conflicts: pain and pleasure, muteness and screaming, fasting and overeating. In the closed environment of the small middle- and upper-class convent of Maria Medingen, she must have been a major nuisance to all the other nuns. Indeed, she does record that all but one nun shunned her at first. Later, her reputation as a visionary holy woman was such that she was accorded respect and attention rather than a cold shoulder.

Her illness first manifested itself as pain, followed by a gradual loss of sensory capabilities. First, a great pain in her chest prevented her from breathing ("My breathing could be heard from far away"), then the pain moved to her eyes, affecting her vision, and finally to her hands, which she could no longer control. Only her hearing, she noted, remained unimpaired.[35] When headaches attacked her during the first three years, she laughed and cried continuously for four or more days.[36] At first, she sought medical advice to recover her health. At the advice of the only nun who spoke with her, she came to accept her pains as a gift from God, no longer seeking health. To the contrary, she prayed for continuous illness, and her prayers were answered in full.[37] By the third year, she was completely paralyzed and could not move at all. For thirty weeks, she said, she lay immobile, as if dead, neither eating nor drinking.[38] This state was followed by twenty weeks of copious sweating. After this she grew better, but the illness recurred when she was thirty.

For half a year she lay in bed in great pain, unable to speak. It was at this stage that her pains were finally rewarded with visions, which were to accompany her for the rest of her life. Instead of speaking, she wept profusely, earning only the scorn of her sisters, which made her sicker. She needed no self-mortification (and therefore was excused most of the convent routine), for God in his goodness had given her illness.[39] Nevertheless, she ardently wished to recite her Pater Noster. When unable to do so, the frustration made her all the sicker. All her entries in her diary of revelations are marked by date during the liturgical year and the monastic *horarium*, but her participation in communal rituals, including fasting, was sporadic at best. Gradually, her sisters came to respect her. Eventually, the preacher Heinrich of Nördlingen (God's friend, as she referred to him) heard of her and began a long, intimate correspondence with her. Indeed, it was at his urging that she wrote her work. The fame of her visions spread beyond the convent, and she is known to have corresponded with several other people.[40]

For the rest of her life, Margaretha Ebner displayed a variety of symptoms. She was often struck mute for months at a time, "bound silent" (*gebunden swige*). At such times, she was known to break out in screams. Her bout of silence and screaming during Lent of 1345 is perhaps the one described in most detail, but something similar occurred almost every year. On Monday, 12 March, during matins, she was stricken with great pains in the heart and could not pray. For two days she lay in bed, alone, then the loud screaming began. From the early hours of Wednesday, 14 March (she began during matins), she screamed "*owe*" continuously, so loudly that she could be heard throughout the convent and as far as the town. At the same time, she attempted to beat her breast so hard that three women were needed to hold her down. The loud screaming, accompanied by loud weeping, recurred several times during the following days, invariably beginning either after compline or before matins. This situation lasted for two weeks, until Easter (29 March), when God forcibly closed her mouth, reducing her once more to silence. Despite all the pain of the episode, Ebner noted that after each screaming bout she experienced a sweet taste in her mouth.[41] This bout was preceded by eating disorders. First, before Lent, she could not eat or drink at all, noting (in Latin), "Augustinus ad alimentum sicut ad tormentum ivit et Bernardus similiter." But as of 18 February 1345, she felt a compulsive need to eat and drink and did not observe the fast that year. As usual, she was allowed to do as she wished, for nobody could know or understand the forces that compelled her.[42]

Ebner saw her pains as a gift from God, and so ultimately did the entire convent. What emerges from her account is the intense conflict of internal and external forces that buffeted her back and forth while she struggled to stay afloat. Indeed, the words "inward" (*inwendeclichen*) and "outward" (*uzwendenlichen*) recur throughout her book. It is not clear whether she perceived her pains as attacking her from the outside or stemming from her soul. She had no words to express her agony; she could only scream and beat her breast. As Ebner tells it, she had no choice in the matter. She did, however, have a choice when writing her tale, and she chose to tell of noisy display.

This summary, of course, does gross injustice to Ebner's entire work.[43] Though constantly embattled within herself, she built an entire mystical life around a cross and a Christ doll that she carried with her, described her frequent visions, was passionately interested in imperial politics, and maintained her correspondence with Heinrich of Nördlingen. Furthermore, though her German was far from literary, she did attempt to convey her revelations in writing, as her confessor and friend had suggested.[44] Ebner in pain is only one aspect of the life, but she saw fit to grant it a central place in her work, before and after she came to associate pain with God, and to candidly describe her behavior during her attacks. She clearly saw no reason to be ashamed of her behavior or to try and moderate it. At no point did Ebner describe herself as going mad. We have no idea what her sisters thought of two weeks' worth of continuous screaming, but she herself invariably diagnosed her behavior as ordained by God. As she tells it, she was gripped by forces far greater than herself and could not have done otherwise, even had she wished to. Judging by her sisters' initial reaction to her, such actions were unusual and unacceptable unless sanctioned by divine forces. And yet, within the mystically inclined Dominican communities, unusual behavior was understood. It received sanction both inside the convent and from external confessors, Dominican or otherwise.

Ebner's account forms part of an entire literature produced by southern German Dominican nuns in the fourteenth century, the *Nonnenbücher*; other mystics within this tradition also described their visions, but not such behavior as hers.[45] The fullest account of such visions is the testimony of Elisabeth Stagel of Töss. Stagel presumably wrote the *vitae* of her sister nuns, while their confessor wrote her *vita*.[46] What emerges from all these biographies and from what Heinrich Suso, her correspondent and adviser, tells of Stagel is the constant practice of self-inflicted pain, visions, but no indication concerning behavior. Stagel, too, suffered from frail health, but she persisted in mortifying herself, which in male eyes was questionable. Stagel was destined to confront Suso twice.[47] The first time was when he discovered, much to his displeasure, that Stagel had been secretly writing his biography. The irate Suso, according to his own testimony, promptly destroyed part of her work and sat down to write his *Exemplar*—his own version of his devotional biography.[48] The second confrontation took place in writing, when Suso rebuked Stagel for her extreme austerities. When she pointed out that he practiced the same, he insisted that men were stronger and therefore better able to bear self-inflicted pain.[49] Neither of them, though, spoke of vocal complaints but of the practice of self-flagellation. Thus, in the same area and at the same time two Dominican spiritual advisers, Heinrich of Nördlingen and Heinrich Suso, adopted different positions concerning the spiritual and bodily suffering of nuns.

The dearth of men in this analysis is not deliberate. It is the result of the male authors' tendency to portray women's mysticism in terms of bodily suffering, even if the women in their own writings mentioned no such thing.[50] There was no lack of male mystics and visionaries in the later Middle Ages. Other than Heinrich Suso, already mentioned as both mystic and adviser of female mystics, one can easily think of Meister Eckhardt, Jan Ruusbroec, Pierre d'Ailly, Denis the Carthusian, and several others. Most of those men were erudite Latin and vernacular writers who have left many tomes of well-preserved meditations, visions, and treatises. Nevertheless, they very rarely bothered to set down what they felt while undergoing their experiences. In this sense, Suso is unusual, both for writing his autobiography and for recording his sensations in it.

Lives of male living saints present a less extreme picture than those of women. Jacob Griesinger sighed deeply and moaned while meditating on the Passion.[51] Richard Rolle's meditations on the Passion thank Christ for each pain the meditator receives, but there is no word concerning expressivity. Furthermore, Rolle's text is very much a carefully structured literary artifact.[52] Meditational texts also advise empathy and weeping during the process, but there is no further evidence of overt expression of pain among men, willing or unwilling. We have no evidence that holy men in religious orders were ever criticized for weeping publicly. To the contrary: St. Francis of Assisi was praised in his *vitae* for his constant crying. Preachers, by all accounts, did so, encouraging the audience to join them.[53]

The lack of such records for men can be explained in two different, opposing manners. One is to argue that, since extroverted public pain behavior was acceptable for men, it aroused neither comment nor animosity. It might well have taken place, but nobody recorded it. This answer, of course, begs the question of autobiographical sources that avoid mentioning the performance of pain. Conversely, one could argue that men indeed avoided extravagant pain behavior due to gendered behavior codes. This answer is equally unsatisfactory: as we shall see in the case of ill pilgrims, it was not considered shameful for men to weep and writhe with pain in public. Why should a man have wept in a restrained fashion while meditating upon the Passion? Why, with the exception of Francis of Assisi, did no man receive stigmata and so few men record sufferings motivated by empathy with the Passion?

The only remaining answer is that our sources are genre scripted as well as gender scripted. Overt pain behavior—or any behavior interpreted as un-restrained—did not add dignity to the performer. Women had to dispense with dignity in order to gain power. Holy men could have both; they did not need to weaken their dignity by overt pain behavior because they already had the power of charisma. Writing about such experiences—which is all the evidence we possess—followed the same norms: women had to have a written record of their empathetic pain with Christ, but men did not.

In marked contrast to this norm is the tale of Rulman Merswin, mer-chant of Strasbourg, in his account of the first four years following his ini-tial revelation. Merswin was a layman who had never considered devoting himself wholeheartedly to a spiritual life until the age of forty, when his first revelation came upon him. Like Augustine's, it took place in a garden. Though he understood from the first that he would have to face great trials to achieve unwavering faith, he did not foresee how difficult it would be. Merswin practiced self-mortification to subdue his temptations, but dur-ing the following four years he struggled against doubts, temptations, and illness. He perceived the illness as a shameful expression of his unwanted temptations. His entire body became swollen and he suffered such severe "shameful" pains (though he did not specify their placement) that he be-came bedridden. While he may have fought his temptations, he succumbed to his illness quite freely. He lay in bed, he screamed and prayed for Christ to help him, and went nowhere. Thanks to the Virgin, he was cured on Ascension Day, though temptation continued to plague him for two more years.[54]

Merswin's account is unusual in its condemnation of bodily frailty and sickness without any attempt to sanctify them as an imitation of Christ. The sickness was part of his body's battle against his soul's progress, not a cleansing instrument or a shower of grace. That a fourteenth-century vi-sionary should have seen his illness as an attack on his enlightened self rather than an aid to purification does suggest that not all mystics wel-comed disease and pain.

But Merswin was not, properly speaking, a candidate for visible holiness. He eventually joined the *Gottesfreunde* movement but remained a layman for life. Though he did write down his revelations and prophecies, his pains were not part of those spiritual enlightenments. Hence, the broadcasting of his suffering would have done nothing to enhance his nonexistent sanctity. Conversely, pains of living saints that presaged or were part of visionary exaltation merited the widest possible publicity.[55]

When was it improper for a self-proclaimed holy woman to scream and cry for religious reasons? The answer seems to lie in the situation of the woman involved. Almost all the women we have surveyed were members of religious orders and were of good families and standing. Abbesses, like Douceline and Colette, aroused no criticism. A middle-class simple nun like Ebner eventually transcended antagonism. Another woman of similar background, Stagel, was apparently not challenged within her convent for self-mortification, but we do not know much about her actual behavior in pain. Finally, a peasant laywoman was long classified as a madwoman before achieving respect, as can be seen in the biography of Christina Mirabilis.

Between the two extremes one finds a great many holy women. There were two main geographical foci of women's pain and blood mysticism: one was the Beguine movement that began with Mary of Oignies in the Low Countries and the Rheinland, and the other consisted of individual saints in thirteenth- and fourteenth-century northern Italy. Angela of Foligno, Catherine of Siena in the south, and Christina of Stommeln, Christina Mirabilis, Mary of Oignies, and several others in the north, all practiced public self-mortification.[56] In addition, there were many whose main affective performance consisted of weeping. The best known are Margaret of Cortona (1247–97) and Margery Kempe (ca. 1373–1438). Kempe's emotional outbursts of crying in empathy for Christ acutely embarrassed both the townspeople of Lynn and her fellow pilgrims on the way to the Holy Land.[57] Kempe was one of a long series of weeping saints, both male and female, but none of them was described as weeping because of physical pain. The emblematic weeper was one who wept in contrition and for love of Christ, not because of bodily aches and pains.[58] Judging from their *vitae*, emblematic religious figures were expected to weep publicly in paroxysms of religious grief or in ecstatic fits but to hide the physical pain of illness.

Living saints were not models of public behavior for the laity (or the clergy, for that matter) to copy. The extraordinary behavior of those acknowledged as saints was accepted, but anyone else (like Margery Kempe) suffered hostility and condemnation for similar actions. Nevertheless, ecstatic saints had their own code to follow. Furthermore, following this code could result in the identification of the visionary as a genuine saint. Since living sanctity, unlike royalty or childbirth, was a fuzzy category, how some-one behaved while experiencing pain could very well help legitimize that person as a genuine saint.

Women in Childbirth

Childbirth is one of those situations in which we know, beyond all doubt, that pain is present. As we have seen already, Colette suffered worse than any parturient woman, and Christina Mirabilis howled like one. Preachers compared the pains of hell to those of childbirth, and some women actually lost their minds due to the pain. It was therefore a given that women giving birth were in pain. Did the pain dictate any specific behavior? Misogynist literature mocked women for making a great fuss over childbirth to defraud and fool the innocent husband, but nobody took the topos seriously.[59]

Medical texts contain very little advice on how a parturient woman should behave. Michele Savonarola wrote a vernacular tractate of gynecol-ogy for the women of Ferrara. The entire tractate is addressed to the young woman and describes the stages of her life in a sympathetic, helpful manner. When the young woman reaches childbirth, Savonarola's advice (addressed to the parturient, not the midwife) is clearly spelled out: "At such a time, with such pains and changes, you must be governed like a gravely ill woman."[60] Savonarola goes on to say that the physician's (or midwife's) actions should be guided, among other things, by the strength or weakness of the pains. The pain might complicate the delivery, for women insist on walking around during contractions, "not wishing to suffer the pains." When the parturient woman felt her pains in front and descending near the pubis, then she would know that delivery was near. The physician's most startling piece of advice to the woman was to scream loudly, even if her pains were not yet severe, so that all present, her husband included, would take pity on her.[61]

A detailed record of a specific delivery is practically unique. Such a sin-gular case happened in Zaragoza in 1490. Isabel de la Cavallería was the recent widow of Pedro de Francia, lord of Bureta, and was worried about her forthcoming baby's inheritance. To ensure that nobody would raise the claim of a substituted baby or a fake birth, she had a notary and witnesses present in the delivery chamber throughout her labor, to testify and de-clare that this was the baby born of her body, and that no fraud had been practiced. The notary recorded everything that happened from the moment Isabel went into labor until the male baby was properly wrapped in a cloth and identified by all present. All present, including notary, witnesses, and midwives, were named and recorded. The notary also made sure that no other baby was hidden anywhere in the chamber, having been ordered to conduct a body search of the midwives and a thorough search of all bedding and curtains, in case a girl was born.[62]

The narrative is painstakingly detailed. Following the search, both midwives were made to kneel at a statue of Christ and swear upon the icon and a Gospel to "administer well and without any fraud or trick the labour of the aforesaid Isabel." Indeed, the women were watched "with the deliberate intent to prevent that they did not and could not do any trick in bringing any baby and changing one for another." The parturient woman lay supported in the arms of "the magnificent lord Martín Gil de Palomar y de Gurrea, lord of the town of Argavieso," in whose house she was giving birth. The notary took careful note of every detail of the process of childbirth, including amniotic fluids, blood, and placenta. All of these are minutely recorded as proofs of a genuine birth process.[63]

The notary and his clients also considered labor pains an integral part of the delivery's legitimacy. The formulaic phrases "complaining about suffering from the pain of her pregnancy," "continuously complaining about her suffering and proceeding to go into labor," "complaining about the pains of her labor," and "after very many big pains that the aforesaid Isabel de la Cavallería was suffering" occur in all the appropriate places in the narrative—first, when Isabel was just beginning her labor, and then interspersed at all the key points.

These statements were of crucial importance. It was essential that the notary and witnesses be absolutely sure that this was not a counterfeit delivery, that Isabel had indeed been pregnant when her husband died, that she had born a child, and that the child born to her was indeed male and her husband's true progeny. For the latter part of the assurance, they needed to see the baby born and identify it. For the first part—to ensure that indeed Isabel was really delivering a child—they had to know that she was truly in labor, and for that, her complaints of pain were an integral part of the verisimilitude of the birth scene. Had she not complained loudly throughout the delivery, the birth would presumably have remained suspect. Indeed, crying out in labor was a required part of the delivery. In sixteenth-century Germany, a woman was reported to the authorities for "not having acted during her labor as she should," and other women were also censured for not crying during childbirth.[64] The German sources show that the norm could be occasionally violated, but that this violation earned public disapproval. Isabel's account is probably as near as one can get to the actual expressions of childbirth. Nevertheless, it once more bears the suspicion of scripted events. The norm for childbirth was crying out; it was therefore necessary to enact the norm and to register the enactment. Is one therefore to believe only those cases in which the norm was honored in its breach? I tend to assume that norms and reality had a great deal of common ground, if only because people often behaved as expected from them. Women who did not do so were likely to be suspected at best of misbehavior and at worst of faking the delivery. In any case, they would not receive all the sympathy they required. It may be a truism that European women cry out during childbirth, but this fact does not diminish the pain.

Pilgrims Begging for a Cure

What was a young noblewoman to do if she suddenly stubbed her toe or even broke her arm? Was she to behave in a manner markedly different from that of her male counterpart or female inferior? Would the reaction differ in different places? We know very little about what people did when injured or sick and in pain. Medical texts almost never describe the behavior of people under those circumstances.[65] A rare exception appears in the writings of Gilbertus Anglicus, who mentioned a case he had treated with phlebotomy: "I will tell you also what I myself saw in a woman suffering and screaming with pain in her right wrist."[66] Most medical texts, though, do not speak of the patients' behavior. Paradoxically, we discover the mundane when we investigate the miraculous. Descriptions of cures effected by saints often added details of sensations and behavior before the cure.

The world of the later Middle Ages was rife with miracles. Even leaving aside the miracle that took place every time the Eucharist was consecrated, all sorts of supernatural events could happen: souls of the dead haunted cemeteries,[67] sinners were struck down in the midst of their evil deeds, and devils walked about and even entered churches and monasteries, eavesdropping on women's gossip and tempting monks.[68] Most miraculous events, however, took place only upon request to a specific saint. Dead mules did not come back to life and paralytics did not walk unless saintly intercession was provoked by tears, prayers, and requests.

Since thaumaturgic cures usually took place at pilgrimage centers, in a big crowd, it is as well to describe the scene. The ill, congregating around the grave, slept there all night in the hope of an overnight miracle. "You could hear, during the first hour of the night, among the crowd of the infirm the creaking of bones, the rustle of nerves stretching in sleep, the whispers of the possessed, and the loud wailing of various sick people."[69] This was public space with a vengeance.

Saints could perform any kind of miracle, but as of the twelfth century, the greater part of the miracles recorded were those that had taken place at the shrine, mostly thaumaturgic miracles. At every shrine, the local registrar recorded the local miracles. The registrar selecting those miracles worth publicizing would naturally weigh his stories according to specific criteria. Would miracles relating to children or peasants be important enough to include; would they impress their readers and potential donors? Conversely, would the shrine benefit more from stories telling of the punishing might of the patron saint, who exacted revenge on misbehaving visitors? The types of *miraculés* (i.e., people who have been miraculously cured) change from shrine to shrine and from period to period. Similarly, the way the story was told also changed. One registrar might simply record illness and cure; another might add a detailed account of the patient's suffering prior to the cure or even during the healing.

The manner in which miraculous cures were told reflected contemporary sensitivities. Rarely did a registrar simply record a miracle without giving some details as to the subject's gender and status (especially if the latter were prominent). Details of the healing were even more central, including the disease and the manner of its cure. Pain is interwoven in many of these narratives. People arrived writhing in pain and screaming or weeping so hard that they could not even speak. Sometimes they had to be restrained, and even the cure was sometimes sensed as a flash of pain. Here we encounter the close identification of pain behavior with insanity behavior. Registrars seeking a way to describe the behavior of people in pain very often resorted to the simile of madness with its attendant flamboyant behavior.

The prompt cure of a visibly afflicted person, without any medical intervention, was a powerful spectacle. In most medieval stories of thaumaturgic cures, the miracle takes place in the full glare of publicity and involves highly visible diseases: dropsy, leprosy, or insanity, to say nothing of impediments to mobility (paralysis, limping, etc.) or sensory handicaps.[70] A cure had to be visible, and for this to happen, the prior disease had to be just as visible or audible. Though there are also records of gradual cures, most of the records speak of instantaneous public healing. Consequently, the sufferer's demeanor before the cure was a central element. A sufferer who cried, complained, twisted and turned, begged for help aloud, or screamed was a sufferer whose healing could be authenticated. Stiff-upper-lip patients provided no drama. Miraculous healings were thus some of the few situations in which loud complaints of pain, regardless of gender or status, were highly prized. It is not clear how much of this recorded behavior stems from a model of recording or from a performative model of behavior. It is most probable that both elements were at play simultaneously. Miraculous cures had to be recorded as dramatic reversals; both the registrar of miracles and the sufferer knew this, and either one or both articulated pain and disease to the best of their ability and according to their role.

At the same time, the culture of pain transcended disciplinary boundaries. Every cure narrative began with a diagnosed illness, and the diagnoses of miracle narrators (though far more emotional than recipes or medical treatises) in many cases accorded with medical descriptions. Thus, both physicians and narrators determined that headache and toothache were diseases in and of themselves rather than symptoms of another illness.[71] That some pains were independent illnesses was a commonly held truth that nobody queried, similar to the diagnosis of paralysis or blindness.

Severe pain in thaumaturgic narratives appears as part of the out-of-the-ordinary world. Therefore, when pain is included in narratives of miraculous cures, it is dramatic, superlative, unbearable, extremely harsh. And only under such circumstances would people deviate from their usual behavior sufficiently for their digression to merit comment and description.

Pain behavior at shrines belonged in the realm of behavior under extraordinary circumstances. Was vocalization of pain at home improper? The place to seek an answer is in prescriptive manuals of behavior, except that they never mention pain directly. Late medieval manuals were heavily religious in content, full of moralistic examples culled from ancient mythology and more recent exemplary lives. The best known at the time was undoubtedly the *Le livre du chevalier de la Tour Landry pour l'enseignement de ses filles*, translated into English and German within a century of its appearance and reprinted many times.[72] Neither the *chevalier* nor other authors of behavior manuals for women or for men thought it necessary to discourse on behavior when in pain.[73] Presumably, the standard injunction of modest and restrained behavior (urged upon both genders but required of the female) held also for behavior under any kind of stress, and pain was not something to expatiate upon when prescribing a regimen of living. Women walked abroad and young knights faced court society on a daily basis, so downcast eyes and courtly body language were necessarily mentioned, but pain was not part of this rigid behavioral scheme. Sermons *ad status* addressed to women in the later Middle Ages castigate vanity and public appearances but not uncontrolled pain behavior.[74] Somewhat in the manner of medical textbooks, prescriptive manuals dealt with general patterns, not specific situations.

However, here and there miracle narratives describe behavior at home: people like the proverbial young noblewoman, hurt at home, who prayed to the saint and was healed without having recourse to the shrine. In those cases, status was the paramount consideration. Priests, noblemen and no-blewomen, and even young girls of good family who suffered extreme pain at home were praised for their restraint and ability to hide pain. The texts speak of modesty, shame, embarrassment, and fear of criticism as hindering expression.[75] Sometimes, however, pain was an excuse to subvert normal codes of behavior. The theme of insane behavior when in pain occurs time and again in public thaumaturgic miracles throughout the ages.

To appreciate the extraordinary violence of the pain, the attendant be-havior, and the cure, it is well to view a concrete case. The one cited here is extremely early, coming from the miracles of St. Otmar, first abbot of St. Gallen (d. 759). It concerns a young man from Orléans whose entire body was contracted and twisted, and who traveled from place to place by propel-ling himself in a small cart. He had traveled all the way to Rome seeking a cure, in vain, and then crossed the Alps to St. Gallen. The worn wheels of his cart and his calloused hands stood witness to his impossible journey:

> The youth, when first entering the basilica to the body of Saint Otmar, as the binding of his joints stretched, falls on the floor when descending from his cart and assaults the church roof with a horrendous scream, im-pelled by a pain beyond measure, *to which the unheard-of noise testifies* [my italics]. Our abbot, in those days Grimaldus, who at the time was standing outside the basilica under the cloister, heard the unprecedented racket, and bringing with him Bishop Salomo and the abbot of Reichenau (who happened to be present by chance on that day) he enters the church to determine the cause of such a frightful and unusual clamor. What more can be said? The abbots, together with the bishop, come, notice the pitiful weeping of the youth twisting about on the floor, and see him forcing and wounding his own fingers, almost tearing them apart. After a long ordeal, the left hand, contracted into a fist, stretches out, the curved neck straightens . . . the sole of the right foot, which was embedded in his buttocks, straightens, while the bishop sings "Te Deum laudamus," with the breaking of the knee and a great effusion of flowing blood.[76]

This description was taken down in late-eighth-century St. Gallen, but it hardly differs from much later ones. The long, heroic journey, the provi-dential presence of venerable witnesses, and the ritual prayers of thanks are typical.

Many other cases concern people who had lost their minds as a result of pain and people whose behavior in pain led others to believe they had lost their minds. A merchant who had tried to profit from the pilgrim trade at Conques was punished by St. Foy with fire: "You would have been astonished at his horrible bellowings as the flames drove him mad, at the noises he emitted as he kicked, at the grating of his teeth, at his wildly rolling eyes and the uncontrolled contortions of his whole body. In his unbearable pain, the wretch seemed to be propelled back and forth in headlong movement."[77] A toothache sufferer with a swollen jaw was brought to St. Thomas's tomb at Canterbury, restrained by several people, to be cured of madness, as his cries and gestures had indicated insanity. Another young sufferer came to the tomb "twisting, turning, and screaming; falling over, rising but unable to stay straight." A headache sufferer, cured by St. Louis of Anjou (d. 1297) had indeed lost his senses from pain. He was deprived of sight and hearing, recognized nobody and talked nonsense.[78] Women during childbirth could go mad with pain. The concubine of a priest actually lost her mind from pain during labor, but drinking water from St. Thomas's well gave her an hour's sleep before the delivery.[79]

The most eloquent descriptions of people driven mad by pain come from fifteenth-century Flanders. Emotive piety, it seems, went hand in hand there with extravagant gesturing and crying. Several women became almost mad (*quasi furibunda*) or frenzied (*penitus rabida*) with aches and pains. An eminent Franciscan, Brother Petrus, was suffering from a migraine during his visit to the convent of St. Peter in Ghent. It had been plaguing him "for a year and a half already, with horrible and inexpressible affliction. He often got up from the table, wandered around the garden wailing and crying piteously, not hearing those who tried to speak to him because of the pain."[80] Taken as manuals of behavior for people in a state of sickness, miracle stories provided a range of expression far beyond any that daily aches and pains may have called forth. At the most extreme, at the border of the miraculous, people were not expected to show modesty and restraint. They were supposed to express their sensations loudly and visibly, by gesture and clamor (*gestu et clamore*).

Outside the drama of the miraculous, most texts speaking of illness say little of people's behavior. One literary example is Boccaccio's terrifying description of the onset of the Black Death in Florence. He tells of healthy people whose terror moved them either to fervent penitence or to a life of vice and luxuriousness. As to the ill and the dying, he merely says that people would fall ill suddenly, writhe for a few minutes, and die. The sick and dying in the *Decameron* were no more than a lurid background against which to set the motives and actions of the living.[81] Most other accounts of the plague are no more informative. They speak of pain during the short agony of the infected but say nothing about how pain may have affected behavior.[82] Once again, Stalin's dictum proves true: the death of one man is a tragedy and the death of a million people is a statistic.

A totally different description of epidemic victims, however irrelevant to western Europe in the later Middle Ages, is still worth examining. When Procopius described the plague in sixth-century Constantinople, he spoke also of the dying, not only of those who had to dispose of them: the disease, he said, began as a fever, continued with the eruption of buboes, and subsequently developed in different ways:

> For there ensued with some a deep coma, with others a violent delirium, and in either case they suffered the characteristic symptoms of the disease. . . . But those who were seized with delirium suffered from insomnia and were victims of a distorted imagination. [Those who cared for them were to be pitied], for when the patients fell from their beds and lay rolling upon the floor, they kept putting them back in place, and when they were struggling to rush headlong out of their houses, they would force them back by shoving and pulling against them. And when water chanced to be near, they wished to fall into it, not so much because of a desire for drink (for the most of them rushed into the sea), but the cause was to be found chiefly in the diseased state of their minds. . . . And in those cases where neither coma nor delirium came on, the bubonic swelling became mortified and the sufferer, no longer able to endure the pain, died. And one would suppose that in all cases the same thing would have been true, but since they were not at all in their senses, some were quite unable to feel the pain; for owing to the troubled condition of their minds they lost all sense of feeling.[83]

Here Procopius put his finger on an unusual, inherent connection between madness and pain. Those who suffered pain and retained their sanity died of the pain. But he also assumed that all those whose buboes had burst had been quite literally driven out of their senses by the pain; their senses having abandoned them, they must have become immune to pain.[84] No parallel description exists in the West in which sufferers driven mad by pain lost only their minds but not their sensitivity to pain. On the contrary, as we shall see, medical science claimed that ill people who felt no pain when they ought to were mad.[85] Normative descriptions of illness that did not include a miraculous cure usually excluded madness unless the illness was the final one.

Men on Their Deathbeds

Ill people could clamor for health, but once the die was cast and death approached, it was incumbent upon the dying person and his or her friends to relinquish any attempts for a cure and prepare for death. As we have seen in chapter 1, from the thirteenth century onward there was a tradition that no longer identified salvation (*salus*) with health and life but with an appropriate death. Jean Gerson had counseled the friends of the dying to direct their thoughts away from health and toward heaven.[86] Gerson's work, though, was merely the tip of the iceberg. The "good death" literature was extensive and graphic, adorned with woodcuts, showing the ill man (it was almost invariably a man)[87] in bed, surrounded by angels and devils fighting over the soon-to-be-liberated soul (see fig. 4). Who would carry the day really depended upon the dying person: one must not lose hope, for despair was a sin, but one must not be too sure and vainglorious; one must genuinely repent all previous sins and make amends for what one could. Finally, it was crucial to confess, be shriven, and receive the viaticum. The consequences of dying unprepared could be terrible: either purgatory or aimless wandering on earth, seeking help, awaited those who did not die properly.[88]

Did the good death include any pain? According to the manuals and sermons, pain had no useful place at the bedside of the dying. One was too busy preparing for the big transition to pay any attention to pain. Nor did advice on the good death include any specific suggestions about suppressing pain. Presumably, the authors assumed that this was a subject best glossed over in silence. If one was to weep, it was in penitence, not pain. As we have no information from those who were about to die, we cannot tell whether pain formed any part of their experience. Accounts of near-death experiences, subsequently recounted as prologues to descriptions of the afterworld, do not include pain as part of the (unfinished) passage.[89] Possibly, narrators' imagination, too, focused upon other subjects at that microsecond.

Pain could crop up, though, as an impediment to the good death. The anonymous treatise on good death attributed to either Albert the Great (1193/1206–1280), Matthew of Cracow (1335–1410), or Domenico Capranica (1400–1458) acknowledges that death is the most terrible experience of all but claims that those wishing to die do so easily.[90] Pain is one of the tools the devil uses to induce despair, and the sufferer (*infirmus*) must think of Christ on the cross in order to belittle his own pains. The presence of pain, which the treatise acknowledges as almost inevitable at death, might cause impatience, which is another temptation of the devil. Once more, we find here the observation that pain can drive people, even on their deathbeds,

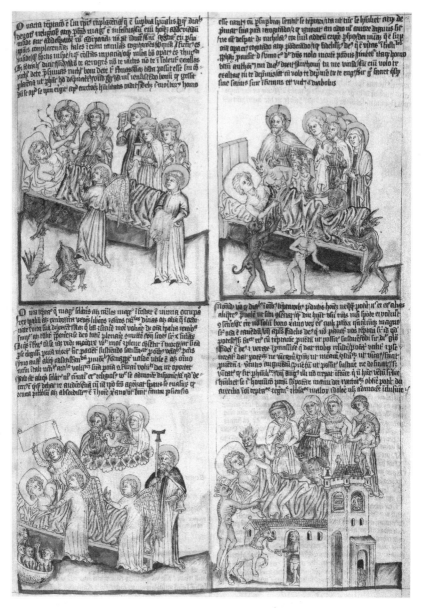

Figure 4. Deathbed scene. From "Apocalypsis S. Johannis cum glossis et vita S. Johannis;
ars moriendi, etc." (ca. 1420–30). Wellcome Library, London, MS 49, fol. 30r.

to madness and hence to despair.[91] Those who wish for an easy passage heavenward must steel themselves against the pain and not allow it to disturb their concentration upon penitence, prayers, and hope. On a difficult and hazardous journey, the almost inevitable pain of dying was a dangerous distraction that might cause the traveler to lose his footing and tumble into the abyss of hell. Pain, that useful tool of virtue throughout life, metamorphosed at death into a menace.

Those were the norms inculcated into any dying Christian. Did those norms apply exactly in the same manner to dying kings? On the face of it, the answer is overwhelmingly positive. Good kings who died a good death did so according to all the prescribed Christian rules: atoning for their sins, confessing, preparing their souls.[92] Still, rulers, more than anybody else, had different codes for different occasions. Johan Huizinga deduced from the seemingly impetuous behavior of late medieval Burgundian dukes that medieval people were childlike in their uncontrolled display of emotions.[93] This view gained a much-needed review in the work of Gerd Althoff, who showed that the anger of the king, *ira regis*, had its place in ritualized court behavior during the High Middle Ages: German emperors openly displayed anger when the occasion so warranted.[94] Both authors, almost a century apart, extrapolated their findings to all medieval Western rulers. Presumably, there was more than one way of displaying anger, and the range between raising one's voice and drumming one's feet while lying on the floor and screaming is quite wide. Nevertheless, when it comes to self-control and impassivity during pain, the range is much narrower. At most, a hagiographer might describe a dying martyr either as completely immobile or as showing a smiling face. When it came to deathbed behavior, the rules were stricter: deathbed behavior epitomized the essence of the dying person, reflecting in one instant all that the sufferer had been in life and all that awaited her posthumously. Thus, the good death of a king was more important than the good death of any of his subjects. Indeed, throughout medieval history those labeled "good kings" died well, whereas bad kings did not. Should any reader doubt the true nature of the historical personage in question, the deathbed scene sealed the characterization for all time. Occasionally, narratives of the death of the great followed a pattern somewhat different from the one advised by the manuals: it was a clear pattern of suppression of pain.

We can see a concrete example in the biography of King Charles V of France (1338–80), *Le livre des faits et bonnes moeurs du roi Charles V le Sage,* which Christine de Pizan wrote at the request of Duke Philip of Burgundy in 1404. The king had been dead for nearly a quarter of a century by the time the book was written, and it was indeed meant to eulogize and display an ideal of Christian kingship. As was fit, Charles had made a good death, entrusting his soul to God, hoping for salvation, and concentrating on his devotion. One of the key elements in his behavior was his suppression of any manifestation of pain. Despite his great pains, he insisted upon arising every day and getting washed and dressed. On the day before his death, "one could see the signs of approaching death, and nevertheless nobody knew the torture he endured, because he continued not to show the least sign of suffering."[95]

It is impossible to know what Charles V actually felt on his penultimate day on earth. What we do know is that the memory of his death was scripted in the same manner as that of his life: an exemplary Christian and an exemplary king. Kings were not supposed to cry and scream when in pain. The contrast between the model descriptions of Charles "the wise" and his son Charles "the mad" insist on the difference between someone who could govern his behavior regardless of his senses and someone who could govern neither his senses nor his behavior: the first manifestation of Charles VI's madness was his sudden unbridled attack upon his entourage, thinking them all enemies.[96]

The suppressed suffering of dying kings goes back a long way. It may have had its origins in Roman ideas of decorum, but the earliest medieval ruler whose memory gives any insight to the subject is a Merovingian. As Gregory of Tours records, King Chlotar, on his deathbed, was "miffed at the King of Heaven for failing to show any professional courtesy by allowing other great kings such as himself to die in pain."[97] Chlotar (d. 561), apparently, could not master the art of appearing to suppress his suffering while broadcasting it and required true surcease to be able to die as a king should. Interestingly, just before falling ill he had visited the shrine of St. Martin, where he had prayed with great sobbing (cum grande gemitu), which was perfectly acceptable. Conversely, when Charlemagne was dying, insisted Einhard, though he suffered from the pain of pleurisy, he still fasted and did not complain.[98] Emperor Henry II (973–1024) suffered terrible pains when visiting Monte Cassino, but the worst of his pain expression was failing to fall asleep.[99] It is worthy of note that the biographers found it important to record that these rulers had not cried in pain.

Prelates were likely to follow the same pattern. Thus, Adam of Bremen tells of the death of Archbishop Adalbert in 1072: "It was said that already on the third day before his death he knew that he would not arise from his bed. But such was the fortitude of his soul that while in gravest illness he wished for no help and never gave voice to his pain."[100] The lordly example was spoiled only by the devout regrets of a worldly prelate who at the end wished he had spent more time in affairs of the soul. While the pattern seems most obvious in high medieval Germany, it did affect biographies of rulers all over Europe. Some were destined to follow this model—at least in their biographies—throughout the Middle Ages.

Conclusion

One of the first codes established by Christianity was that of behavior while experiencing pain in public. Remarkably, this code was clearly distinct from all the descriptions of Christ's behavior on the cross. Martyrs did not weep, nor did they forgive. They fought, they argued, they denied, they refused. Either actively or passively, they were passionately antagonistic to their judges. What they absolutely did not do is manifest pain. Late medieval Christianity inherited this double standard: Christ's overt manifestation of pain, which was definitely not a lack of control, as opposed to the bellicose suppression of pain in the martyrological writings. The behavior of holy men and women could thus be modeled upon an entire spectrum of possibilities. As we have seen, there was no one standard, and the codes depended very much upon the specific situation the holy person found herself in. In this, saintly codes were identical to those of the rest of society: where, when, and why dictated how.

Norms of behavior are fine-tuned codes, more often tacit than openly laid down. The infinite variety ranging from the intolerable, to the barely permissible, to the perfectly laudable form of behavior depends upon an enormous number of nuances that cannot be conveyed in writing. Presumably, a properly weeping pilgrim in a shrine who complained in a broad lower-class accent, or whose gesticulations resembled dancing too much for the clergy's taste, would not end up as an emblematic *miraculé*. Such a man would be very much in the category of the silent parturient or the screaming moribund person. As we have seen, manuals of conduct have nothing to say about behavior while experiencing pain, but miracle narratives do yield up some standards.

Clearly, there was a common denominator between the emblematic and the anonymous. Rarely do we hear of control and suppression: most of the texts speak of people in the grasp of irresistible forces. Whether it is a nun in the grip of a vision or an epileptic in the grip of a seizure, or merely a headache sufferer who could take no more—all were described as having no choice in their mode of behavior. Pain, the originator of madness, stood as the opposite of reason and human choice. This is precisely why the usefulness of pain was inverted upon the approach of death. If ever people needed to be clear-headed in order to make the choice of salvation, that was the time. Pain brought about impatience, despair, and madness, all of them harbingers of damnation.

Tracking back, one can work from the identification of pain with madness to the descriptions left by recorders of thaumaturgic miracles. If a registrar needed to describe someone suffering from severe pain and due for miraculous healing, the best way was to describe the sufferer as acting like a mad person. And everybody knew how mad people were supposed to behave, with uncontrolled gestures, screams, and contortions. Although Procopius had assumed that madness desensitized people to pain, nobody in the West thought so. Madness and pain were one, and pain could be decoded through the dance of madness.

PART II

Knowledge from Pain

Pain was a source of salvation and punishment, said theologians. Pain was a source of justice and truth, said jurists. Pain was a source of weakness and death, said physicians. Pain, properly enacted and presented, was a source of power. The last statement was never openly made, but it can most certainly be deduced from the public actions of sufferers.[1]

At the basis of these mostly positive assertions regarding pain lies a very obvious truth—namely, that to suffer one must be both one's own subject and one's own object. As Murat Aydede puts it, if one perceives an apple, the apple is there also for other people's perception. However, if one perceives a pain, the pain is not perceptible to others by its own nature.[2] The pain is inherent in the individual and has no existence outside her.

This very basic truth has been obscured by a number of factors. Prime among them is linguistic usage, which very often characterizes pain as an external force that attacks, bludgeons, pricks, stings, and so on. The use of transitive verbs to describe pain and its effects endows pain with a spurious individuality. "It" does those things to people or animals rather than being an intrinsic part of the entity. Another cause for perceiving pain as an independent, external force derives from the fact that most of the writing about it comes from the pens of observers, not sufferers. As we have seen, even self-descriptive texts are culture bound, adopting the style of an external observer. The observer regards pain as a phenomenon fraught with meanings, and perhaps the most central of those meanings is that pain is a sign, waiting to be interpreted and understood before it is managed.

Observers of pain have wrought our perceptions, and they are also often the managers of pain. Scholars and theologians may only have reflected upon the subject, but their reflections endowed the past pain of Christ with significance. The same people, acting in pastoral roles, provided the sufferings

of their flock with other meanings. Mystics, meditating upon similar subjects, gave pain a transcendental aura. The most active interpreters of pain,
however, were the practical managers of pain: physicians and torturers.

What could people in the later Middle Ages learn from another's pain?
The knowledge depends upon two factors. First is the subject-object relationship. Who is suffering? Who is interpreting the pain? Second, what is
the aim of observation? Is it the eliciting of facts or the investigation of
truth? Of course, the categories are not mutually exclusive: sufferers may
also have been the interpreters of their pain, and interrogators may have
inflicted pain in order to elicit facts leading to guilt.

In the following chapters we will investigate how interpreters of pain
used taxonomy and language as bridges between sufferer and observer, and
then we will delve into the transcendental meanings that medieval culture
and people attached to human pain, in their own past and in their own present. The interpretation of words and the interpretations of the holy past
interacted in the explanation of pain.

CHAPTER FIVE

The Vocabulary and Typology of Pain

Specific human situations create the vocabularies necessary for them. Medieval French has half a dozen words for "horse," such as *destrier* (warhorse) and *somier* (packhorse). When it comes to pain, however, both Latin and vernacular Western languages are extremely poor. None of them has different nouns to denote different types or different degrees of pain, and this dearth is probably indicative of the powerlessness of Western culture when dealing with pain.

Two groups of professionals at least were in absolute need for words describing pains and their results: physicians, who used pain as a diagnostic, and jurists, who ordered suspects to be tortured. Both had to be connoisseurs of pain and its variants lest their patients die. The word "patient" is derived from the Latin root that denotes, among other things, suffering (*pati*). It is thus of prime importance to examine the linguistic usages of both groups. Neither group invented new terms. Rather, they relied upon tradition to provide them with words, the semantic fields of which they could transform for their own uses.

Physicians in need of specific descriptors resorted, as did their Greek, Roman, and Arabic predecessors, to synesthetic devices. Faced with nameless sensations, they borrowed words from different sensory fields for their descriptors. As there seems to be general agreement concerning the taste and smell of sweetness, for example, it is possible to apply the term to other senses. In like manner, a pain could be described as sharp or throbbing, though it was neither a knife nor a heart. Such semantic transitions had become so common that one had no need ever to think about the original usage of the terms.[1] Unlike physicians, jurists solved the problem by circumlocution. One could speak of constant men who could resist torture in their certainty of innocence or of fortitude under torture but never of pain.

Jurists' vocabulary was partially culled from Roman law, which is even poorer in such terms than medieval Latin. But much of it was borrowed, in a surprising twist of meaning, from late antique martyrological narratives, which told of judicial torture from an entirely nonjudicial point of view.

The two opposed attitudes—attaching descriptors to every possible type of pain and completely avoiding any mention of it—are two aspects of the same coin. Pain is intransmissible, indescribable, immeasurable. And yet it must be transmitted, described, and measured, or the manipulators of pain are helpless. Easing of pain depended first of all upon language and ideas, with the practices emerging from those ideas.

Medical Usage

Painlessness in situations and places in which a patient ought to feel pain was an ominous sign. Pain sensations in a wounded limb indicated first of all that it was alive. Dead limbs felt no pain, and when amputating a gangrenous limb, the surgeon must cut above the corruption, where an inserted probe would find firm flesh and pain.[2] Some internal organs simply felt no pain, even in illness. In cases where pain had been present and then vanished spontaneously, this might not necessarily be a sign of health. Quite the contrary, it could herald worse developments. Since pain could be the indicator of an ongoing process—a change of "complexion" (the combination of humors in the body) from healthy to pathological, from balanced to unbalanced—the disappearance of pain while the illness remained signaled the victory of corruption over the entire body. Henceforth, the sufferer had a fully unbalanced complexion, with all the resultant dire consequences.[3] Furthermore, lack of pain sensitivity could also indicate madness. Hippocrates had already noted that those who fail to feel pain when they ought to are sick in their minds, and the aphorism on this subject was often cited in later centuries: "When people ailing in body sense no pain, they are sick in their minds."[4] Impassibility in illness could therefore mean death, either of soul or of body. If pain resided in the mind or the soul (which medieval intellectuals sometimes conflated), then senselessness and lack of sensation could be the same. Finally, there was the possibility of misleading pain. Sometimes, said Avicenna, the patient felt the pain of a secondary illness, while the primary illness did not manifest itself through pain.[5] In these cases the physician had to study the patient's complexion, for pain was not a sufficient sign. As a rule, since pain signified present or future illness, the lack of pain when other symptoms indicated an illness was the worst sign of all.

If one were to list, in descending order of importance, the signs of ill-ness considered meaningful by late medieval healers, pain would not top the list. The color, consistency, and taste of the patient's urine were un-doubtedly more important, as were pulse and fever. Those were easier to determine than pain, for they did not depend upon the patient's testimony. Nevertheless, different types of pain also indicated the causes of illness. A most explicit author in this sense was Gilbertus Anglicus, who tells in his *Compendium medicinae* how he diagnosed various illnesses through ques-tioning the patient and finding out where the pain resided:

> The escape of blood in the urine is due sometimes to the liver, some-times to the bile, sometimes to the kidneys and loins, sometimes to the bladder. If the blood is pure and clear, in large quantity, mixed perfectly with the urine *and accompanied by pain in the right hypochondrium,*[6] it comes from the liver. Such urine presents scarcely any sediment. If the blood comes from the *Irili* vein, it is also rather pure, but less pure than in the former case, nor is the quantity so great, *while pain is felt over the region of the seventh vertebra, counting from below.* If it comes from the kidneys, it is scanty and pure as it leaves the bladder, but soon coagulates and forms a dark deposit in the vessel, *while pain is felt in the pubes and peritoneum.*[7] (my italics)

Similarly, an infection in a wound was noted by the burning sensation in it, and cardiac illnesses were spotted by "excessive pain," among other symptoms.[8]

Later physicians on the Continent were more sophisticated. By Gilber-tus's time, the translation of Avicenna's *Canon of Medicine* had become common in the West. Gilbertus himself had no professional medical train-ing, but students in Paris and Montpellier knew already Avicenna's detailed description of fifteen types of pain and their meanings.[9] Though not all the humors Avicenna blamed for different pains appeared in Galen's writings, the use of humoral terminology embedded Avicenna's different types of pain within the traditional conceptual matrix. University-trained physi-cians learned to view pain more as a sign than a symptom. None of these humors was in itself an illness, but the result of illness. In interpreting pain, one had to consider a variety of factors: the nature, strength, and location of the pain. For this task, it was necessary to create and use consistent catego-ries, providing them with clear, unambiguous names.

In her book on the history of pain, Roselyne Rey had argued that the presence of a rich vocabulary (in the Hippocratic corpus) of pain terms and descriptors was proof of, at least, a clear consideration of its diagnostic and prognostic importance in ancient Greek medicine.[10] I would argue that the existence of a stable vocabulary of pain was the first requirement for any sort of functional discussion on pain. As pain by its own nature is intransmissible, the indispensable basis for both its treatment and its use was for a medical practitioner to be able to explain to another what pain denoted which illness.

The conservatism of pain vocabulary lies in its functions. If the patient sensed pain and could transmit the precise knowledge of the type and location of this sensation to the physician, both diagnosis and prognosis might be easier. When it came to the description of symptoms, it made little sense for physicians to pioneer a new vocabulary or be creative with the literary forms of language. Speech models and similes are at the basis of communication between people. Unless both sides share the same concepts, the power of a simile is lost. The transmission of diagnostic knowledge especially requires that all sides be unanimous in attributing the same meanings to words, and medieval physicians were conscious of this necessity. We therefore have a reasonably coherent and continuous vocabulary of pain in use during the later Middle Ages. The analysis of this vocabulary provides a window into the minds of physicians confronting pain.[11]

Any such analysis must be conjoined with the examination of named and organized categories and subcategories of pain. Taxonomy is an extremely important source for past frames of mind. Zoologists could choose whether to classify animals by their consumption value to humans (as edible or inedible) or by their skeletal formations (as vertebrate or invertebrate); from these two starting points, they could proceed to subdivide their categories into domestic edible animals and wild edible animals or, among the vertebrates, into mammals, reptiles, and avians. Similarly, different taxonomies could simultaneously apply to pain. Sufferers might classify pain as tolerable or intolerable, strong or weak.[12] Physicians, however, were more interested in pain as a set of clues, to be interpreted for diagnostic purposes. Medical categories of pain were based upon perception and sensation. To determine what had caused the pain, physicians queried patients' perception and description of pain. To decide whether the pain was sharp and localized or extensive, diffuse, and hard to locate, one had to ask as well as examine the patient.[13] The more detailed the description of pain given by the patient, the clearer the evidence. Pain could be a burning sensation, "so that it seems to him that occasionally a flame passes through his shoulders."[14] Sufferers of gout cannot walk or sleep, lose their appetite, constantly vomit, need medication, can neither drink nor have sex, are constantly feverish—

all because of their pain.[15] Such descriptions of pain were geared toward the subjective, personal experience of the sufferer, which provided a basis for the diagnosis.

The genealogy of medieval pain descriptors and categories begins with Galen. Galen's most detailed work on pain, *Of the Affected Parts (De interioribus)*, includes a vitriolic diatribe against the Syrian physician Archigenes (ca. 75–ca. 129), who had tried to build a clear descriptive taxonomy of pains in a book of the same title as Galen's, with the aim of creating a foolproof diagnostic tool. Archigenes's goal, it seems, was to create a table of equivalences: a sharp pain denoted one disease; a diffuse pain, another. The gist of Galen's objection to Archigenes was that it is impossible to categorize types of pain autonomously from the specific organ in which the pain resides, so that categorizing pain independently was useless. Galen insisted that, since pains could move from place to place, the important classificatory criterion was the location, not the type of pain. Moreover, he maintained that, pain being ineffable and intransmissible, the only person who could write knowledgeably about all the types was a properly trained physician who had felt them all personally, possessed all the qualities needed to analyze them, and had conducted his research by thoughtful observation and without any self-pity or subjectivity. Galen himself confessed to having failed this test. He had once suffered a severe piercing abdominal pain, which he diagnosed as a bladder stone, because the pain was located deep in his abdomen, where he knew the ureters descend from the kidneys to the bladder. He applied an enema, which produced almost immediately, with great pain, a bowel movement with a transparent humor. However, the pain soon subsided and no stone came out, which proved that his pain had come from the intestines.[16]

Archigenes had committed every possible error in classifying pain. The adjectives he had used to describe pain were *nomina absurda*, wrongly placed, obscure, and meaningless. What exactly, rhetorically asked the indignant Galen, did Archigenes mean by comparatives like *dulcior, imbecillior, obtusior*, or *minus molestum*? And what precisely was the meaning of *dolor ulcerosus, punctorius, infixus*, or *lacerans*? As far as Galen could make it out, all attributions, if comprehensible at all, were diagnostically wrong. Thus, Archigenes had most carefully described liver pain as *tractorius et inherens et stupidus [est], atque atrocius urgens*, which made no sense to Galen and gave him no clue as to the disease behind the pain. As far as Galen was concerned, he might as well have described pain as red or blue.[17]

Arnau de Villanova took up this invective more than a millennium later. Arnau's *Doctrina Galieni* is an elaboration on Galen, and when it comes to criticizing Archigenes for his use of descriptors, Arnau was far more explicit and even more vicious than Galen. After listing all of Archigenes's descriptions of pain (including several Galen had not cited), Arnau pithily adds:

> Even if it is useful to name things not only according to the fashion of the learned but also as the lay name it, it still does not exempt Archigenes from having erred. Even if some patients call a certain pain furious or acute, nobody would describe himself as suffering an oily, salty, or viscous pain, or anything similar. If indeed he had used these descriptors because of a poverty of names for describing types of pain, he was still guilty of inadequate usage. Even if pain accompanied by a greater or lesser constriction could be described by synesthesia as sharp or astringent taste, nevertheless by no stretch of similarity can pain be described as sweet,[18] for all pain afflicts rather than causes pleasure. If he called a less powerful pain sweet, it would have been better to name it weak.[19]

Arnau's expansion of Galen makes the most basic point about descriptive similes: if they are to work in the medical field, they should not excite the listener's imagination. They are meant to convey information, and Archigenes's flowery poetic flights did nothing of the sort. His problem was not poverty of vocabulary but the opposite, an embarrassment of adjectives. His similes merely misled everyone, patients and physicians alike.

Given Galen's objection to a fixed description of pain types and the practical bent of early medieval medicine, his casual descriptors did not really fall into clear-cut categories. What physicians of Arnau's period did, though, was not to eschew all similes (which was impossible) but to restrict them to a workable, commonly held list. Medieval authors liked to quote Galen's terse words (in his commentary on the Hippocratic aphorisms) concerning how the numerous kinds of pain can all be subsumed under three or four main categories,[20] but such statements still left the field open to various different systems.

Mindful of Galen, several authors attempted to adapt their classification of pain to the rest of the body's anatomy. However, the Galenic idea that pain must independently relate to each organ was too complex. Thus, several authors came up with the correlation of pains with humors. Constantine the African had a simple fourfold division. He was very likely relying, as he did in all of his work, upon an Arabic tradition,[21] but his division had no following in the West. His starting point, as that of almost all medieval physicians, was that pain resulted from a sudden change. The change, consequently, was inevitably a humoral alteration. Thus, his first two categories,

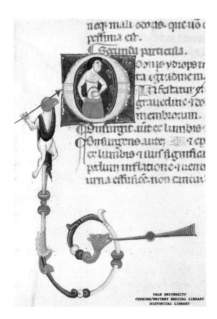

Figure 5. Abdominal dropsy (ascites) shown in initial *O*. A brown-haired male, nude to the waist and with orange drapery over his lower body, frowns and places his left hand on his abdomen. MS 28, Paneth Codex, fol. 17, Bologna (ca. 1300). Courtesy of the Cushing/Whitney Medical Library, Yale University.

gravis and *tensivus*, both resulted from a plethora of cold humors—black bile and phlegm—and a thinning of the blood. Conversely, *calefactivus* and *dolorosus* pains were the opposite, the result of an imbalance in favor of acute, fiery humors: choler and blood. The hot and dry humors generated a great motion of fluids, resulting in heat and pain and sometimes in fever. If the humors boiled and did not putrefy, the pain was merely *dolorosus*, not *calefactivus*, manifesting itself as acute pain in the entire surface, as in the pain of a wound.[22]

Constantine lived in Monte Cassino, and his work was closely tied to the dominant nearby center of prescholastic medical learning in Salerno. It is thus logical to find the same attempt at correlation in the Salernitan school, in the late-twelfth-century work of Maurus of Salerno. Maurus counted six types of pain, four of them directly connected to the four humors: *infixivus*, *pungitivus*, *aggravativus*, *extensivus*, *deambulativus*, and *congelativus*. The first four types resulted directly from specific humors, respectively blood, choler, phlegm, and black bile, while the latter two stemmed from ventosity and cold.[23] Presumably, the addition of the latter two categories came from clinical observation, which did not necessarily fit

in with theoretical humoral frameworks. Salernitan masters prided themselves on being practicing physicians as well as academics, and the result
was a compound list that might not have made much philosophical sense
but that did fit practical experience.[24]

Following generations took different routes. By the time Maurus was
writing his works in Salerno, the translations of Gerard of Cremona, among
them the Latin *Canon* of Avicenna, began reaching Western universities.
The list of pains in the Latin Avicenna looks as though Gerard of Cremona
had plumbed the depths of his synonym thesaurus, having had great trouble
transposing pain categories from Arabic to Latin. What he produced was no
fewer than fifteen categories: "*Pruritivus, asperativus, pungitivus, compres-
sivus, extensivus, concussivus, frangitivus, laxativus, perforativus, acualis,
stupefactivus, pulsativus, gravativus, fatigativus, mordicativus.*"[25] After
listing these categories, Avicenna went on to explain each one's meaning,
though the explanations are sometimes as obscure as his definitions. He
provided no hierarchies of taxonomy, no rationale or order for his list. No
wonder Arnau de Villanova was later to accuse him of doing nothing but
confusing Latin physicians.[26]

It is possible to risk translating some of these terms, assuming that a
throbbing or spreading pain is the same now as it was in the first or in the
eleventh century. It is doubtful, however, that we can achieve a precise
rendering that would explain a diagnosis based upon such translations. One
might well argue that the incomprehension is ours, stemming from distance in time and too many linguistic transitions. Galen had faced the same
problem within the Hellenistic Greek tradition, across only a few decades
of usage between Archigenes and himself, and had ended up rejecting the
entire method. Many terms, after all, lose or change their meaning with
time, translation, and transmission.[27] The usages of late medieval Latin
physicians indicate that one linguistic transition, from Arabic to Latin, was
already one too many. Pain was not an elusive eastern import. It was there,
and needed comprehensible names. Clearly, medieval physicians found the
full list puzzling at best or meaningless at worst. Of the fifteen, I have found
only five in consistent use by late medieval physicians and surgeons, either
in textbooks or in *consilia: extensivus, gravativus, mordicativus, pruritivus,* and *pungitivus*—categories that obviously meant something to Latin
writers of medicine. Avicenna's list was both overcrowded with categories
rendered obscure by translation and inadequate. Western authors who discarded his list nevertheless came up with their own terms: *inflativus, congelativus, calefactivus, corrosivus, infixivus,* and several more.

The difference might have been cultural as well as semantic. Different linguistic groups possess descriptors for different types of pain that do not exist in Latin. What made sense in Persian and Arabic medicine made no sense in Latin. Bernard de Gordon discarded most of Avicenna (at least as far as categories go), listing four categories of pain and using several new terms:

> There are many types of pain according to Avicenna. According to Galen, they can be reduced to three or four, as he says in the [commentary on the Hippocratic] aphorism *Spontaneous lassitude indicates disease* and in his book *Regimen of Health.* There is a pain called sharp [*acutus*], stabbing [*pungitivus*], ulcerative pain; there is another [called] stretching [*extensivus*] pain; another is *inflativus* and another *gravativus* or apostemous. If there are other kinds, they can be reduced to these.[28]

In Bologna, Bartolomeo da Varignana, Bernard's almost exact contemporary (ca. 1260–1318), completely ignored both Galen and Avicenna, citing three main categories: *congelativus, pulsativus,* and *aggravativus.* In addition, he also mentioned *perforativus, corrosivus, pungitivus,* and *mordicativus.*[29] Though Bartolomeo, like Bernard, was a scholastic physician, he ignored conflicting traditions for the sake of clarity. His categories are faintly reminiscent of Maurus's division; these are the only two classifications to specify cold (*congelativus*) pain as a category. All of the other descriptors were already in Avicenna's work except for *corrosivus,* which was Bartolomeo's one contribution to the typology of pain.

What stands out in these attempts is the refusal to follow past traditions, be they classical or Arab, blindly and an insistence on trying to form a coherent, serviceable vocabulary. Furthermore, like his contemporary in Montpellier and like any well-trained scholastic, Bartolomeo da Varignana formed his knowledge into a hierarchy of main categories, resorting to secondary descriptors only as phenomena, not types. This sort of flexibility allowed one to use many names without assuming that they were absolute keys to a diagnosis.

Both southern French and Bolognese schools of medicine simplified the vocabulary of pain through a hierarchy of primary and secondary descriptors, and the system worked. Henri de Mondeville used the categories of Bernard de Gordon, and Michele Savonarola used those of Bartolomeo da Varignana.[30] Bernard did imply that there were also other descriptors, but that they could be subsumed under the four main headings and were of no ontological value. Moreover, he did not consider those subcategories worth listing in detail. Possibly, he thought they were unimportant, imprecise synonyms for the same phenomena rather than meaningful classifications. Mondeville, surgeon rather than academic, used descriptors freely and profusely, as needed for each case: *tolerabilis, intolerabilis, fortis, ventosus, furiosus, inflammativus, ponderosus, deambulativus* (a clearly clinical distinction for a pain that prevents the patient from being mobile), *intercutaneus*, and so forth. He could describe a certain type of pain as "a pain that comes from the blood, piercing, tolerable, noninflammative," which phlebotomy could cure. In contrast, a paralyzing, intercutaneous, stabbing, and itching pain came from an excess of bile.[31] Again, one sees the surgeon's more clinically focused attitude. His descriptions (rather than categories) were far more diverse and fluid than Bernard de Gordon's, aimed not so much at a taxonomical hierarchy but at practical, accurate description.

Medical discourse was largely borrowed from standard usage. All the terms above could be, and were, used in nonmedical discourse. In one unusual case, the same term was adopted in different senses in medical and theological discourse. The sympathetic pain felt in a body part of a person at the injury of that body part in another was the same as what the soul felt when the body was injured, *condolentia*, or suffering together.[32] Until the twelfth century, the term was used frequently to express sympathy and sharing a grief. Alain de Lille transposed it to mean what the Virgin felt during the Crucifixion, though later authors preferred to refer to that feeling by the term *compassio*.[33] The idea that perception of another's pain might actually be transmuted from a cerebral apprehension to sharing in the feeling was originally a religious idea, but a late medieval physician could use the term in a purely physiological sense.

Bernard de Gordon's fourfold scheme had several other advantages beyond its simplicity and clarity. First, two of his four categories are explicitly connected with specific ills: ulcers and apostemes. A categorization that linked symptoms directly with specific syndromes was far more useful than a long vague list. Second, it created a hierarchy of categories and subcategories of pain, which Avicenna had failed to do, that was also useful for diagnostic purposes. A coherent hierarchy of perception, attributing a descending scale of importance to different sensations, was the most useful tool practitioners could have.

Finally, in a conceptual world that saw four as the constitutive number of seasons, compass points, elements, and corporeal humors,[34] a fourfold division of pains made sense. Though after Constantine and Maurus the attempt to equate specific pains with corresponding humors was rare, such a division linked sensations, pain especially, with the entire framework of the body and the universe. It broke down neatly into two dichotomies: just as there was dryness and humidity, north and south, so the categories of pain were acute as opposed to extensive and inflative as opposed to gravative. In *consilia* one can see how this division worked in descriptions of pain. The description used was often *gravativus et extensivus* or *pungitivus et mordicativus*.[35] It could also consist of only a single descriptor, but never both gravative and inflative, for they were opposites within the same category, and such a description was an oxymoron. Thus, Avicenna's cumbersome list had shrunk to two main categories, one denoting the localization of pain and the other its nature. Each category comprised the two opposite manifestations, localized or diffuse, swelling or concentrating. This was a systematic hierarchy, which made sense of pain while mirroring other universal and anatomical schemes.

It is impossible to generalize from so few writers to the entire corpus of medical literature. Mondeville and Chauliac, the two main surgeon writers, were exceptions to the usual run of surgeons rather than the rule. Besides, surgeons who wrote manuals with theoretical digressions on pain were one step away from trespassing into the medical field.[36]

All of this vocabulary, however, was in Latin, while the contacts between physicians and patients were conducted in vernacular languages. Was there a parallel vocabulary for daily clinical use? A glance at the Middle English work of surgeon John Arderne (fl. 1370) shows a total lack of any kind of pain vocabulary. All he uses is synonyms: *ake, anguysch,* and *suffre*.[37] Since Middle English is hardly devoid of pain descriptors, both Latinate and Anglo-Saxon, one can only attribute this sparse language to Arderne himself. Indeed, the vernacular translations of Henri de Mondeville rendered his neutral "corrosion" of cancer in far more imaginative language: "The torment of a gnawing tumor was underscored in the vernacular translations, which preferred 'ronger,' 'fretting,' or 'fressen' over the Latinate 'corrosion.'"[38]

Chiara Crisciani, researching the work of Michele Savonarola (1385–1462), has shown that vernacular Italian versions of medical and surgical texts could be far richer in metaphors and imaginative language of pain than the tradition-bound Latin ones.[39] Instead of writing a standard treatise on gout, Savonarola used an anthropomorphic ploy, a dialogue between gout and medicine. Gout (Madonna Gotta), daughter of Messer Lamentable (Rincrescieuile) and sister of Spider (Ragnolo) and Rat (Topo), is a magnificent queen and ruler. She has come a long way from her humble beginnings. Being a daughter, she says, she inherited from her father only the countryside but found the peasants much too active and healthy for developing gout. Her brothers had fared no better: the spider found his webs in wealthy houses swept twice a day, and the rat could not reach the food for fear of cats and traps.[40] When the three met again, bewailing their various fates, Gout suggested they change places, so that she got all the sedentary people, "the great masters, popes, cardinals, lords, knights, gentlemen, etc." The dialogue develops, Medicine giving learned speeches about the reasons for gout and pain, with declarations concerning the nature and types of pain, quoting all the standard wisdom on the subject.[41] Not to be outdone, Gout has a band of soldiers under her command, and Medicine has an army too and intends to fight her. Gout considers herself a ruler, has a court and ambassadors who warn the noblemen of her imminent arrival, a lady-in-waiting, fever, and faithful chamberlains—the seven types of pain. The lords who suffer from gout can tell them apart, for each type of pain wears its lady's livery. Her magnificent captain is coitus, and his squad commanders are all the things that cause gout—bad air, too much food or drink, sleep in the middle of the day. Her words are law and she enacts statutes. Those who transgress her prohibitions are punished with pain. She discusses at length, for the benefit of her *brigata*, the lifestyle necessary to ease the pains of illness, so that her army would know whom not to attack.

Savonarola knew his Galenic and Avicennian definitions but chose another set of seven pains: *extendente, comprimente, frangente, stupido, pulsante, fatigante, mordicante*.[42] They appear in various types of gout, all according to the humoral complexion of the patient: the sanguine will suffer extending pain, and the choleric will suffer acute or mordicative pain. Since the author was dealing with a specific illness, he could concentrate upon each type of pain with a detailed description, but the most one can say about this list is that none of the terms was new. They were all part of a fairly flexible vocabulary based on four general types but often including several others. There is no clear-cut methodological taxonomy, but the repetition of certain terms does indicate that they were inculcated as technical, professional terms rather than lay descriptors, such as "vehement" or "strong" pain. Furthermore, the general need to list types of pain, despite Galen's furious objections, does indicate that the idea of pain description was indeed prevalent.

Savonarola wrote his entire tractate as a parody of court life (it is dedicated to Savonarola's patron Niccolo d'Este, marquis of Ferrara). It is also a *consilium* for the marquis, who suffered from gout. Not surprisingly, it contains far more metaphoric language than any impersonal text. The lack of an obligatory linguistic tradition, then, could work both ways; to an imagi-

native, articulate, and expressive writer like Savonarola, it could be an inspiration to enliven his writing beyond what the learned tradition allowed.
But to an inarticulate surgeon like Arderne the freedom from traditional descriptors meant doing without any at all. Pain was pain. One could employ
the occasional synonym but nothing else.

Two texts in two different languages are not enough to build theories of
vernacular expression.[43] I might argue, though, that for descriptors to be of
any use they needed to be backed by a tradition to infuse them with significance. A medical writer might have felt impelled to add many inventive descriptions of pain to his work, but unless his writing was based upon a long,
widely understood tradition of descriptors, his work would be as useless in
the later Middle Ages as that of Archigenes was in the second century.

The entire question of pain description and descriptors had arisen
largely because different types of pain presumably indicated different diseases. Most of the academic writing on pain was concerned not so much
with the alleviation of pain, which belonged more commonly to recipe collections, but with the analysis and understanding of pain as a sign of specific
illnesses. Naturally, this meant categorizing not only the locality of pain
(not always so obviously simple) but also the type of pain. Galen, in his fury
at Archigenes, had thrown out the baby with the bathwater, giving as diagnostic examples only those cases in which he could reduce the statements
of his antagonist to absurdity. Thus, throbbing, which Archigenes had seen
as the constant symptom of an aposteme, was no such thing, for the pulse
throbbed continuously also in health. Contrary to Archigenes, the feeling of
having a nail hammered into one is never sensed in the liver; and liver pain
is not furious but heavy.[44] Inadvertently, Galen thus did assign some meanings to pain. In addition, he (and Arnau in his wake) noted that sometimes
pain was more of a precursor than a symptom, disappearing once the real
illness had arrived. Quoting the Hippocratic prognoses, he described certain
types of fever that began with a headache, dancing spots before the eyes, and
stomachaches—all before the real illness was made manifest.[45]

In his long list of pains Avicenna tried to assign causes: "the cause of
extensivus pain is either *ventositas* or a humor that stretches a nerve or a
muscle as far as possible . . . and the cause of shattering [*frangitivus*] pain
is either matter or *ventositas* between the bone and enveloping tissue or a
cold that strongly constricts the membrane." An itching pain was caused by
a pungent, sharp, and salty humor; a stabbing pain came from a humor that
stretched tissues sideways; and so on.[46] Such explanations were not very
helpful. While the general discussion of pain took place in the first book
of the *Canon*, Avicenna relegated the precise types of pain relevant to each

disease to book 3, which deals with illnesses organ by organ, from head to foot. The specific pain appears, where appropriate, among the signs for each illness. For a practitioner looking for a diagnosis, it meant that first one had to have at least a tentative diagnosis in order to verify the signs. Given that pain was only one of the categories of symptoms, this is understandable, albeit again not very helpful.

Maurus of Salerno gave far more concrete indications than Avicenna. When dealing with an aposteme, a clear problem of humoral imbalance, the physician had to verify whether the pain was *infixivus, pungitivus, aggravativus,* or *extensivus.* In the first case, the swelling was expected to burst before the twentieth day; if the pain was *extensivus,* on the twentieth; if *pungitivus,* on the fortieth; and if *aggravativus,* on the sixtieth. The different prognoses were derived from the specific humoral character of each aposteme and each pain: a phlegmatic aposteme was signaled by extensive pain, a choleric one by stabbing pain, and so forth. Thus, the type of pain provided the physician with both a diagnosis and a prognosis. An aposteme in the throat might cause a swelling of the uvula, in which case pain and color will give the answer: if the pain was *infixivus* and the uvula was red and, blood was the guilty humor; if the pain was stretching (*extensivus*) and the uvula whitish, it was phlegm; and so on. In cases of acute fevers, said Maurus, the pain's location would also provide a diagnosis. The time of the pain's onset in tertian fevers predicted the course of the illness. Headache sometimes appeared on the first day; then one must expect it to worsen on the fourth and fifth days, and the healing crisis will come on the seventh. The later the headache appeared, the more stubborn the disease, and the more indigestible the corrupt matter that caused it. If the headache appeared only on the fifth day, the crisis was to be expected only in another nine days.[47] In later centuries, the same principle appeared in more detail in the work of Bernard de Gordon:

> if one feels a crushing, aggravating [sensation], as though one was pierced with needles or stung with nettles, or feels a stabbing [*pungitivus*], itchy [*pruritivus*], or boring [*perforativus*] movement between the skin and the flesh, it indicates that the humors dominating in the body are choleric, hot, sharp, or salty and, when melted in steam, go to the sensitive members and induce acute pain. If, though, one feels a stretching [*extensio*] in a member, and it is rigid and tense as a bowstring, then they [i.e., the humors] are melancholic or windy [*ventosi*], and nature cannot dominate them. If indeed the pain endures, it is caused by humors. If it is *deambulativus,* it is windy. If heavy [*gravativus*], as when one feels a

great weight so that one dares not move, it is a sign of many evil humors. The first pain means evil humors; the second [means] many; the third both. The fourth type of pain may be called inflammative pain, for a man feels as though a flame was passing across his shoulders, as happens to those sensitive to putrid fevers, especially in the blood, and for such a pain—heavy, crushing [*confractivus*], and inflammative—one must immediately perform a phlebotomy.[48]

Despite Bernard's earlier thoroughgoing condemnation of Avicenna's categories, one can hear those categories and their causes reverberating in his work.

Pain, for both Maurus of Salerno and Bernard de Gordon, was a harbinger of disease. One could forestall a fever by deciphering the type of pain and taking preventive action. All physicians agreed with the principle that a physician ought to be able to decode pain. Even Arnau de Villanova, devotedly commenting upon Galen, asserted in his own voice that, if one wished to effect a cure, one had to identify the illness, and pain was an effective indicator. When it came to the inner organs, which one could neither see nor touch, it was necessary to judge by the effects of the illness—either by discharges (such as urine) or by the exterior quality of the body (in the case of tumors) or by the different types of pain.[49] Unfortunately, as Arnau was writing a commentary, he never did fulfill his promise to give a table of meanings for types of pain.

In practical medicine, case descriptions normally place pain in a long list of symptoms that, taken together, indicate a diagnosis. Bartolomeo Montagnana described in each *consilium* a multiplicity of symptoms and diseases, which strongly suggests that these cases were putative. One famous lady suffered, in addition to migraine and other headaches, pains in the muscles and tissues of the face, a decline of sight and hearing (the latter accompanied by tinnitus), damage to her interior senses, drowsiness, and difficulties in moving her arms and hands. The entire list of symptoms stemmed from "mala complexio frigida et humida substantie cerebri" (an evil, cold and humid complexion of the brain matter).[50] When Arnau de Villanova was presented with a knight who had fallen off his horse, he pounced on him joyously. Everything possible was wrong with this man. To begin with, he was badly formed: his neck was too long, his shoulders were bent, his chest was hairy, and his muscles were weak. There had been several other problems before his accident, most of them having to do with heavy drinking and late hours. When he got a cold, he started spitting blood, suffered pains in the neck, shoulders, chest, spleen, and other (unspecified) organs, on both sides of the body, especially in his left nipple, and had difficulty breathing. He also suffered from hemorrhoids, and then the fall injured his back.[51] It is not clear at which stage Arnau had been called in (if indeed the case was real), but obviously his main concern was not the fall, but the man's life-style, which called for a drastic change and purgation. Thus, the pains in his chest and the injuries to his back were of secondary importance. The back injuries were apparently no worse than contusions, and the doctor prescribed only anodynes (soothing medication) rather than anesthetics. The gist of Arnau's instructions was a healthy regimen of life.

The general impression resulting from these diagnoses is that pain was important but hardly ranked first among symptoms. Whatever vocabulary physicians chose to use, they could not be sure the *vulgus* (as Arnau called them)[52] understood them or used the same words. This was especially true for a Latin vocabulary meant to be a basis for vernacular communication between doctor and patient. The very tradition that allowed a vocabulary of pain put the same vocabulary beyond the reach of many patients.

We cannot therefore estimate the real usefulness of the medical vocabu-lary of pain for interpretation. What can indeed be deduced from it is that the issue both interested and challenged physicians, and that they attrib-uted sufficient importance to pain typology to create not only descriptors but also theoretical categories of pain. The same cannot be said of jurists.

Legal Usage

The evolution of the judicial vocabulary of pain infliction differed from that of medicine. The medical-vocabulary tradition began in Greek and ab-sorbed Arabic influences during the Latinate Middle Ages, but judicial writ-ing began and remained for the most part in Latin. Treatises of customary law, written in vernacular languages, had no influence upon the tradition of learned and practical *ius commune*, or the practical application of the learned evolution of Roman law. When jurists began glossing and teaching Roman law, they based themselves strictly upon the *Corpus iuris civilis* of Justinian and, to the best of their abilities, tried to remain within its vocabulary. When new terms became necessary, jurists looked back to late antique Christian sources to find them. Thus, the problem of a vague, in-definite vocabulary did not exist for jurists. They relied upon a universally acknowledged set of terms, all of them carrying a legitimate long history.

Unlike physicians, jurists quite systematically avoided words that de-scribed how pain felt. Given that the declared aim of torture was to extort a confession, pain was measured not by its character but by degree of severity. Judges and jurists accepted the medical opinion that severe pain could damage and kill people, but their main problem was not how to alleviate pain but how to cause the exact degree necessary for producing a confession without causing "excessive" damage. Certainly, a dead unconfessed suspect was the judge's greatest nightmare, for the judge might then be tried for homicide.[53] How does one speak of pain infliction almost without using words for pain? Jurists—both ancient and medieval—used the resultant actions instead of descriptors of pain. The suspect displayed fortitude or obstinacy (duritia), confessed, remained constant, persevered in his confession, and so forth. On very rare occasions, pain perforce did creep from the dungeon into the text.

The most common noun for torture in the *Digest* is *quaestio*. So common is the usage throughout the sections dealing with torture that one cannot speak even of circumlocution or euphemisms. Clearly, *quaestio* did not mean posing polite questions. Nevertheless, when speaking of the act of torturing, the classical text is usually even less covert, speaking clearly of *torquere* or *tormentum*. One peculiarity of classical torture was the occasional insistence that it affected both mind (or soul) and body, and the power to withstand it came from both physical endurance and the human will. Given that most of the texts dealing with torture refer to slaves, this insistence is remarkable. Thus, *tormentum* was endowed with the spurious etymology of *torquere mentem* (torture, or twist, the mind), and several variants spoke of *cordis dolor* (pain of the heart) rather than *corporis dolor* (pain of the body); similarly, a suspect who resisted torture was said to have steeled both his body and his spirit.[54]

Roman jurists were aware of the effects of torture—hence the provision that youths under fourteen were exempt and hence the insistence that the suspect not be killed: "so that the slave will be whole, either to [achieve] innocence or to face the death sentence."[55] Hence, too, the advice of Paulus (which Accursius [ca. 1182–1263] tracks back to Gaius) that, if several people are to be tortured in one case, one ought to begin with the youngest or the most easily frightened.[56] In a very rare example, a jurist was willing to admit to the harshness of torture (*asperitatem questionis*) when speaking of the exception granted to minors.[57] This is a meager harvest of indirect admissions to the horror of torture. The greatest part of the argument about torture in the *Digest* revolves around the question of slave ownership: presumably, a tortured slave was as good as dead, and the jurists debated the range of cases in which other masters' slaves might be tortured.

The earliest glosses, compiled by Accursius in the *Ordinary Gloss*, added nothing to the vocabulary of torture. Late medieval torture literature,

beginning with the *Tractatus de tormentis* and Albertus Gandinus, did add
the vocabulary of Roman-canonical procedure, and this vocabulary was of
remarkably interesting extraction. Medieval jurists, following their Roman predecessors, avoided speaking of pain. All the same, they were not
torturing slaves but free people, and killing a suspect had become a paramount danger. Apparently, the problem was greater in those areas that had
recourse to the strappado as standard procedure. In northern France, where
the standard torture of criminal suspects was stretching and pouring water
into their mouths, the danger was far less.[58] While many broke down and
confessed, they were not permanently crippled by the procedure. In Italy,
where the strappado was standard and judges were most commonly urban,
not royal, employees, the danger was graver.[59]

Many medieval jurists avoided the term *quaestio,* using *tortura* instead.
This was probably the result of the growth in Europe of inquisitorial procedures, which might or might not use torture to gain information. But
like their Roman predecessors, late medieval jurists insisted that torture
affected the mind as well as the body. In fact, Paulus Grillandus went even
farther when adapting torture to the questioning of heretics and witches:
"Broadly put, it is possible to say, improperly, that the term 'torture,' as
some describe it, is taken from causing fear [*a terrendo*] . . . or you can say
that, even if the body is not really tortured, nevertheless the spirit [*animus*] is well and truly tortured, and the suspect suffers from fear; thus, one
can define torture loosely."[60] Nevertheless, there was a clear distinction
between courage and physical survival. In torture tractates the technical
term for the ability to survive torture was *fortitudo.* In the later Middle
Ages *patientia* became associated with Christ and could thus not be used
in legal texts. While the ancient meaning of "fortitude" almost invariably
referred to strength of mind rather than body, between the second and the
thirteenth century its semantic field had shifted. Beginning with martyrdom
narratives, fortitude became the virtue of martyrs. It had little or nothing to
do with physical strength or endurance. Thus, Jerome juxtaposes fortitude
with temerity—the one a virtue, the other an excess. Ambrose instanced
St. Lawrence when treating fortitude, which he defined as justly protecting
the homeland from barbarians.[61] Augustine was perhaps the first to stress
St. Vincent's fortitude as his central characteristic, but he was followed by
practically all later hagiographers and sermon writers.[62] The ability to tolerate torture without flinching became identified as fortitude.

By the twelfth century, fortitude was one of the four, and then seven,
virtues. William of Saint-Thierry put it together with prudence, temper-
ance, and justice.[63] Thomas Aquinas listed it as a cardinal virtue, following

up immediately with a section about martyrdom as fortitude's principal act.[64] Throughout history, fortitude was mainly perceived as a virtue of the soul, not a physical talent. The only exception is the late medieval and early modern shift in meaning that comes through torture tractates. In this literature fortitude meant the physical hardihood required merely to survive torture, without any reference to either resistance or confession. Thus, pregnant women and those who had given birth during the previous forty days were exempt from torture because they lacked the fortitude to withstand it.[65] A failure of fortitude did denoted, not fear or wavering, but the suspect's death.

The problem of fortitude in the face of torture came up specifically in the description of the five degrees of torture.[66] Paulus Grillandus, who established the scale of harshness, repeated the need to adjust torture to each suspect's fortitude. Unlike his colleagues, however, he made it clear that what defined degrees of torture was the pain felt by the questioned suspect and her ability to survive it.

The adoption of the term "fortitude" for a legal problem was part of a bigger phenomenon. Many of the terms used in torture proceedings to denote the suspect's actions derived from the same martyrological source, with a similar twist. Thus, martyrdom narratives spoke repeatedly of saints publicly persevering in their refusal to sacrifice to pagan gods. In late medieval legal parlance, however, perseverance meant something else. Since confessions were extracted in the darkness of the semijudicial, indeterminate space of the dungeon, they were invalid unless repeated in open court. Perseverance was the act of publicly repeating the confession. It was no longer a virtue, merely a judicial necessity. As noted before, there was serious doubt as to the validity of a freely offered, self-incriminating confession. Though a freely offered confession was not supposed to incriminate the speaker, it was customary in Italy to incarcerate those who made one.[67] Spontaneous confessions lacked not only the secret interrogation and pain but perseverance. Even in standard cases, most jurists insisted that confessions be repeated in court time and again and not just once. Perseverance became the hallmark of validity, not of truth.[68]

Perseverance was closely tied with the concept of constancy, for perseverance was the act of a constant man. Unlike perseverance, however, constancy had a long, purely judicial history, parallel to that of its martyrological twin. All martyrs, male and female, were endowed with a constancy that allowed them to continue unswerving in their statements before their accusers. But constancy, and the man constant in the face of threats, had appeared already in Roman law.

Why did jurists borrow so much from martyrologies? To modern eyes, it might seem as though medieval jurists were trying to whitewash a very controversial subject by using sacred narratives. Judicial torture, however, was not controversial until the eighteenth century and needed no sacred whitewashing. Nowhere in the literature do jurists actually compare their suspects to the martyrs. The answer is much simpler. Undoubtedly, to anybody untrained in medicine, the torture narratives of the martyrs provided the best and most detailed vocabulary. Although much of it did not fit with Roman-canonical rules of procedure, subtle adaptation could solve the problem.

In sum, the judicial vocabulary is notable for hardly mentioning pain at all. It does speak of degrees and results of pain, but it avoids the thing itself. To fully appreciate this silence, one must remember that pain was not merely an unfortunate but an inevitable corollary of torture and confession. It was the very fear and pain of torture that produced confessions. Had there been no pain, torture would have been useless. Pain thus stood at the center of the practice of interrogatory torture, and yet jurists were extremely careful not to speak of it.

Conclusion

"Language is neither a transparent medium for an accurate representation of a reality nor does it derive its meaning from some purified extralinguistic object or subject."[69] Thus does Joseph Ziegler begin his analysis of the language that Arnau de Villanova employed in his writings, which spanned medicine and religion. Words carry an entire semantic field, often trailing older meanings and associations when they are employed in a new field. In this chapter I have attempted to examine two opposing cases of pain description: physicians, who were heirs to a rich multilingual tradition and who sought to describe pain in the most accurate way, and jurists, who were heirs to a thin, monolingual, and single-source tradition and who were forced to borrow words from another field altogether. The two disciplines stand at opposite ends, one with a confusing wealth of terms and the other with almost none at all.

The heritage of each discipline was suited to its needs. Medicine required detailed description of pain, while law needed words that would draw a veil of ambiguity over the pain of torture. It is thus clear why physicians went about the task of pruning an overluxurious vocabulary to a set of useful, clearly defined terms, while jurists expanded classical legal vocabulary as minimally as possible to suit the new procedural laws. Jurists did need terms, but they needed those clear-cut terms to be euphemistic.

Given the divergent interests of the two professions, their foci on pain are materially distinct. Physicians were mostly concerned about types and locations of pain, jurists about intensity. True, physicians, too, occasionally wrote of a very strong pain, especially when dealing with alleviation, but they did not attempt to create a scale measuring its gravity. In contrast, jurists—who ordered the pain administered—not only knew precisely where each torture would hurt but also had to be careful about its intensity. Calibrating pain as a tool of truth-finding, they had to define precisely how much pain would elicit truth and at which point it would cause either death or a lie.

Both disciplines, however, were acutely aware of the individual character of pain tolerance and of the relative uselessness of words in assessing pain in different people. Jurists, focused more upon intensity than typology, were the ones to stress this individuality more emphatically, but physicians were also aware of the difference in the pain tolerance between men and women, young and old, healthy and sick. Their comments come up in the same context as that of jurists, when dealing with weakening or painful procedures. How old did a patient have to be before one could safely administer a phlebotomy? Healers, however, did not resort to the martyrological vocabulary adopted by jurists.

The usual assumption of research is that vocabularies can percolate from one discourse to another. As Joseph Ziegler and Peter Biller have noted, physicians often resorted to religious terminology, and vice versa.[70] Nevertheless, here we have two scholastic discourses that shared many formal characteristics (such as the genre of *consilia*) but went in totally different directions when it came to the vocabulary of pain. The reasons for this divergence are several. In the first place, pain discourse was not a dominant strain in either discipline and may not have been familiar outside professional boundaries.[71] Second, medieval medicine was heir to a polyglot tradition that enriched language, while law was purely Latin and Roman. But most importantly, the functional identity of each pain cognizance was completely different in law and medicine. Medical typologies would have been of no use to jurists, and vice versa. Consequently, each built its own vocabulary. Pain is elusive and needed different vocabularies for different purposes.

CHAPTER SIX

The Christian History of Humanity

Physicians and jurists treated human pain as describable and measurable. Theologians viewed it as a historical force accompanying humanity from the Fall to the Last Judgment. The question was not how much or what sort of pain, but when and why it attached itself to humans. Pain was thus viewed in theology as a historical force that shaped human destiny in salvation and damnation.

Theology had accompanied Christianity from its earliest centuries.[1] The number of patristic writings produced and preserved since the second century is vast, and many of them concern pain. From Tertullian, who spoke about martyrs, to Augustine, who spoke about souls, to Gregory the Great, who recorded visions of hell, the subject was ubiquitous. Nevertheless, before the thirteenth century it is hard to find a single coherent theory of human pain emerging from all this writing. Given the geographic, chronological, and mental distances separating different thinkers, variety and multivocality are to be expected. Statements were made in different circumstances and in different countries and were formulated against different heresies. But by the twelfth century, agglomerations of scholars were coalescing outside monastic communities in universities, and these scholars conducted constant, lively, and often-acerbic exchanges on all possible topics. More importantly, their discussions and theories were not formed under the pressure of immediate events. Heresies existed in the twelfth and thirteenth centuries, but they were a matter for armies and inquisitors to deal with. Scholastics often had the luxury of thinking issues through in an independent manner, with the result that their answers are far more sophisticated than those of their predecessors.

In any religion that keeps God and humans strictly apart, as Judaism and Islam do, the nature of the human body and human sensations need not necessarily be a subject of intense theological speculation. But in Christianity, the basic idea of God-made humans forced theologians to think very carefully about all aspects of humanity: nature, the relationship between body and soul, the differences between Christ's body and soul and those of the rest of humanity. Consequently, Christian theology, both scholastic and vernacular, made a thorough study of humans and their sensations. How and where on a scale running from the lowest living creatures all the way to divinity one was to place angels, martyrs, humans, and especially Christ was a central theological issue for medieval Christianity. Thus, pain became a subject of importance in the narrated history of humankind.

In the process of dissecting, analyzing, and contextualizing pain, it was sometimes necessary to transpose the phenomenon from the divine, the miraculous, and the eschatological to the simple human plane. It is only by reference to the known and the natural that one can perceive and understand the unknown and the miraculous. Theologians were thus forced to formulate theories of human pain, constructing an entire mental edifice of the human body and soul. In trying to understand Christ, they first and foremost had to define humans, or rather man, for woman was usually seen as a derivate of man. But which man? As all readers of Paul and Augustine knew, the nature of man had changed materially after the Fall. Prelapsarian Adam was far less vulnerable to pain than his own postlapsarian self and his descendants. And yet, pain had existed even before Adam's creation; the rebellious fallen angels were immediately afflicted with eternal torment from the moment of their arrival in hell. Subsequently, God created man and harvested his body for the making of a woman. Did the extraction of the rib hurt? Or would it have hurt had God not put Adam to sleep first?

The answers were chronologically structured according to the human journey from creation to resurrection, from birth to death and afterlife. Each stage bears different distinguishing traits. In fact, one can chart human destiny according to the stages of human reactions to pain. The first significant change after creation was the Fall. Both Adam and Eve had sinned, thus bringing about an irreparable breach in their bodily defenses against sin, illness, pain, and death. Prelapsarian and postlapsarian Adam were therefore two different genera of humanity, and Adam's descendants definitely inherited the traits of the second genus. Next, one followed in the footsteps of Adam's descendants throughout their own individual journeys in life. Scholars pondered why and how people suffered, what they must learn from their pain, and how to benefit from it or—very occasionally—avoid it. These questions properly belong more in didactic literature than in scholastic discourse, but they are relevant here too, since they are intimately tied to the continuation of the journey after death. Who will suffer what pains, whether in purgatory or in hell, for how long, why, and how are all questions that form an important part of scholastic discourse. The human journey, however, does not end until time stands still. Resurrection was perceived as the revival of the body and the sensations. What would postresurrection bodies feel? Would pain still be part of their destiny, or would they revert to the state of prelapsarian impassibility?[2] The history of sensations shifted and changed with the destiny of humanity, mirroring in miniature the entire cosmic history of humankind.

In this chapter I will therefore follow the scholastic method of dealing with pain: first, the general principles, then the careful subdivision that corresponds to the ecclesiastical history of humanity, from creation and fall to redemption, followed by the fate of humanity throughout history. As I will try to show, thirteenth- and fourteenth-century scholastics did create a fairly coherent and well-argued opinion about their cosmic questions, and their opinion pointed flatly in one direction: humanity was irreversibly passible.

Woven together with scholastic discourse, pastoral literature and vernacular theology were also infused with pain. Preachers and confessors traced the same journey as scholastics, beginning with creation and ending with the resurrection. The closeness of the two disciplines is especially important from the thirteenth century onward, when mendicants, both Dominicans and Franciscans, populated academic chairs and pulpits alike, preaching their narrative to the masses. Nevertheless, the same ideas took distinctly different forms when posed as scholastic questions or sermons to the laity. In the following, I will attempt to juxtapose the two forms of pain analysis and description as much as possible. In this chapter I will address the pain of humans as a whole, while in chapter 7 I will place Christ and his pain within the framework of suffering humanity.

Scholastic History

The creation of humanity posited the appearance in God's world of sentient and conscious beings. Though the Fall changed many physical and spiritual characteristics, it did not affect human senses. Adam and Eve's sensitivities in paradise were, agreed most scholars, no different from those of their sin-laden descendants. It was clear to medieval thinkers in the Aristotelian tradition that human beings were by their very nature sensitive to external impressions.[3] The senses were part and parcel of humanity, and remained so after the Fall.[4]

This tradition was based upon late antique patristic writing:

The nature of our bodies is such, that when endowed with life and feeling by conjunction with a sentient soul, they become something more than inert, insensate matter. They feel when touched, suffer when pricked, shiver with cold, feel pleasure in warmth, waste with hunger, and grow fat with food. By a certain transfusion of the soul, which supports and penetrates them, they feel pleasure or pain according to the surrounding circumstances. When the body is pricked or pierced, it is the soul which pervades it that is conscious, and suffers pain.[5]

These words were written in the fourth century, in the midst of the Arian controversy. Hilary of Poitiers (ca. 315–ca. 367) was a bitter and persistent opponent of Arianism. Consequently, in his book on the Trinity he did his best to distance the figure of Christ as much as possible from humanity. If Arians were attempting to humanize Christ, insisting that he was not of the same nature as God the father, Hilary was going to pull orthodoxy in the opposite direction. To illustrate the basic difference between man and Christ, he described the process by which pain affects humans: their bodies are in conjunction with their souls, and when the body is touched, the soul senses it. Human bodies, therefore, suffer through the agency of "a certain transfusion of the soul." Human suffering, in sum, was somatic, the soul simply being a sensory agent. Naturally, such an explanation put Christ in a completely different category of sufferers from the rest of humanity.

A few decades later, in another part of the Roman Empire, Augustine of Hippo was facing different controversies. In fighting what he considered heresies, he reversed some of Hilary's insights. It was no longer bodies that suffered through the agency of the soul, but souls that suffered through the agency of the body.[6] Augustine's argument was mostly concerned with the fate of souls after death, but within this argument, he revived the old Aristotelian claim that sensations formed part of the soul, and pain belonged to the sense of touch. The generations of scholars who followed were very much aware of the two thinkers' writings, common opinion leaning on the whole toward Augustine's position. Sensations, pain among them, formed part of the human soul. The balance tipped more sharply than ever in the Augustinian direction with the rise of Monophysite ideas in the fifth and sixth centuries. The Monophysites, who seceded from the Catholic Church after the Council of Chalcedon (451) asserted that there was but one nature in Christ, and that nature divine and pain free. If the latest heresy claimed that Christ was all God, it was the duty of orthodoxy to reaffirm the human suffering of Christ, and therefore humanity must suffer through its soul.

Little of what was written after Augustine in the West interested late
medieval scholastics. The writings of Pope Gregory the Great on the fate
of souls in hell are an exception, but even those did not address the basic
issues argued in scholastic circles. The one formative influence came from
the East, carrying bits of Greek philosophy in its wake. John of Damascus
(675–749) had been a well-known scholar and monk, a pillar of orthodoxy,
the terror of Monophysites and iconoclasts in eighth-century Damascus.
His *De fide orthodoxa*, translated from Greek into Arabic, Church Slavonic,
and Georgian, was disseminated in the East as the standard theological
summa.[7] Like his intellectual forebears, John wrote within the context of
theological controversy and the need to define orthodoxy. Like the writings of other Eastern church fathers, his work was destined to influence
Western thinking long after the original controversy had become forgotten
and irrelevant in the West. Though he neither cited nor named Aristotle,
John probably knew that he was repeating pagan philosophy in a Christian
guise. His twelfth-century Western readers, however, saw John's work as
pure orthodoxy, not a controversial philosophical question (and Aristotle
was still controversial in the twelfth century). Thus, the embattled, contentious Eastern monk's words were turned in the West from questionable
theories to incontestable facts. His writings had the same status as patristic
authorities or biblical glosses. As much as creation or the existence of four
humors within the body, John's words were a basis one could build upon
without fear of controversy, heterodoxy, or question.

John's view of the human species is a case in point. The narrative follows
the book of Genesis faithfully up to a point. Creation, paradise, and the
tree of life are all there. Man, however (*homo*, not Adam), departs from this
model. He is both prelapsarian Adam and humanity in its general, unchang-
ing aspect, a microcosm of the universe and a body-soul continuum.[8] In this
classical mode, man was made of the four humors, corresponding to the
four elements of the universe, while the soul was a spectrum ranging from
the most rational qualities, governed by nature, to irrational/emotional faculties which might be controlled by the will: the passions of sensing joy,
sadness, fear, anger. The senses, too, were faculties of the soul, but the same
soul also contained the rational faculties: thought, memory, imagination,
and speech.[9]

The Latin version of *De fide orthodoxa* made hardly any mention of
pain. Burgundio of Pisa, the translator, used the term *dolor* explicitly only
when dealing with the double meaning of "passion," which could be "corporeal, as in sickness and wounds," or the incorporeal, soul-centered (*animalis*) sense of emotion. But even when contemplating sensory pain, John

carefully distinguished passion from sensation: "therefore, passion is not pain, but the sensation of pain."[10] Pain as sensation had very little room in John's classical man.

Though scholastics shared a universe of ideas and a common theological heritage, occasionally borrowing each other's arguments without so much as an acknowledgment, their theories on such a wide subject as pain inevitably spanned a wide range of differing opinions. Some things were basic: such as the canonical ruling that Christ had a human, as well as a divine, nature and had truly suffered at the Crucifixion. Augustine's view, that pain was sensed in the soul and not in the body, was also widely accepted. Beyond that there was no one single tradition. Instead, the various threads mesh into a tapestry of divergent, sometimes-contrasting ideas.

Pain emerges from most discussions as a negative deviation from the natural state. Following an Augustinian tradition,[11] the term *dissensio* and the basic reluctance to suffer recur time and again.[12] Pain is a force, a corrupting process working *against* the natural, *against* our will. Unwillingness—negation in general and negation of the human will in particular—is its very essence. Thirteenth- and fourteenth-century scholars argued about the precise type of internal comprehension necessary for sensing pain without ever considering that external forces could be the cause. To the contrary, it was the self's reaction to those forces that caused pain. Underlying this argument was the assumption that pain was apprehended in the soul and therefore was born there. The idea that it might be an external physical force, acting upon a physical organism, never even arose.[13] Alexander of Hales (ca. 1185–1245) defined pain in bodily terms, claiming to cite Aristotle, "pain is the [dis]solution of continuity," or, in modern terms, a breach in the wholeness of the body.[14] This definition, presumably born in the realm of philosophy, was taken in the thirteenth century from the world of medicine and transposed into the scholastic world, which saw pain as unrelated to the purely bodily realm. But even Alexander went on to embed pain within the world of feeling, perception, and knowledge. In other words, he returned it to the soul. His contemporary William of Auvergne agreed with him. He, too, insisted upon the ensoulment of pain, disproving the pseudo-Aristotelian tradition by a simple distortion. He claimed that Aristotle had defined pain as "solution of quantity," evidently a corruption of "continuity." Demolishing a nonsense statement was an easy job, and William could triumphantly reiterate that the soul pervaded all sensitive organs of the body, and all sensation resided in the soul.[15]

The intuitive rejection of pain existed side by side with theological views valorizing pain. The purifying forces of purgatorial (and purgative) pain, the punitive power of hellfire, the sanctifying effects of martyrdom, and, above all, Christ's Passion and the resultant salvation of humanity—all these were part of the scholastic perception of pain. Human beings might seek to avoid pain, but given human tendencies toward sin, that did not make pain any less salutary. Pain was adjudged odious, not evil. Sometimes it was salutary, sometimes destructive, but it was always inevitable for passible humanity.

This tradition made it impossible for theologians to ignore somatic medical perceptions of the human body. These perceptions referred to the body as related to the soul, not to the soul alone. While the traditional view argued for a simple, unified soul, by the thirteenth century those who followed the newly discovered Greek learning saw the soul as a hierarchy of different interacting parts, culminating with the rational soul.[16] Though there is some ambiguity on this point, most authors agreed that all parts of the soul might not immediately react to passions, but they all shared in sensing pain. Some identified the sensual soul with the lower reason as the part vulnerable to sensation.[17] Others saw the *ratio inferior* as a middle stage between the sensual soul and superior reason, which was the cognitive capacity.[18] While all parts of the soul shared in pain, the cognitive powers received the idea, rather than the sensation, of pain.[19]

This perception dictated the control of mind over body. Thomas Aquinas noted that fear could make people blush or pale, and shame also caused blushing. This was due to the activities of the humors around the heart, the center of life.[20] For Walter Chatton (ca. 1290–1343), delving into Christ's feelings before the Crucifixion, a vivid imagination could cause even more than fear of approaching pain: it could cause the humors to move around the heart in such a way as to provoke not only fear but even fever.[21] By the mid–fourteenth century, pain was credited with a purely metaphysical ancestry. It was born of cognition, memory, imagination—anything but stones and blows.

By the time Aristotelian and medical ideas had been incorporated into the Western fields of knowledge, another independent tradition had come into being. The Parisian master and bishop Peter Lombard (ca. 1100–ca. 1160/64) wrote and published his *Sentences* around the middle of the twelfth century, and the text became central to all subsequent theology. When discussing pain, almost all subsequent scholastics referred to Peter Lombard's discussion of Christ's nature in book 3 of his work. Since almost every self-respecting, university-based scholar had at some time during his career taught the *Sentences* and written a commentary (or even simply a gloss) on it, the commentary tradition referring to Christ's nature and passibility is exceedingly rich.[22] Much of the contents, however, were relevant to humanity in general. Given that Christ partook of the sensibility to pain common to all humans, one had to expatiate upon pain sensibility in general. The definitions of pain were all presented within this framework.

In addition to those commentaries, most scholastics devoted either a question or a whole section in *summae* and quodlibetal questions to pain. In these sources the question of pain did not necessarily stem from Christ. They incorporated all humanity, from sinners to saints. Startlingly, devils and angels also came in for their share of attention. Thus, Giles of Rome (ca. 1243–1316) placed his entire discussion of pain and its theory under the question of the suffering of devils in hell. The answer, long and learned, is a treasure trove of scholastic theory of pain, though it says next to nothing about devils. Henry of Ghent and William of Ockham (1280–1349) discussed the same questions while examining the human soul and its sufferings in hell. The multifarious fields in which pain was embedded, naturally or artificially, are evidence for the all-embracing interest in the topic.

The scholastic *homo* was a composite of several traditions: philosophical, theological, and medical. From the thirteenth century onward all these traditions were integrated in scholastic writings, for scholasticism was primarily the science of human beings. All scholastics stressed the unity and necessary harmony of all components. Body and soul were tied together until death, and sensations flowed from one to the other, affecting all parts of the soul.

Throughout those discussions, the reader is aware of the scholastic effort to appropriate and master pain. Had the masters ever seriously entertained the idea that pain might also result from external causes, as medical authorities asserted? If so, it was only to dismiss it. The same blow would hurt the soul governed by a highly intelligent, subtle mind much more sharply and longer than it would hurt the simple mind. The trajectory from the prefatory dread of imagination to the stick that hit the head to the mind or from the fire that burned the hand to the feeling that registered the injury, to the memory that recorded it, to the understanding that shrank from further injury and dwelt upon the former—this was what shaped human pain. And this trajectory was totally subjective and individual. The stick and the fire were unimportant. The manner in which their impact was internalized was all that mattered.

Prelapsarian Adam

Scholastic theories were an integral part of the ecclesiastical history of mankind. The gallery of sufferers included several figures; first came Adam, before and after his fall. He was followed in turn by his descendants, living and dead, by Christ, by martyred saints, and by the resuscitated glorious bodies at the end of days. All such analyses began with the creation of Adam. Adam, not necessarily Eve.

Was Adam before the Fall intrinsically different both from his own post-lapsarian self and from his descendants?[23] Augustine had thought so. As he said, in paradise man had possessed the possibility of immortality. There, man had been both mortal and immortal, because he could potentially have died and he could potentially have avoided dying—a choice he no longer possessed after the Fall.[24] Following Paul, Augustine's interest centered primarily upon the moral effects of the Fall, which caused mankind to become vulnerable to perturbations of the spirit, especially to lust. But the prelapsarian immunity from passions implies also an immunity from dis-ease and pain. When speaking of Adam's impassibility in paradise,[25] Augus-tine concentrated upon the absence of sadness and loss, not upon corporeal sensation. Nevertheless, in his mind, pain, sadness, and sickness were all closely connected.[26]

Was Adam then immune from all possible pains? Hugh of Saint Victor was the first to speculate on the subject. Adam, he said, was potentially passible by nature even before the Fall, but as long as he did not sin, he avoided suffering.[27] Hugh's contemporary Anselm of Laon also asserted that *primus homo* had had the potential to be both immortal and impassible, free of change, corruption, and passion and, consequently, free of pain.[28] The first thinker to connect Adam's freedom from pain with his physical constitution, though, was not a scholastic. Hildegard of Bingen, who was both visionary and physician, connected Adam's perfect health and freedom from pain with his perfect humoral balance.[29]

By the thirteenth century, Adam was commonly credited with the pos-session of an equal complexion—the perfect balance of humors. His immu-nity, however, stemmed from spiritual factors. Just as pain was a quality of the soul, so was impassibility. The subject was largely a Franciscan concern. Both Bonaventure (1221–74) and Alexander of Hales developed prelapsar-ian anthropology to a highly sophisticated degree. Under their scrutiny, Adam's immunity to pain began to disintegrate. Bonaventure insisted that impassibility was not freedom from pain but freedom from the overwhelm-ing mastery passions held over men's souls. Adam did know and feel pas-sion, but passion was subject both to his nature and to his will (which then tended toward the good). Consequently, passions could then be mastered and prevented from causing pain. In contrast, postlapsarian man, whose nature and will are enslaved by passions, cannot avoid pain.[30] This line of

reasoning continued in Franciscan scholarship with Matthew of Acquasparta (fl. 1245), who ascribed the postlapsarian soul's vulnerability to pain
to the disordered nature of postlapsarian human will.[31]

The most important discussions of prelapsarian Adam, undoubtedly,
are the *quaestio disputata* that Alexander of Hales devoted to the subject
and the chapter his students dedicated to it in the *Summa theologica* they
published under his name.[32] Adam in paradise was already passible, in the
sense that he was naturally subject to change and exterior influences. He
received impressions, saw and reacted to things, and changed with external
influences. He had sensations and was moved by desire. His soul was vulnerable to temptation. He was influenced by the stars. He was even subject
to those passions necessary for survival, the generative and nutritive forces.
They made sure that he ate, slept, and (potentially) generated children, albeit without lust.

Furthermore, Adam's corporeal sensations were like those of his descendants. Though protected while innocent, he had the potential to suffer and
change. He was susceptible to pain, for he did require sleep while undergoing the extraction of his rib. It appears that even the Creator had to resort
to anesthesia to prevent pain during such surgery. Adam could theoretically also have been wounded by stones, since his flesh, like ours, was soft.
Had he been mutilated, he would indeed have felt it. Had he been killed in
paradise, he would have suffered in all innocence.[33] Adam's freedom from
pain, therefore, hinged not upon his impassible nature, but primarily upon
the absence of nocive elements in paradise. Adam had lived in a protected
environment. Changes there were not necessarily painful, nor were natural
functions a fault. In a perfect environment, Adam had no need to be perfect
to avoid suffering.

There is one hint, as early as Augustine's writings, that Adam could
have felt pain, or perhaps *ought* to have felt pain, even in paradise. Adam
was the prefiguration of Christ, and Adam's sleep, during which God extracted a rib to make Eve, was the prefiguration of the Crucifixion. The
wound in Adam's side was likened to the wound in Christ's side: "Eve out
of the side of the sleeper, the Church out of the side of the sufferer." Could
God not have taken the rib painlessly without putting Adam to sleep? In
fact, remarked the pain-wise Augustine, sleep was not much use as an anesthetic during surgery. Any sleeper would have woken up during such an
operation. In consequence, he concluded, God could have done it without
putting Adam to sleep, for it was not sleep but God who prevented his
pain. However, the prefiguration of the suffering Christ required it.[34] By the
twelfth century, Adam's painlessness during surgery had assumed a more

natural, less miraculous quality, being likened to the drugged slumber of a man under anesthetics.[35]

Neither Augustine nor his twelfth-century successors ever paid much attention to Eve. Eve, who had tempted Adam and been explicitly punished with labor pains, ought to have been the ultimate focus of any discussion concerning the connection between the Fall and suffering. Yet she is glaringly absent from scholastic discussions.[36] In all the rich literature dealing with Adam in paradise, very few raised the hypothetical question of potential labor pains in paradise. Copulation (though without concupiscence) and childbirth, said Augustine, would indeed have taken place in paradise had Adam and Eve not sinned, but he had no opinion on Eve's possible labor pains. Honorius Augustodunensis devoted two lines to the subject: "How would she have given birth?" inquires the disciple, and the master tersely answers, "painlessly and immaculately."[37] Honorius used precisely these words later to describe the virgin birth of Christ, and so his description of Eve's parturition seems likely to have been borrowed from Mary's.[38] Clearly, prelapsarian Eve was of little interest.

What made Eve and the pains of childbirth vanish from sight? Was she simply dismissed as irrelevant until she was tempted by the snake? Indeed, in most paradise narratives and speculations, between her creation and the Fall Eve earns little mention. She is completely subsumed in Adam and his sensations, as though before her sin she had had no prior existence. I believe that Eve's absence was no mere oversight. It was possible to extrapolate from man to woman, since woman was a faulty version of the male model, but the opposite was impossible. One could not extrapolate from Eve's potential childbirth experience to that of "humanity," synonymous with man. And since interest centered upon the gendered male as man, any extra discomfort women might endure because of their faulty nature was not relevant. Nor did Eve's invisibility change in the following centuries. Throughout the Middle Ages, it seems that Eve had only one purpose in paradise—to get Adam expelled from the Garden of Eden. Her humanity and passibility were never topics of discussion.

Postlapsarian Humanity

To the mind of twelfth- and thirteenth-century theologians, the expulsion from paradise was one of the most momentous events in human history. The most influential insight into the consequences of the Fall was Anselm of Canterbury's *Why God Became a Man*, written more than a century before the Franciscan discussions of Adam in paradise. After several centuries in which the question had lain dormant, Anselm reaffirmed the need of Christ's human suffering for the redemption of fallen humanity.[39] Though Anselm was far more interested in Christ than in Adam and his sin, he opened the door to discussions of the Fall and its effect upon all of humankind.

A century later, the changes affected all the parts of man, both soul and body. The most notable change, according to Bonaventure, was the transformation in the hierarchy of forces operating within man. The defenses against the extraparadisiacal, hostile environment were breached. Any attack upon man's integrity provoked an onslaught of uncontrollable passions in him. And once the passions took over, sensing pain became inevitable. Man was now equally vulnerable to mental and sensual perturbations, such as anger. His soul was the battleground on which will and nature fought the passions: "we are made up of contraries, of actors and patients, so that there is a constant compromise in our bodies. . . . We therefore suffer [are subject to passions], whether we wish to or not."[40]

In putting the Fall in terms of the loss of free will, Bonaventure was going back to what he saw as Augustine's definitions of pain. Augustine most certainly had seen pain as unwilling subjection: "pain is dissent from those things that happen to us *against our will*" (my italics).[41] Thus, postlapsarian man had lost his will: he could only contemplate his own corruption, sense it, and bemoan it.[42] The breaches were not purely spiritual, for bodily integrity was damaged as well. If Adam was originally created from a very special clay, after the Fall his flesh came to resemble common earth and became poisoned, and thus vulnerable to disease and pain.[43]

Scholastic literature tended to couple death and pain as human postlapsarian attributes. Where death existed, so did pain. The Fall had corrupted the balance of Adam's perfect complexion, and man had lost the possibility of freedom from pain. He had become subject to change: aging, disease, pain, and death.[44] Though Genesis mentioned only childbirth pain for women and hard labor for men as penalties, Christian exegesis extended the vulnerability to pain to men.[45]

Postlapsarian nature stood in contrast to both Christ's and prelapsarian Adam's nature. Scholastic discussions of Christ's passibility very often included speculation on precisely how much of man's faulty nature he had assumed. Inevitably, such discussions cataloged human faults, if only to ascertain which of them Christ had not needed to take on. Postlapsarian man suffered from hunger, thirst, fatigue, sickness, and age. He was susceptible to all the forces, inner and outer, that could attack humanity, and he had neither the complexion to repel them or the will to resist.

There is a striking difference between theoretical and historical views of pain. No matter how far scholastics went in theory to stress the internal generation of human pain, the Fall clearly let the hostile environment in. Being postlapsarian, being passible, meant that humans were vulnerable to those same forces that could only harm the mind and soul left open to their impact. The theoretical discussion of pain did not view humans as previously impregnable fortresses, now irreversibly damaged. To the contrary, it considered only humanity as its subject, obliterating the Fall from discussion. In this argument, human beings were nurseries of self-generated pain. Discussions of the Fall and its consequences shifted the causes to the external world. Before one could apprehend pain, fear it, and remember it, one had to be burned by the fire or hit by the stick, neither of which could happen in paradise. In the grim reality that followed the Fall, sticks and fires were there to hurt, and human beings could receive and perceive that hurt. Nevertheless, nothing on earth compared to what was waiting for people after death. The few elect righteous ones might go to heaven, to spend eternity singing in one of the nine choirs, but most of humanity was headed for a much worse fate. At best, it was purgatory. At worst, it was hell.

Postmortem Humanity

The pains of purgatory and hell have been surveyed already from the point of view of their utility in frightening people away from sin. Not only preachers but scholars, too, dealt with the subject. The utter incomparability between human experience of pain and postmortem sufferings posed a problem to all those who attempted to analyze it. Despite the inconceivable gap between worlds, preachers resorted to comparisons culled from daily life, but scholastics were bound by their disciplinary rules to avoid hyperbole. How scholastics went about analyzing and describing the impossible and inconceivable afterworld highlights the different concerns of scholars and preachers.

Postmortem sufferings cropped up quite often in scholastic debates. What manner of suffering that was and how it accorded with the principles of physics and human nature laid down by Aristotle were points of doctrine and theology, and scholars could hardly avoid treating them. Nevertheless, had anybody wished to reconstruct what purgatory and hell looked like to medieval people, scholastic sources would have given scant help. Scholars were interested in specific problems: the nature of the fire and the nature of the souls' pain. The central problem of scholars was one of essence, not feeling. If what suffered in afterlife was a soul, how could the sufferings be

sensory? Furthermore, was the fire purely conceptual, or was it a real, corporeal fire? And how did such a fire affect human souls? Finally, did devils
partake in the suffering? In all their discussions, scholastics were forced
to rely upon visionary materials—the *Dialogues* of Gregory the Great, the
Purgatory of Saint Patrick, and similar (presumably dubious) sources. While
these did provide some useful details, they left a great deal unknown. The
gradual introduction of purgatory into the picture, naturally, complicated
theological questions, though not greatly. For the most part, what was valid
for hell was valid for purgatory.

One question that several early visions had answered was the locality
of hell. Early medieval authors had pointed to Mount Aetna in Sicily and
to St. Patrick's purgatory in Ireland, but secondhand stories were not the
stuff that scholastics unquestioningly accepted. Henry of Ghent, asked in
a disputation whether hell was in the center of the earth, constructed an
entire geography.[46] Relying upon the accounts of visions, those of Gregory
the Great among others (the veracity of which he openly doubted), he con-
ceded that hell was as far underneath the earth as possible, but whether it
was at the center or at the edge he could not tell. Decades earlier, William
of Auvergne had already discussed the question,[47] concluding that hell was
indeed in the middle of the earth. Henry refused to answer this point, but he
did add that there were four divisions (*interclusurae*) in hell: the lowest was
the *interclusura* of the damned; above it was purgatory; then came the two
limbos—that of unbaptized babies and, on the top, that of the patriarchs.[48]

Though the most important issue was the suffering of disembodied
souls, that suffering hinged upon the nature of hell, the fire, and the inflic-
tors: the devils. Here the source of discussion was Gregory the Great's assertion that the same fire punished different sinners to different degrees.[49] Even
in hell pain was relative, not absolute. But the difference, insisted Gregory,
lay not in the perceptive powers of greater and lesser sinners (how could
lesser sinners possibly be less perceptive?) but in the miraculous nature of
hellfire, which was indeed real but different from all other fires.

A fire that was real but disobeyed the laws of nature was something
for thirteenth-century scholastics to worry about. The pain it caused was
relative but hurt infinitely more than earthly fire. Hellfire was perpetual,
it gave no light, and it worked upon incorporeal entities. How could that
be? It was not even necessary. After all, dreamers could suffer pains from
their dreams alone, needing no real fire to cause their pain. Nonetheless, affirmed William of Auvergne, God would not stoop to the fictive sensations
of dreams. Hell was real, and so was the fire. If souls felt that fire in a subjective manner, it still did not alter the veritable reality of the fire.

The nature of hellfire came into question in the next generation, too. Thomas Aquinas, ever the champion of natural phenomena, maintained that there was nothing miraculous or supernatural about the action of corporeal hellfire upon incorporeal souls. This he maintained in contradiction to "some" (aliqui), who claimed that, as an instrument of divine justice, hellfire was beyond the laws of nature. According to Thomas Aquinas, the fire was indeed an instrument of divine justice, but it acted according to the laws of nature. This was going too far, and Thomas himself was not certain on the latter point, reversing himself later.[50] Indeed, the natural character of hellfire was problematic. Henry of Ghent challenged this point fifteen years later, arguing that a natural fire would affect all souls equally, lesser and greater sinners alike. On the authority of Gregory the Great, he said, we know that each soul is afflicted according to its degree of guilt.[51] The fire, consequently, was beyond the laws of nature.

Whether the fire was natural or not, it was unquestionably real. Despite the overwhelming importance of perception of pain in life, hell remained real, purgatory remained real, the fire was real, and so was the pain. During the thirteenth and fourteenth centuries, scholastic culture shaped and placed hell and purgatory in a very real context. Sporadically, the idea that suffering was mostly intangible and incorporeal came up, only to be rejected. Regrets might gnaw the souls of denizens of purgatory and hell, but they were hardly comparable to the real pains endured there. As William of Auvergne, one of the earliest of these scholars, put it: "the fire really and truly tortures the bodies of the souls."[52]

By contrast, Thomas Aquinas had severe doubts about hellfire (undoubtedly corporeal) really torturing souls. To his mind, human souls ranked higher in the hierarchy of the universe than an element like fire and therefore could not suffer from it, real though it might be. So real was the fire that other inhabitants of hell, devils included, also felt it.[53] Like much else, the sources for this position lie in Augustine's writings. Augustine had used the argument of diabolical pain to prove that incorporeal entities could indeed suffer from a real, veritable fire. If devils suffered, so could disembodied souls.

Devils had received scant attention before the twelfth century. They occasionally appeared to the living in visions and unsuccessfully tried to invade churches or tempt the thoughtless to sin. But until the thirteenth century nobody had bothered to prove or analyze their pains. Again, it was William of Auvergne who did so, claiming that both angels and devils, though lacking carnal bodies, were susceptible to passions[54] and hence to pain. Indeed, when one gave it thought, devils necessarily had to suffer in hell. After all, they were fallen angels, eternally punished for their sin of pride. What was the point of relegating them to hell if they only enjoyed themselves there? Of all the intricate fauna of hell described in visions—monsters, toads, serpents, worms—none came in for such discussions, being deemed instruments only, devoid of cognition. Devils were different.[55]

But the central subject of hell was the human beings who populated it after their death and who would populate it forever after the final judgment. The first to leave a lasting imprint upon the discussion was Augustine. Both in his literal exegesis of Genesis and in the *City of God,* the bishop of Hippo confronted the basic question of souls really burning in real fire and suffering bodily pain. His answer, destined to be quoted for the following millennium by scholars, was clear-cut:

> Moreover, if we attend to the matter a little more closely, we see that what is called bodily pain is rather to be referred to the soul. For it is the soul, not the body, which is pained, even when the pain originates with the body, the soul feeling pain at the point where the body is hurt. As then we speak of bodies feeling and living, though the feeling and life of the body are from the soul, so also we speak of bodies being pained, though no pain can be suffered by the body apart from the soul. The soul, then, is pained with the body in that part where something occurs to hurt it; and it is pained alone, though it be in the body, when some invisible cause distresses it, while the body is safe and sound. Even when not associated with the body it is pained.[56]

Augustine's theory of pain was known, cited, and reaffirmed for centuries to come. Whatever contrary theory cropped up in any generation, it was invariably rebutted with reference to Augustine.[57] From *summae* to sermons, from questions to dialogues, all authors considered Augustine's words as the basic source for understanding posthumous punishment.[58]

The problem became more complex with the gradual increase in discussion about purgatory.[59] Augustine's unquestionably real painful fire became attenuated into an abstract idea for twelfth-century Neoplatonists. According to Honorius Augustodunensis, souls in purgatory had not yet faced their final judgment (which would only come on doomsday) and therefore suffered only the sadness of deprivation from divine glory. This theory, which goes back to the ideas of John Scotus Erigena in the ninth century, was also present in Richard of Saint Victor's thinking and later in Thomas Aquinas's.[60] While souls in no way relinquished their lost bodies as tools of sensation, their suffering became tenuous and unreal. Subsequent scholastic discussions of purgatory and hell still turned upon the problem of the reality of pain but adopted the opposite approach. Souls well and truly suffered in hell. Furthermore, their lack of body was put in doubt, for to many scholars it seemed as though the souls still possessed some sort of body. When William of Auvergne discussed hell, his analysis of suffering souls echoed much of what Hugh of Saint Victor had said about the power of memory to create pain but also predicated the presence of ensouled bodies:[61]

> Therefore, the human soul is only witness to its burning, since it has no heat in it. . . . Why would it be wonderful, given that the fire burns in it purely by force of imagination, and the soul judges itself to be burning, for imagination is closer to the soul's substance than the senses and is purely spiritual . . . ? This appears so to [the soul] because of the extremely strong conjunction and union between it and the body, and thus it seems to it and it considers itself suffering what the body suffers, as it is not only [the soul that is] in the body, but the body, as many philosophers say, is rather in [the soul]. . . . it is not the soul that really suffers from these passions as though they were its own, but rather as empathizing with those of another.[62]

The reality of suffering in purgatory and hell was predicated upon the ineluctable connection between soul and body, a connection that death did not really sever.[63] Souls still bore the image of the body imprinted upon them; they still felt the passions inflicted on them. This view accorded perfectly with thirteenth- and fourteenth-century views of pain in general. It required little or no external stimulus. It was born almost exclusively in the soul, with the body serving as an excuse for feelings. Apprehension was the foundation of sensation, and if the soul in hell perceived itself as suffering, it did in reality suffer. As it is, the corporeal fire seems almost unnecessary, though William did insist upon its existence.

The connection of body and soul after death invariably led to speculations about their relationship before death. Thomas Aquinas treated the question three times at least—twice in *questiones disputatae* and once in a quodlibetal question.[64] He inevitably referred to Augustine as their starting point. Unlike his predecessors, Thomas added a great deal of subtlety to the topic. He was the first to apply the polysemous nature of *passio* to the question at hand. "Passivity," as the antonym of "activity," was one meaning. The act of receiving upon one's self somebody else's action was another. The spiritual movement, or emotion, aroused in the recipient was the third, most common meaning.[65] This was what caused in the object, the *patiens,* alterations and corruption and, as such, could affect only living bodies, not souls separated from the body. Subsequently, this meaning had evolved into anything that was contrary to and prevented the object's comfort. In this sense, souls could indeed suffer.[66] This analysis enabled Thomas to reject the Augustinian explanation that the soul possessed a certain *similitudo corporis*—an imprinted perception of the body and its sensations—and that this was the sufferer. His conclusion was that, since cognition was essential for suffering, souls could suffer in hell by way of sadness and a recognition of the fire's harmful effects, but not physically: "in no way does the soul suffer from corporeal fire." Furthermore, hellfire will, after the resurrection of the body, well and truly afflict the sinners' bodies.[67]

But how could souls that received no external input be aware of the fire and suffer from it? Henry of Ghent, a few years younger than Thomas, was familiar with the parts of the soul, and as a result he did have a problem with the suffering of incorporeal souls. The soul suffered through its sensitive force, and this force was lost once body and soul parted company, for senses were fed information through bodily organs. His answer to this problem was that souls still potentially retained sensitive forces, which enabled them to suffer in hell. Though his answer was more technical and more Aristotelian than William of Auvergne's impassioned words, in principle he had changed little, for his souls still felt sensations.[68]

Henry's contemporary Matthew of Acquasparta treated the subject more carefully. Rather than answering a quodlibetal question, he devoted a question to the subject at his own initiative, and his treatment is the most exhaustive of all. He debated no fewer than twenty-one objections to the separated soul's punitive suffering.[69] Like Thomas shortly before him, Matthew hinged his interpretation upon the polysemous nature of *passio.* The meanings he attributed to the term, however, were subtly different. He completely ignored "passivity," starting with the sensory and intellectual reception of external stimuli. "Passion," however, could also be construed as the changes wrought by such stimuli. Finally, "passion" could mean anything contrary to our will "for example, being tied up or imprisoned," or, in other words, suffering.[70] Only in this third sense did "passion" apply to the souls of the damned. They were detained in hell against their will, as in a jail. Nevertheless, Matthew, too, rejected the Augustinian explanation that souls carried with them an image of the body after death. If the pain were no more than a figment of imagination and memory, there was no need for real fire, and for the latter's existence he had Gregory the Great's own authority. He equally objected to the proposition that discorporate souls suffered by apprehension, so that the souls only perceived the fire as burning them. How, he demanded, could a fictitious fire deceive and inflict pain upon the demons, who were known for their perspicacity and acuteness? And it was well known that demons also suffered in hell. The fire, therefore, was real.[71]

Having taken this extreme realist position, Matthew was left with very little with which to explain hell. Fire was real, but it could only affect souls as an instrument of divine justice, miraculously, since material fire could not affect immaterial souls. Like Henry of Ghent, he credited separated souls with senses, but real, not potential, senses. Furthermore, since souls used bodies only as conductors of sensation, the separated soul, rid of intermediaries, sensed pain directly and immediately, more vividly than the living one.[72] The power of imagination—the same power that could make Christ sweat blood simply by envisioning his upcoming crucifixion—could certainly make souls suffer in hell.[73]

All the same, realism had its limits. Like Thomas, Matthew was aware of the physical effects of emotion, and it was totally inconceivable that an incorporeal soul would be able to produce a blush of shame. Indeed, in his rebuttals, Matthew admitted that the separated soul could not suffer from passions originating from its union with the body. Consequently, he said, it could not suffer pain in the medical sense (*sensus divisionis continui*), although hellfire did cause suffering from other passions, such as guilt.[74] This barely acknowledged contradiction was simply avoided by the same scholastic trick of polysemy. *Dolor* could mean sensory pain, sadness, or both at the same time, and here Matthew came full circle, returning stealthily to a more abstract perception of hell.[75] For, in addition to the fire, there was the worm of regret, and Matthew claimed that the pains of regret far exceeded those of the fire.[76]

There was no single theory of suffering in hell. Hell was real, the fire was real, and the devils were real, but it was not clear what provoked the suffering. Did souls have bodies or not? Did they suffer sensory pains or a mental reflection of unbearable loss and sadness? These questions were important, but they were far more important to those engaged in pastoral work than to masters of theology. While scholars could debate the topic at leisure, preachers needed hard and fast descriptions for their flocks. And while theologians were not particularly interested in enumerating and describing the different penalties of hell, preachers most certainly were.[77] The same author, pondering a scholastic question and addressing an audience (especially a lay one), was certain to come up with different narratives.

Human Pain in the Culture of Devotion

In one of his Lenten sermons, Jacobus of Voragine defined the three greatest pains in the world: "This pain is similar to torture, childbirth pangs, and the pain of those weeping for [the death of] an only child. These are the three greatest pains one can find."[78] He was speaking, of course, of Christ's sufferings, but the need to make ultimate pain comprehensible to mere mortals forced him to have recourse to similes culled from human experience. Significantly, Jacobus made no distinction between sensory and emotional pain, for he did not grasp them as essentially different.

Devotional beliefs and practices that encompassed pain in one form or another exist in many religions.[79] These beliefs often include illness as punishment, postmortem penalties for sinners, and the sufferings of gods and heroes. Given the all-inclusive preoccupation of Christianity with pain, the devotional interpretations of the topic are extensive. They range from painting and music to ascetic practices and mystical visions. I have concentrated here upon the written and spoken word: preachers' manuals, sermons, and visionary literature. Those were the most accessible messages for believers, and their impact, though immeasurable, remains unquestioned.

This is not to say that all experiences of religious pain were filtered through a single unifying imaginative and expressive norm. The devotional practices of Elisabeth Stagel, Heinrich Suso, and Margaretha Ebner, all stemming from the German Dominican devotional trend, show a marked dissimilarity.[80] Here we have three people who practiced intense Christocentric Passion devotion and were in touch with each other, and yet, there are three different types of pain experiences here: illness (Ebner), self-inflicted ascetic practice (Suso), and frustrated yearning for such a forbidden practice (Stagel). Devotional attitudes toward pain, then, were individual as well as communal.

Illness

The interpretation of illness during the later Middle Ages was double-edged, usually meaning one of two opposites. On the one hand, illness was a metaphor for sin, from which Christ had cured humanity. On the other hand, illness was viewed as a salutary tool for encouraging people to forgo worldly pleasures and concentrate upon otherworldly destinies. I have already mentioned that William of Auvergne praised illness as his prime defense against temptations.[81] His rich metaphorical language, evoking harsh cleansers and kilns that burn human clay, however, was not meant for public consumption.

Some of his ideas did permeate his sermons, but most of them remained within *De universo*, a treatise not meant to be read beyond the boundaries of contemporary academe.

For the most part, until the fourteenth century thinkers tended to opt for the first position. In one of his Lenten sermons, Jacobus de Voragine discussed the verse "Totum hominem sanum feci in sabbato."[82] The sermon is a summary of the belief in *Christus medicus*, in the inherent illness of humanity that only Christ can cure, and is modeled after a medical diagnosis.[83] There are four causes for human illness of mind and body: overeating, cold, corruption of the blood, and corruption of the humors. Each one of these causes has its own interpretation. Gluttony was the cause of Adam's fall, which rendered him vulnerable to illness. Many die of it, because the fat prevents blood from flowing and strangles the inner heat. Cold is another name for mortal sin, the nature of which is cold since it extinguishes divine love. Corrupt blood is wealth, which leads to lust. Corrupt humors are simply vices. Only the first cause, gluttony, can be cured by keeping a Lenten fast. The rest are cured by Christ: cold by the heat of his sweat, corrupt blood by his own bleeding (here named *minutio*, i.e., phlebotomy), and corrupt humors by the bitter medicine of the gall he was given to drink on the cross.

The sermon continues its medical metaphor with a discussion of health and its signs. The sermon draws a clear correspondence between bodily illness, as defined in medical terms, and illnesses of the soul. The idea was hardly new in the thirteenth century, but at that time it appeared clad in the new scholastic medical terminology. Still, Jacobus speaks of pain only in one context: the bitterness that Christ swallowed on the cross. The sick patients—humanity—suffer no pain in illness; only Christ who cures them suffers.

This attitude is typical of most preachers' attitudes toward earthly sickness. First, it is the patient's fault for indulging herself. Second, it needs to be cured, but the pains attendant upon the sickness are not relevant. In fact, as captives of metaphor, preachers drew a picture of "ill" sinners enjoying their sins rather than suffering for them. The suffering would come only later, after death. Terrestrial pains, as we shall see, appear as metaphors for infernal ones, but in themselves they merited little attention.

The opposite view, that illness was a salvific gift, gained strength during the fourteenth and fifteenth centuries. The charismatic presence of living saints, most of whom were said to have suffered a multitude of illnesses with great patience, bolstered this view. As we have seen, the *artes bene moriendi* hesitated between praising illness as a harbinger of death and deprecating the distracting effects of pain upon the sufferer.[84] Delivering a public sermon on the value of pain was perhaps conceivable only in the fifteenth century. A few decades after Gerson wrote his treatise on the good death, the Dominican Johannes Herolt (d. 1468), whose model sermons were extremely popular for more than a century after his death, devoted one to the subject.[85] While far less emotional than William of Auvergne, Herolt adduced even more reasons for embracing and welcoming illness, putting together all of the previous arguments. All sickness, even a headache or toothache, was a harbinger of death sent by Christ to encourage people to prepare for leaving the world. Furthermore, suffering purged people from previous sins (though not as drastically as William of Auvergne had envisaged), strengthening the soul at the body's expense. Thus, the sick find no pleasure in the vanities of life but concentrate on confession and penitence. It is God's special gift to some people and will shorten their stay in purgatory. Finally, and most importantly, it is a guarantee of eternal salvation, a door to heaven, and a form of *imitatio Christi.*

In praising sickness and pain, it was essential to acknowledge that sickness was salutary precisely because it made people suffer, which people did not wish to do. One way to make them accept illness was to point out the future advantages: any illness on earth would compensate in advance for much worse sufferings in the future. Illness thus stood for the sum of all earthly pains: its evil was good, its life was death. In trying to make sense out of a very common and prevalent phenomenon in contemporary life, late medieval preachers had found a way to valorize involuntary pain. They advised penitence and virtue; they did not advise the laity actively to seek pain. Flagellants and lay ascetics were more suspect than welcome to the clergy.

While the similarity between William of Auvergne and Johannes Herolt is apparent, so is the difference. William was careful not to interpret unsolicited pain as *imitatio Christi,* whereas Herolt did so, granting the lay sick the dignity of imitators of Christ. Two centuries of discussions and sermons about pain produced a change: the importance of personal suffering grew to the point that it was seen as *imitatio Christi.*

Hell

When St. Francesca Bussa de' Ponziani, also known as Santa Francesca Romana, dictated her detailed visions of hell to her confessor, she was already a known ascetic and founder of an order of nuns. But she was no scholar: her education had been that of a noble Roman matron, and she was neither particularly literate nor intellectual. She knew the Bible, Jacobus de Vora-gine's *Legenda aurea*, and some of the twelfth- and thirteenth-century vi-sions of hell.[86] The same might be said of Bridget of Sweden (ca. 1303–73), also a visionary who had visited hell. These women were both aristocratic and—once widowed—economically independent, but their visions hardly manifested deep learning. What they knew of the topography of hell was what every devout layperson knew.

Visionaries were as well versed in the paths and labyrinths of hell as any priest or monk and could probably have found their way there and back without the help of the ever-present guiding saint or angel. They knew what the different parts of hell looked and smelled like; they knew whom they would find in each section, what kind of fire to expect, and where Lucifer sat. Most importantly, they told what the tortured souls felt, what they shrieked, what they hoped for despite their hopelessness. One would be hard put to grow up in any late medieval city without familiarizing oneself with hell as intimately as with local geography. Everyone who went to hear sermons knew these things. The difference was that one could learn to be-ware certain pitfalls in a city; once in hell, there was no avoiding them.

Most modern readers visualize hell through the words of Dante. Dante, however, was uniquely different from earlier and subsequent visionaries who described hell. In fact, he stood outside a tradition of venerable an-tiquity.[87] Visions of hell were a common literary genre dating back to late antiquity.[88] The central motif in all of these visions was the narrator—a living person plucked out of his or her environment and plunged with scant warning into the afterlife.[89] The traveler invariably toured hell, purgatory (as of the twelfth century), and heaven, though the last part of the trip was often truncated. The narrator usually lay as one dead for three days or so, thereafter returning to life in order to impart the story to all listeners.

The purpose of this tour was twofold. In the first place, the vision-ary—if not already devoted to a life of penitence—invariably converted to the religious life afterward.[90] Second, and more important, was the narra-tion. Indeed, the tale was written, copied, transmitted, authenticated, and translated into vernacular languages repeatedly, from Ireland to Austria and beyond. Some tales, like the vision of St. Jehan Paulus, were originally writ-ten in the vernacular.[91] Abbreviated "visits to hell," in which the returned tourist could vouch for the real horrors, appear frequently in exempla.[92]

The topography of the imaginary landscape of hell varied somewhat from one vision to another.[93] Some late visitors, like Dante Alighieri and Francesca Romana, saw a hell divided up by the type of sin: the hell of the sodomites, the hell of the usurers, the hell of the heretics, and so forth.

Earlier descriptions stuck to topography: first a place of darkness, then of noise, then a fire or a wheel, a freezing lake or river with a horrible beast in it, a mountain, a bridge, and finally the pit of hell, where Lucifer resided.[94] In all cases, the saint or angel stood by the visitor's side, providing a verbal exegesis of the vision.[95]

Some motifs recur throughout the vision literature. One is the suffocatingly crowded nature of hell, the enormous number of sinners stuck cheek by jowl. Others are darkness, noise, the contrast of intolerable heat and unbearable cold, iron hooks, cauldrons, and monstrous beasts which constantly swallow and expel (by either birth or defecation) the miserable souls. Devils were omnipresent; according to Santa Francesca, each sinner had two devils, one to torture and one to revile.[96] Everywhere could be heard the screams of tortured souls, either begging for mercy (occasionally even appealing to saints, as the monk of Evesham noted) or cursing and blaspheming.[97]

All visions insisted upon the embodiment of suffering. Despite the constant reiteration that those were indeed souls, every guiding angel explained that these souls had bodily, sensory organs to incorporate the pain. The tradition that hell and hellfire were *really* sensed, and that souls suffered in a corporeal form from a real fire, goes back to the late antique Apocalypse of Paul.[98] The corporeality of the afterlife was explicitly stressed in the introduction to the treatise *Purgatory of Saint Patrick*:

> In these [stories] nothing is told that is not corporeal, or similar to it: rivers, flames, bridges, ships, houses, groves, meadows, flowers, black and white men, and other things such as exist in this world [created] either to be loved for joy or to be feared for torture; he, too [i.e., the knight Owen], tells that those [souls] freed from their bodies were pulled by the hands, led by the feet, hung by the neck, whipped, hurled down, and many other things hardly strange to nature.[99]

So the world of the afterlife looked, felt, and smelled very much like life. Human beings had corporeal souls to suffer with, souls that possessed all the organs of the live body. Moreover, they had all five senses: they suffered by seeing, smelling, being touched and burned, and hearing.[100] They even tasted the pitch and sulfur in their mouths. In addition, they had voices to scream with and limbs to be tortured. Souls were also fully gendered. When Tnugdal witnessed the impregnated souls unnaturally giving birth in an icy swamp to serpents that ate up their progenitors, he insisted several times that both male and female souls had suffered the same monstrous rape and pregnancy.[101] They also possessed all the accoutrements and characteristics of their lifelike bodies, since visionaries sometimes recognized specific familiar sufferers.

Tours of hell provided readers and listeners with both knowledge and vicarious thrills. As in suspense novels, one knew from the beginning that the hero would emerge at least physically unscathed in order to tell the piteous and horrifying tale of others who had remained behind. Visions were pain at two or more removes: usually the narrator had only seen but not felt the suffering, and his or her story came through various written and preached versions to the audience.

Was this sufficiently terrifying to frighten listeners into repentance? The wailing and gnashing of teeth and eternal darkness provided no more than a backdrop to the hero's adventures. The real sufferers were rarely allowed to speak in those tales, for normally the dialogue was between the hero and the guide. Readers or listeners to such tales would hardly feel the liquid pitch and sulfur creeping up to their knees, the snakes and toads eating their entrails. They would be watching all of this through the hero's horrified gaze, sure of an eventual return to the world. The writhing masses could screech their pain and anger, but they rarely had either names or identities.[102]

A certain tedious repetitiousness must also have made the stories less than frightening over time. If we take, for example, Santa Francesca's vision, most of it is divided up by sins. She begins with the *limbo puerorum* but is promptly translated to the sodomites' hell. The description is horrifying, including all the required details: devils, iron hooks, and the variety of pains. The usurers' section adds cooking pots full of liquid gold and silver, screams, blasphemy, and anger. By the third and fourth sections (traitors and murderers), the author cuts off her repetitious description with "and they also had all the other general pains,"[103] a statement appended to several other chapters. Fifteen sins or so later, when the various souls have all been speared, torn apart, thrown into cauldrons filled with various noxious substances, ingested and regurgitated, the narrative does begin to lose its hold. As Jérôme Baschet has noted, the fierceness of torture in visions increased significantly after 1330.[104] The damned in hell are described being pierced, flayed, torn apart, and decapitated. This trend conforms with the general trends of accentuating and describing pain in overt, even extravagant terms. The tortures, as we shall see, are parallel to those that martyrs in thirteenth-century legendaries underwent.[105]

Medieval preachers also seemed to find visions ineffective and—though drawing upon them—took a far more explicit tone when describing hell. What we have are only the written versions of their verbal messages, but these do differ in some material ways from the visions. This is perhaps why sermons dealing with hell and purgatory rarely spent time retelling the popular stories of the visions, other than in a short exemplum here or there. Very often hell was not the subject of the sermon but was merely mentioned as the destination of whoever succumbed to some specific temptation. An exemplum inveighing against the pleasures of games simply told the story of a monk who, while on a short visit to hell, saw there a very virtuous knight whose one fault in life had been his inclination toward hawking and chess. Another, exhorting people to confess regularly, spoke of a dead woman appearing in a vision to monks and telling of her terrible fate because she had not confessed her sin. Similar fates awaited those addicted to dancing or other worldly pleasures.[106]

Preachers also used mnemonic devices to make sure people did not forget. The nine pains of hell were such a device. They go back to twelfth-century theology, to the writings of Honorius Augustodunensis and the sermons of Bernard of Clairvaux, and inversely parallel the nine choirs of angels.[107] Thomas of Chobham added several other pains to the original nine, for all five senses were to be affected.[108] Caesarius of Heisterbach and Stephen of Bourbon made up mnemonic verses for the various pain-causing penalties.[109] The rough impression is that preachers relied upon a stock of "physical" penalties first and then tried to add psychological elements, which they considered essential but not part of the basic menu.

Upon this skeleton preachers built the most terrifying picture possible. The main source for suffering differed from author to author: one said it was the fire, another the extremes of hot and cold to which the souls were subjected, and a third insisted that the worst was the deprivation of divine vision. Thomas of Chobham insisted that there was neither distinction nor gradation: all torments happened simultaneously and worked to a similar degree.[110] By contrast, Bromyard insisted that hell was a sort of merry-go-round where one went from one set of torturing devils to another, so that by the time one came back to the first set, its torments had already been submerged in the later penalties, and the old ones seemed forever new again.[111]

The individuality of human pain melted in the infernal fires of this picture, losing its power to terrorize individuals with individual sins. The fine distinctions between sinners seemed to fade in the glare of eternal darkness and fire. To personalize the picture, preachers used exempla that referred to specific people with specific pains. A recurrent story, going from Gregory the Great to Bede and thence to thirteenth-century preachers' manuals is that of the hermit who lived alone, subjecting himself to constant sharp changes of boiling-hot baths and icy rivers. Whenever questioned about his ascetic practices, he responded that, had his interlocutors seen what he had seen, they would do likewise. He had been a solid paterfamilias before his visit to hell, but after his return he gave away all of his property and retired to the desert, concentrating on self-mortification.[112] Going beyond the anonymous hermit, Caesarius of Heisterbach concentrated upon people known and named to his readers. He could tell precisely what had happened in hell to Landgraf Ludwig or to Wilhelm, count of Jülich.[113] Several other preachers told about revenants from hell who explained in detail what they were suffering.[114] One need not have been anything special to earn a visit to hell; even a woman who simply wanted to know what most displeased God was wafted there for a short view of the torments of an acquaintance, a virtuous and charitable woman unfortunately addicted to feminine vanity.[115]

Preachers tried to relate the pains of hell to familiar everyday experiences, calling upon imagination and memory—the experience and knowledge of one's own physical pain. In one exemplum, a dead scholar was revealed in a vision to his erstwhile master. The scholar, who was in hell, dripped a single drop of sweat upon his live master's hand, and the corrosive drop ate through the hand. Ever afterward, says the story, the master was left with a hole in his hand.[116] The best illustration was probably Pseudo-Augustine's, who had said that purgatorial fire bore the same relation to worldly fire as the latter bore to a wall painting of fire. In this world, the painting has little sensory impact other than sight. Should one thrust a hand into a painted fire, one would feel nothing. But a hand burning in terrestrial fire pales into insignificance compared with the experience of purgatory. In fact, no worldly penalty whatsoever could in any way compare with the pains of purgatorial fire. Imagine therefore how much worse were the fires of hell![117] The latter statement was repeated by several scholastic authors writing about purgatory. Bernard of Clairvaux was reputed to have added that one spark of hellfire hurt more than a thousand years of labor pains, another comparison that should have spoken eloquently at least to the female half of his audience.[118] When illustrating the pain of transition from extremes of heat and cold in hell, Stephen of Bourbon remarked that experienced washerwomen, who went to warm up at the fire after washing the laundry in the frozen river, were familiar with the feeling of sudden change.[119]

When John Bromyard tried to explain how the same hellfire affected different types of sinners differently, he borrowed his examples from secular penology and civil law. In the world of the living, too, punishment affected the rich and the poor differently. For a rich man, a fine of ten shillings was less than a ten-penny fine for a poor one. Conversely, those used to poverty suffered less than the greedy rich from prison, blows, hunger, and thirst.

Nor would they feel humiliation, since they had never received respect.[120] The very existence of hell could be inferred from life's experience, claimed Stephen. Every king had a palace, "a most beautiful and most honorable place" (*pulcherrimus et honestissimus locus*), a service section comprising kitchen and stables, "lower and less respectable" (*magis infimus et minus decens*), and the lowest, most secret place of all—a dungeon. Thus, the universe comprises heaven, the world, and hell.[121] Thomas of Chobham used a similar institutional simile when trying to worry people about the Last Judgment. Here on earth the judge, the prosecutor, the witness, and the advocate were different people. At the final judgment, God would fulfill all functions, and there would be no escape.[122] Other pains of hell also resembled personal experience; hunger was perpetual: "So much so that flesh is consumed. . . . So much so that hunger sits between their ribs, and there it is perpetual, since it cannot come out of their ribs. . . . So much so that they gnaw their own tongues. . . . So much so that they devour their own and other people's arms. . . . So much so that just for hunger they curse the devil and God."[123] The stench was the smell of burning corpses, pitch, and sulfur, familiar to all who had survived the plague and the mass burials that took place wherever it hit. The screams were those of *homines tribulati*, who cry in the vulgar tongue, *ve, ve, ve*, bewailing their fate.[124] Finally, while in this world there were distractions from pain; in the next, there were none.[125]

In addition to personal experience, preachers relied on a comparative scale of pain. The fire of hell was the worst conceivable experience beyond personal life. Nothing the martyrs had ever suffered, not even what Christ had undergone, in any way approached what one felt in hell.[126] This was said to people who, every saint's day, heard what Vincent, Lawrence, Katherine, or Ursula had suffered in exquisite, agonizing detail. This was addressed to people who heard all the details of Christ's Passion every Easter and presumably knew all about his pains. During Easter week they were told that, insofar as Christ was above them, so his sufferings were beyond them, a pinnacle of sensation they could not reach. And now the preacher broke it to them that they were destined to suffer worse—worse than the martyrs, whose deeds they knew by heart and whose fortitude they lacked; worse than Christ, who was more than human and more sensitive to pain than all humans. The impact of these comparisons must have stunned many listeners into total belief. By dint of dwelling on the familiar and the comparable, people were made to create in their minds the future sensations of penalty and pain.

But hell was definitely not only about physical agony. The absence of the vision of God stood among the nine pains of hell. In some descriptions the damned were first led to a glimpse of heaven, so that they could spend eternity regretting what they would never have. Sermons, too, dwelt upon despair, self-loathing, anger, regret, and a constant wish to die and vanish into oblivion and loss of identity, although one no longer had that option.[127] In many accounts, fear itself formed one of the pains of hell; Gregory the Great had already maintained that, while in this world fear preceded pain, in hell they coexisted.[128] Together with fear came a constant feeling of loss and self-accusation. The whole universe joined in accusing the sinners in hell: angels, demons, their own sins, the very four elements joined to accuse them.[129]

"Afterlife" is a term invented by modern sensibilities. The assumption that anything beyond the watershed of death, if existent, was materially different from the present life crystallized slowly in the last few centuries. To medieval awareness, continued existence beyond the grave bore remarkable similarity to life. The landscapes of hell were composed of known visual images—mountains, rivers, ice, and fire. Eternity hung as heavily as time upon the sufferers. Disembodied souls felt and suffered all that embodied ones could feel: noise, stench, darkness, and pain. The pains were pains one had either experienced or heard of, and as in the world, they were also punitive. The only difference was that in purgatory or hell it was too late to do anything about it, and nobody needed a priest to explain why one suffered: they all knew why.

Conclusion

The varieties of painful human experience are well exhibited in the clear distinction between scholastic and devotional writing. Scholastic writing turned its spotlight upon human history and the manner in which it affected the present. Paradise, the Fall, and its consequences were the central foci of scholastic inquiry. Even when scholars turned their attention to hell, it was in order to discuss such abstruse subjects as the exact location of hell, the suffering of demons, and the particular divisions in hell. When it came to pain, they contented themselves with repeating Augustine and Gregory the Great. The significant addition was the extra stress upon the soul's role in sensing pain. The original idea, however, was not new.

In contrast, devotional literature is full of imaginative and creative depictions of hell. Little time was spent upon Adam and Eve, paradise, and the Fall. After all, spilt milk helped nobody avoid the terrible future awaiting most of humanity. Describing hell in the most terrifying manner possible, weighing pain upon pain, preachers pointed their spotlight elsewhere. They addressed the living, and their interest lay in the future, not the past. Some did describe different partitions and sections in hell, as visionaries had, but their main emphasis was the suffering of the people involved.

The two different foci cover respectively the past and the future, with some comments upon the pains of present life. But scholars were intent upon explaining the phenomenon, while preachers were more interested in instilling in their audiences the impact of the past upon their own personal future. This is not to say that there was no mixing of the two streams of writing: after all, the same people were often involved in both activities.

The focus was the main, but not the only, difference between the two disciplines. When scholars discussed pain, they sought in the Aristotelian manner to achieve a general understanding of a universal phenomenon. Pain might be stronger or weaker, be of different types, and have different effects, but all scholars, be they lawyers, theologians, or physicians, axiomatically assumed that when they spoke of pain they were all sharing the same idea. In religious experience, the opposite was true; no two pains even belonged to one category. Each pain was unique, and so was each sufferer—hence the patient enumeration of sections and punishments in hell, hence the personal element introduced by visitors. Preaching treatises (and, presumably, the preachers in their wake) treated pain as laypeople had always felt it: intransmissible, unique, personal. The objective voice saw generalities; the subjective one, the individual.

CHAPTER SEVEN

Human and Divine Passion

The incarnation of Christ, son of God and the New Adam, betokened the creation of a new, unique type of man. His form and essence were destined never to be replicated, nor was his pain. However, all postincarnational history of human sensations was colored by his experience. His was the perfect body with the perfect, most sharply tuned sensations. All that preceded or followed was no more than a pale simulacrum, to be measured against the absolute yardstick of the Crucifixion. Even martyrdom, to say nothing of more widely experienced human sufferings, paled in comparison. When it came to pain, the Passion was the ultimate extreme of living agony. Only the pangs of hell were worse.

In the following, I shall survey and analyze two trends of writing concerning Christ's pain. The first, scholastic thinking, has received little attention until now. In contrast, devotional thoughts, emotions, and meditation practices concerning the Crucifixion have already been studied in detail, and I rely upon previous work as well as my own reading of the sources. It is important to stress that these were not two disparate spiritual concerns despite the fact that most outstanding popular preachers were not professional scholars, and there were many concerns and ideas that belonged specifically to one realm or another. The sermons of Bernardino of Siena, for example, owed little or nothing to the tradition of the schools. Nevertheless, what we have is more in the nature of a spectrum than a clear division. Among the multiplicity of forms and ideas, the figure of the suffering Christ, as known to the later Middle Ages, coalesced in forms unknown to previous centuries.

In each discipline, writers attempted to outdo their predecessors in detailed and vivid imagining of the pain of Christ's Passion. Thirteenth-century generalizations grew into fifteenth-century comprehensive listings of pains, stretching back into Christ's life from the very moment of his conception. Devotional works show the gradual growth of Christ's pain far more explicitly than scholastic works, the latter being more prone to careful adherence to sources and traditions.

Scholasticism

Although arguments concerning Christ's nature formed the basis of some of the most acrimonious disputes in late antiquity, the question did not exercise the minds of many thinkers before the twelfth century. To a large extent, scholastic thought grew out of commentaries upon Peter Lombard's *Sententiae*. Specifically, the discussion centered on book 3, questions 15–16, which concerned those human defects that Christ had assumed upon incarnation. In addition, numerous questions, both disputed (*disputatae*) and quodlibetal, treated the nature of Christ, his senses, his body, and his Passion. The material of both these types of arguments forms the basis of this section.[1]

The early medieval argument about Christ and his suffering had to do with incarnation rather than Passion. The argument was resolved in the West quite decisively during the fifth century, and Monophysite heresies were no longer pertinent there. But incarnation meant a great deal more than mere enfleshment. It meant real and total embodiment. Learned discussions included details of Christ's anatomy, such as nerves, bones, and muscles. For scholars who dealt extensively with what pain meant to human beings, the growing stress on Christ's humanity during the later Middle Ages posed numerous problems.

While devotion to the suffering Christ seems to have been part of monastic spirituality already in the eleventh century, theological arguments were another matter. Philip of Harveng (d. 1183) was probably one of the first to wrestle with the full meaning of Christ's human passibility. Philip was troubled by the same issues that were to plague Peter Lombard, namely, the problematic patristic heritage. Specifically, this meant Hilary of Poitiers's anti-Arian arguments, which negated any real suffering on the part of Christ.[2] Philip defended Hilary's position, mainly by stressing the one element that became crucial in the West: namely, the full willingness of Christ to suffer. At the same time, Philip insisted that Christ's passibility was fully human, albeit his divine freedom from the passions could have ensured his impassibility. Here is where Christ's will came into play: had he not willed to suffer, he would not have suffered. All the same, Philip insisted upon the extraordinary nature of Christ's humanity: human he might have been, but he was also a God and miraculously born of a virgin. Consequently, Philip saw Christ's suffering as an extranatural miracle.[3] These issues remained constant points of argument in the following centuries.

Philip was an obscure twelfth-century Premonstratensian abbot, and his ideas had little impact. The systematic theology of Christ's human and divine pain begins with the writings of Anselm of Canterbury. As Gillian Evans has shown, Anselm was one of a group of contemporary monastic writers who composed prayers and meditations.[4] Anselm's work spans the gap between monastic devotional meditation and the early scholastic analysis.[5] In *Cur Deus homo* Anselm redefined the debt that humanity owed Christ for his sacrifice. His work was vastly influential not only in practices of prayer but in academic arguments defining orthodox theology. The treatise spells out fully Christ's consent and free will in suffering crucifixion, as well as Christ's potential and real passibility.[6]

Hugh of Saint Victor also wrestled with Christ's passibility, but from another point of view. Given that Christ had divine knowledge and will, why did he recoil from his ordeal? Hugh's answer relied on the four different wills that existed in Christ, among them the human will, identified with the weakness of the flesh.[7] Altogether, most twelfth-century thinkers were not very deeply involved in the question of Christ's pain. Anselm's ideas caught on mainly in the realm of devotion, not of theology. The great arguments concerning Christ's suffering belonged to the second half of the thirteenth and the first half of the fourteenth century and were ignited not by Anselm's thought but by the work of Peter Lombard.

When Peter Lombard (ca. 1100–ca. 1160/64) wrote his *Sententiae* around the middle of the twelfth century, he produced the first systematic and comprehensive text of medieval Western theology. The book was written in the burgeoning milieu of Parisian *studia* and had become the standard textbook for theology students by the thirteenth century. Within half a century, writing on this subject crystallized around the questions that the Lombard had raised, thus providing us with a solidly connected debate on the subject for two centuries. The same questions arose also in disputed questions and treatises, and all of them form a coherent corpus. Here I concentrate on a small number, mostly from significant authors who were quoted by their students and successors. The repetition of the same arguments across the centuries is one indicator of the growing attention paid by scholasticism to Christ's pain.

In simple humans, it is the soul that suffers. What about Christ? Did an incarnate God feel pain as humans did? To answer this sort of question, scholars were forced into a thorough discussion of Christ's nature, his soul,

his will, and his body. But first of all, they needed to determine how precisely human Christ was. These questions were more than simple speculations. For example, if one had celebrated the Eucharist during the *triduum*,
did the Eucharistic miracle take place? How could the bread and wine
become Christ's body and blood when that same body was dead in a grave?
    These questions gained a new urgency between the middle of the thir-
teenth and the middle of the fourteenth century. Scholars debated them
within the double context of the newly gained knowledge of Aristotelian
divisions of the human soul and the tradition of the Lombard. Beginning
with William of Auvergne's *De anima*, which stressed the complete unity
of body and soul,[8] continuing with the monumental midcentury works of
Thomas Aquinas, Alexander of Hales, Bonaventure, and Peter of Tarentaise
(1225–1276)—all near contemporaries—and culminating with the great
controversy of the turn of the century fought by John Pecham and his students, the debates concerning Christ's human suffering form a key element
in late medieval scholasticism. The same issues were continued among the
English nominalists and their Continental contemporaries in the early fourteenth century. In fact, they were still going on at the end of the fifteenth
century.
    By the latter decades of the thirteenth century the question had got-
ten touchy. The last decades of the thirteenth century saw at least four
condemnations of different scholastic opinions, two in Paris and two in
London.[9] In 1286 Archbishop John Pecham of Canterbury pronounced an
excommunication of any scholars who held that Christ's body—and all
bodies—remained substantially unaltered in life and death. If the human
body (Adam's, Christ's, or Pecham's) had a unique form, ineluctably tied to
its substance, what happened to dead bodies in their disintegration? What
happened at resurrection? All these arguments impinged upon the questions
of Christ's death and resurrection. The controversy raged on both sides of
the Channel, and Paris scholars became reluctant to discuss the question in
open debates.[10] Given the similarity of the arguments enunciated in commentaries, *summae*, and debates, many of which cited one another, it is
almost impossible to trace any coherent chronological development. In the
following, therefore, I shall treat the subject as a medieval scholar would
have done: by topic and argument rather than by strict periodization.
    In book 3, distinction 15, Peter Lombard asserted that Christ had taken
upon himself defects of the body and defects of the soul, but not all of them;
he had not taken on sin. All that Christ had accepted was of his own free
will, for he could presumably have taken on human form without its defects. Christ had taken on a passible soul and a passible body. His body

suffered hunger and thirst, like any other human body. His soul suffered sadness, fear, and pain. Thus, the soul suffered from passions, both directly and through the body.[11]

This particular passage was to have a peculiar history. In the best-established edition, the ability of the soul to suffer pain is inserted as a matter of fact. But thirteenth-century scholars saw a somewhat different version. In Alexander of Hales's glosses the text is much more sharply worded.[12] It had come to include a few sentences quoted from Augustine's literal exegesis of Genesis: "The flesh does not feel, but the soul, using the body as a tool. Just as the soul external to the body sees and hears through the body as if using a messenger to confirm in itself what is sent from outside. Thus, it feels through the body those ills that it would not feel without one, as hunger and thirst."[13] Peter then proceeded to asseverate that Christ had adopted these defects entirely of his own free will. As we shall see, most commentators relied upon a version identical or similar to the one used by Alexander of Hales in his gloss.

At this point Peter Lombard began examining patristic authorities on the subject of Christ's fully human nature. What he found was a series of contradictory opinions. Augustine, Ambrose, and Jerome had espoused both positions at different times.[14] Even assuming that Christ had genuinely suffered, how could he have been genuinely afraid, knowing that he would arise again within three days? The scholastic settlement of discordant sources relied upon a distinction between *propassio* and *passio*. The former was the apprehensive fear that preceded a painful ordeal and that indeed was lacking in Christ. The real pain of the Passion, however, was indeed present in him. His fear was not cowardice nor a yielding to passions but *timor*, an entirely different fear that foresaw and freely accepted the pain.

The following issue confronted Hilary of Poitiers. As we have seen, Hilary's views were a sore point with twelfth-century scholastics. Not only Philip of Harveng but also Peter Abelard brought up his problematic attempt to desensitize Christ's pain through his divinity.[15] Like his contemporaries and predecessors, Peter Lombard flatly denied that the Passion was a simulacrum, as Hilary had suggested. Distinction 16 returns to the voluntary sacrifice of the Crucifixion. There was no necessity for Christ to adopt suffering and death, but he had done so out of his free will.[16]

By the fifteenth century, Christ's humanity and passibility had grown far beyond the Lombard's fairly neutral statement. The influx of Aristotelian writing in the thirteenth century drew a new map of the human soul, raising questions as to which part of his soul Christ had suffered in. The growth of medical knowledge raised the question of his complexion. Most of all, the surge of devotional writing on Christ's life and Passion colored scholastic writing to a considerable extent.

The ones to systematically base the inquiry into Christ's suffering upon general human characteristics were Thomas Aquinas and Alexander of Hales. Both considered that first one needed to establish whether bodies and souls were passible (i.e., subject to passions). While Aquinas considered Christ's sufferings within the context of all souls, dead and alive, Alexander of Hales put Christ in the context of unique persons, together with Adam.[17] In both cases, the scholars began with the polysemous nature of the word *passio*.[18] Given the multiplicity of meanings, one could argue for different types of passibility and impassibility, depending on the meaning attached to the word at any specific time. Thus, when Thomas discussed the passibility of bodies, he argued that only corruptible, changing bodies could be considered passible.[19] There was no question that living souls could undergo *passio* in some inflected meanings, and all that remained to establish was the ability of souls separated from bodies to feel.[20]

The extent of Christ's humanity provided scholars with endless subjects to debate. Could he have been burned at the stake?[21] Godfrey of Fontaines (ca. 1250–1309) firmly maintained that any assertion to the contrary was close to heresy. Furthermore, Christ could have naturally aged, had he lived. Could he have generated progeny?[22] According to Giles of Rome, Christ had a perfect body and could thus have generated children, had such an activity been consonant with his dignity. When speaking of Christ's *body*, was it possible to be speaking of the same thing as when speaking of human bodies in general, or was "*corpus*" as polysemous as "pain"? Henry of Ghent argued this question in a dispute held on Christmas of 1286, and his answer is equivocal. On the one hand, all bodies were bodies, and Christ's body could be compared to Peter's as easily as Peter's to Paul's. All the same, Christ's humanity was not quite identical to all other people's, and his body was unique.[23] The one unusual phenomenon exhibited by Christ's body— sweating blood during the agony in the garden—also eventually received a natural explanation.[24]

The argument, brought up by John Pecham, resonates with contemporary medical ideas. True to Pecham's traditional stance, he asserted that the phenomenon was natural—for Christ, but not for other humans. Blood, too, was polysemous. When one spoke of blood, one referred to two different things: the liquid flowing in one's veins and the humor that made up roughly one-quarter of human complexion.[25] In Christ's case, three forces combined to make him sweat a mixture of both liquid and humor: the intensity of his anguish made blood concentrate around his heart, spread through his limbs, and come out as sweat; the strength of his imagination—and imagination was known to move the humors, especially in someone as supremely sensitive as Christ—caused the effusion. Finally, his noble complexion facilitated evaporation.

The possibility of Christ's soul was sometimes debated, but most often it was taken for granted. Had Christ's soul not been passible, at least in some of its parts, the Crucifixion would have lost its meaning. However, by the middle of the thirteenth century, the human soul had come to possess all the parts with which Aristotle had endowed it, and this, too, was a source of discussion. Did Christ feel the pain in the superior reason, or was it only in the sensitive faculty of the soul? It was Aquinas who provided the subtlest answers. Undoubtedly, all the inferior parts of Christ's soul suffered with the pain of his whole body. All his senses suffered: touch from the pain of the Crucifixion and wounds, sight from seeing his mother and disciple crying, smell from the putrefaction around him, hearing from the curses and laughter hurled at him, taste from the bitterness of the gall and vinegar. But he also suffered in the passions of the soul: the feeling of betrayal and desertion by Judas and Peter, of humiliation at the blasphemies hurled at him and the spoliation of his clothes, of sadness, fear, and weariness.[26] As for the superior reason, subjectively it did suffer, but in its passion for God it did not suffer.[27] Given that Christ's body could suffer, and that Christ's soul was both divinity and flesh, his body was passible, and thus that part of his soul that was tied to the body was equally passible.[28] On the whole, scholastics came down emphatically on the side of the human rather than the divine Christ. Christ had assumed a passible and corruptible human nature. In fact, were it not inconsonant with his dignity, he could just as easily have assumed a female form.[29] When he died, he was dead, truly and naturally, like other men.

But even the most extreme positions encountered the immovable argument that Christ's body was unique, like no other body. This point came up in the discussion of Gethsemane. The final element that made Christ sweat blood was a motif repeated by many other scholars: Christ's complexion. His was the most perfect, the most tender, the most noble complexion. Christ was *optime complexionatus*, of the best and most balanced complexion possible, and this made the effusion of sweaty blood possible. Though all three explanations stay strictly within the boundaries of a natural body, the third one strays dangerously close to those boundaries. Christ was not comparatively better than other humans; he was superlatively and absolutely better.

The perfectly and uniquely equal complexion of Christ recurs often in scholastic writings. Bonaventure and Thomas Aquinas in the thirteenth, Durand de Saint-Pourçain and John Duns Scotus in the fourteenth, and Gabriel Biel (ca. 1420–95) in the fifteenth century all discussed this aspect.[30] The scholars who had originally raised the subject were baffled by the historical (but religiously irrelevant) fact that crucifixion was hardly unique in antiquity, and that several martyrs had died in equally grisly fashions. The explanation for Christ's unique suffering, therefore, had to come from his own nature rather than from the punishment he had suffered.

Since pain came through the sense of touch, which was necessarily aware of humors and changes in the body, equality of complexion was necessary for bodily perfection. The better complexioned the body, the better the soul perceives the pain, and Christ's was the best-complexioned body of all, for it was formed directly by the Holy Ghost. Its human element came only from the Virgin's purest blood.[31] Given that the Virgin, too, had been immaculately conceived, this blood was like no other human blood. Since Christ was also perfectly perceptive, his perception of pain was the most acute of all. The same perfect complexion that had granted Adam his immunity from pain made Christ's pain greater than all other pains in the world.[32] The apparent contradiction between the two bothered nobody, as both Christ and Adam were compounds of nature and will, body and soul, and the hierarchy of forces in each one affected their sensations. Adam's lack of pain stemmed from his immunity to disease. Christ's sensitivity to pain stemmed from the dominance of his will over his sensations, and Christ had willed to suffer. Finally, in addition to an acute perception and a perfect complexion, one had to consider Christ's age at the time of his death. The vigor of a man in his prime exacerbated the pain.

There was more to the disposition for suffering in Christ than the equality of complexion. "It is established that there was something hurtful to the body's temper in Christ, because it was sensed by way of touch, which was most temperate in Christ; therefore, it was followed by real pain," claimed Durand de Saint-Pourçain.[33] If one were to draw a line from prelapsarian Adam to the present, fallen state of humanity, Christ would be in the middle. In Adam, both nature and will controlled the passions, and thus he was impassible. After the Fall, the situation was reversed, and in postlapsarian humanity the passions, including pain, control both nature and will. Christ had voluntarily submitted his nature to pain, but at the same time, his nature did control his will.[34] In the hierarchy of human nature Christ was less perfect than Adam because he had deliberately chosen to be so.

Perfect as he was, Christ possessed human defects. As we have seen, Peter Lombard attributed to Christ a careful selection of defects. The Lombard's followers, however, nuanced his assertions. Thus, Aquinas distinguished between two types of passions: indetractable passions, such as hunger, thirst, fatigue, and pain, could not be affected by grace. Christ did not assume detractable passions, such as a tendency toward evil. Thus far, Thomas had done no more than follow his predecessors. However, he added another category of defects that Christ had avoided: diseases that corrupted the body—leprosy, blindness, fever.[35] When it came to choosing and discarding passions, Thomas added his own insights. Thus, anger had definitely been excluded from Christ's soul, but Thomas insisted that Christ did possess righteous, zealous anger. Similarly, although Christ grieved because of his betrayal, he did not grieve for himself. He also possessed *timor*, in the sense of a virtue, not a vice.[36]

Other contemporary scholastics took up the same problem. Alexander of Hales, Bonaventure, Robert Kilwardby, and Matthew of Acquasparta all discussed the passions of Christ's soul.[37] All of them made subtle distinctions within the different passions, creating an entirely new set of subcategories within the generality of passions. What emerges from this inquiry is a double set of distinctions. The first was a more detailed profile of Christ's soul. Second, these distinctions were valid for human emotions, creating an entirely new vocabulary of emotions that were ethically charged according to intent.

The existence of defects in Christ, as well as his passibility, posed a difficult question for all scholars. Had Christ been purely human, the possession of defects would have been natural. Had he been purely divine, the possession of defects would have been inconceivable. In a faith that claimed full humanity and full divinity, Christ's pain needed to be justified. And the answer lay in the will. The main reason for Christ's total suffering was his will to suffer. Christ had *contracted* defects; he had assumed them voluntarily and selectively. Christ had undertaken nothing against his will. We all suffer whether we wish to or not, but Christ had chosen to do so.[38] Indeed, centuries earlier Hilary's speculation that, since Christ had freely undertaken suffering, "it was as though he had not suffered,"[39] was resoundingly rejected by all his Western interpreters, Peter Lombard first among them. Choice did not ease the pain, for if it did, the whole point of pain would be gone.

Nevertheless, like any other human being, Christ suffered from conflicting wishes. In principle, he acknowledged the need and justice of the Crucifixion, but he could not avoid recoiling from the inevitable pain. Walter

Chatton instanced the case of a merchant at sea who sees a storm coming. He does wish, quite absolutely, to throw his merchandise overboard to save his life, but conditionally, were there no storm, he wishes to keep it. In a case of conflicting absolute and conditional wills, the conflict might be a cause of pain.[40]

The effects of crucifixion upon such a supremely sensitive nature, coupled with a will to suffer, were devastating in their intensity. Nails placed precisely at the nerve centers of hands and feet, "which broke up the continuity of the body parts," the body's weight, and the long agony made his pain worse than that of any of the martyrs. But body and soul were intertwined, and Christ suffered more than bodily agony. Opinions were divided as to whether Christ suffered in his rational, as well as his sensual, soul, but the argument did not minimize his pain in any way. His suffering was caused by total sensual pain in all five senses (not only touch) and by the grief of betrayal.[41] Walter Chatton trenchantly added that Christ suffered a maximum pain, for he was paying the maximum penalty for the ultimate sin.[42]

The demarcation line between sensual and emotional pain always being vague, in this case it disappeared altogether. Even Gabriel Biel, who firmly restricted the meaning of *dolor* to sensual pain, expatiated vividly on Christ's *tristitia*, which definitely touched upon his superior soul—not for his own fate or pains but for the sins and fate of humanity.[43] Thus, Christ suffered in both senses.

By the fifteenth century, Biel could trace Christ's entire life as one long story of pain and misery.[44] Biel's meditation on Christ's life from the point of view of its end is unique in the history of scholastic writing. Rarely did academics apply creative imagination to a commentary on the *Sententiae*. Biel was combining here scholastic analysis with a totally different but connected genre: the biographical meditation on the life of Christ. In fact, Biel the scholar was plagiarizing Biel the preacher. The narrative was taken verbatim from one of his own sermons. What remains remarkable, in the scholastic context, is not the meditation but the fact that Biel transposed it to a scholastic commentary on the *Sententiae*.

The cogitations of some scholars sound bloodless and devoid of sympathy compared to the emotional words of sermons, meditations, and visions. Yet, as in Biel's case, often it was the same men who wrote in both veins. The scholastic discourse was not meant to arouse grief and empathy (*compassio*), it was meant to bring clarification and understanding. Despite the dispassionate tone of scholastic discussions, it is easy to find themes that recur in other types of literature. Some of their thoughts were drawn from medicine; others echoed didactic literature. But one thing remains clear: in attempting to understand Christ and his suffering, scholars had constructed an entire historical human psychology and physiology. From the twelfth to the fifteenth century, Western scholasticism took the theme of Christ's Passion and developed it in minute detail. Every possible option of pain of body and soul was dissected, and every possible descriptor analyzed in every possible meaning. From Adam to the postlapsarian world, scholastics had traced the changes in humanity, placing the startling anomaly of Christ in the middle. Unsurprisingly, the history of human sensations mirrored the history of the world, for man, as everyone knew, was a microcosm.

The great emotional upsurge of Passion devotion during those same centuries was closely linked to the scholastic literature. The science of theology provided the solid basis upon which preachers and mystics could build their own pictures. The proliferation of detail, so typical of scholasticism, was visible first in the written works of meditation and later in the pictorial, literary, and musical works that covered the same theme. Without the scholastic basis, the culture of the Passion could not have grown so coherently.

From Passion to Culture of Pain

The cult of the Passion is the cornerstone of the late medieval culture of pain. The centrality of Christ's suffering in late medieval spirituality is so outstanding, and has been so thoroughly studied in recent decades, that it requires no basic discussion. The research on Passion iconography, Passion literature, Passion meditations, and all other expressions of Western Christian concern with the Crucifixion forms an entire field in and of itself.[45] Whether the cult of the Passion grew out of a general context or was the cause of all other related cultural phenomena, it affected all other fields of emotional, cultural, and scientific production. Even jurists and physicians, whose interest in pain was entirely human and prosaic, always carried within their consciousness the knowledge that there was more than one type of pain, more than the phenomenon they confronted on a daily basis.

Those who thought about the Crucifixion imagined all sorts of sources for Christ's pain. When he was arrested, Christ's hair and beard were pulled. He was so much spat upon that he looked like a leper. While he was carrying the cross, children pelted him with stones. Before being raised on the cross, Christ's entire body had been stretched to fit the prepared nail holes, so that all his bones were dislocated.[46] The nails were driven into the most sensitive nerve centers of his body, and his weight made the pain much worse. Finally, Christ bled profusely, waves and rivers of blood: first from the flagellation, then from the crown of thorns, then from the wounds in his hands and feet, and finally from the wound in his side (though that one had been inflicted after his death). He bled so much that not a drop of blood was left in his body.[47]

This vision of Christ had not always been predominant. Though Christ's human suffering was an integral part of Christian orthodoxy from the fifth century onward, much of the art and poetry written to praise him before the eleventh century portrayed Christ as a majestic, powerful ruler. Even Carolingian crucifixes did not attempt to show suffering.[48] An anonymous fourth-century poetic life of Christ hailed him as king; it lavished a great deal of attention and detail on his royal conception, birth, and ministry. The Crucifixion was mentioned in one line only: "The death of the flesh which he undertook vanquished everyone's death." Five centuries later, Bishop Theodulf of Orléans still voiced the aristocratic views of his circle by repeatedly calling Christ king in his hymns and stressing his royal lineage.[49] The Passion was given short shrift: that Christ had suffered pain and ignominy, and had expressed his feelings, was inconceivable. Though a cult and a theology of the Passion existed in Carolingian times, the Crucifixion was often seen as a victory. "The dominant idea is the triumph of the new Adam revealed in the cross, the tree of life."[50]

As Rachel Fulton has shown in her magisterial book, the cult of the suffering Christ emerged before the thirteenth century. By the eleventh century meditation about the Passion was rife in reform monastic circles, and by the early twelfth century, it had become central to clerical piety.[51] How far it had penetrated lay circles is impossible to tell, however. In the later Middle Ages the suffering Christ appeared even in courtly culture: in illuminated books for royalty, in sermons addressed to rulers and noblemen, and in carefully planned artistic programs of great chapels.[52] Whether high or low, cultural artifacts of the later Middle Ages portrayed a suffering Christ unfamiliar to the earlier centuries.

The new figure was constructed by many forces and ideas. A great deal came from twelfth-century theology, but part of it emerged from the devotional activities of pastors, preachers, and visionary nuns and friars, and much of it, undoubtedly, grew spontaneously among common people, who were now exhorted to interiorize their religion. They did so by connecting with the one sensation they surely shared with Christ: pain. The result was an outpouring of creativity that even Erich Auerbach could not master in one work.[53] The theater, music, literature, and paintings of the Passion are enough to fill entire libraries. Here I am concerned with one topic only: how the sensation of pain was transmitted to readers and audiences through written and spoken means. All such sensations were utterly individual, but Christ, being both human and divine, possessed sensitivities that transcended any human experience or capacity for complete comprehension. Different genres occasionally transmitted different messages, but the new Christocentric religiosity of the later Middle Ages, centered on pain, runs through all of them.

The functions, form, and purpose of the various genres differed from each other. Going from the most public to the most private, one ought ideally to begin with sermons, for they were the most common and most powerful means for delivering Christ's pain to the laity. While we have only the live sermons of a few outstanding figures, preaching manuals formed the connecting link between scholastic theology and sermons. They first appeared in the thirteenth century, proliferating throughout the later Middle Ages.

Authors of manuals usually ignored the chronological order of the Passion narrative in order to concentrate on the points the preacher might later, during the sermon, wish to stress and expand. Thus, they set out the Passion in a strict thematic order. Jacobus de Voragine, who could be quite emotional in his sermons, was factual and restrained in the *Legenda aurea,* a model legendary:

> There were five causes for the pain. First, because the Passion was shameful. This was due to the shamefulness of the place, because criminals were punished on Calvary. Because of the shameful punishment, for he was condemned to a most disgraceful death, as the cross was the penalty of thieves. . . . Because of the shameful company, for he was placed with the disgraced, that is, with thieves. . . . Second, because it was unjust. . . . Third, because it was [due] to his friends. . . . Fourth, because of the tenderness of his body. . . . Fifth, because it was universal, in all parts and all senses.[54]

This division is common throughout Passion literature. It echoes precisely the words of Thomas Aquinas in the *Summa theologiae* on the Passion.[55] Given that Jacobus was a fellow Dominican and that he kept reviewing and editing the *Legenda aurea* until his death, he undoubtedly knew Parisian theology. A century later John Bromyard (d. ca. 1352) echoed the dry manual mode:

> First, the manner is shown. Second, the magnitude. Third, the fittingness or necessity. Fourth, the usefulness or efficacy; fifth, that the evil ultimately lack this usefulness; sixth, that we should show our gratitude

for his suffering and dying for us; seventh, what the thankless resemble; eighth, what extent of punishment is deserved; ninth, some themes are inferred concerning the fittingness of the Passion's timing.[56]

Subjects were discussed by the scholastic question-and-answer method. The *quaestiones* are almost indistinguishable from scholastic texts to preachers' manuals. They were obviously transposed lock, stock, and barrel from one genre to the other. Was Christ's pain the greatest ever suffered? Yes, it was the worst pain ever suffered by a human on earth, but the worst of Christ's suffering was his sorrow for perfidious humanity. Both his body and his soul suffered, and his suffering was exacerbated by two factors: his perfectly balanced complexion and his pure and tender human nature, derived entirely from his virgin mother. Christ had suffered in all his senses and all the parts of his body, and his suffering was essential for human salvation.

Such a text was deliberately dense. It was meant to aid the preacher, not to move the public. Manuals contained a solid theological base and as little emotion as possible. Bromyard's *summa* provided material for dozens of different sermons. In reality, no preacher would have attempted to preach this material without injecting some emotion or exemplum. Anyone wishing to preach on the Passion might have done well to consult Chobham or Bromyard as one would consult an encyclopedia, to get the facts right. At the same time, a sermon based solely on dry facts would promptly have put an audience to sleep. It would have had no emotional appeal and would have evoked no pain or sympathy, and thus, as a tool of oratory and empathy, it would have been useless.

Obviously, much material vanished on its way from manual to actual sermon. Such was the fate, for example, of Christ's perfect complexion. One of the ways of explaining sensations, to this day, is to rely upon "scientific facts." Human sensations, it appears, lie in the province of the experts of the body, or physicians. Consequently, when treating the Passion, preachers' manuals and model sermons often referred to physiological causes for Christ's pain, borrowing his optimal complexion from scholars. However, no real sermons dwelled extensively on Christ's optimal humoral balance as a factor in sensing pain. It was far more appealing to speak in superlatives of a pain nobody else could ever experience than to explicate Galenic medicine. The idea that this pain was unique because of well-balanced humors would hardly have triggered an emotional response.

Another theme that did not survive transition was the uniqueness of Christ's pain in comparison to other crucified victims. Late medieval preachers were speaking to people who had seen various types of executions but nothing remotely resembling a crucifixion or a martyr's death. Unlike scholars familiar with Roman punitive practice, they had no reason to doubt that crucifixion was unique and far worse than any other punitive death. Speaking of physical instruments of the Passion—ropes, hammer, nails, whips—made a great impact. Hence, in sermons to the laity it was unnecessary to stress Christ's uniqueness among a host of crucified sufferers familiar to scholars.

In contrast, the strand that followed the impact of suffering upon each one of Christ's five senses did cross over from scholasticism via manuals to sermons. Since the punishment Christ bore was for all the crimes of humanity, justice demanded that it be paid through all of Christ's body:

> Thus, he made restitution in all his members and parts of his natural body. And just as man sins through all his senses, he who wished to give satisfaction for the sake of humans was punished in all his senses. . . . The head, whose beauty had no end, was crowned with thorns. The face that angels wished to look upon was spat upon by Jews. The ears used to listening to the singing of angels heard the blasphemies of the Jews. Both feet and hands that were joined to the world's ruler were affixed to the cross. His taste was afflicted with gall and his eyes with his mother's pain, so that by suffering he healed the sin our first parents and others had committed in all their senses and parts.[57]

This particular quotation comes from a preachers' manual, but almost exact replicas can be found spanning the spectrum from the scholastic writings of Thomas Aquinas to live Passion sermons of popular preachers.[58] These were the bones upon which a sermon could be structured.

The structure of sermons took a definite shape during the thirteenth century, but the vernacular ones that have survived manage to hide their structure under highly emotional and lively narratives. Most written sermon texts about the life and death of Christ were still fairly close to scholastic models. Jacobus de Voragine's Lenten sermons are typical. They are unemotional expositions of the Gospel texts, citing earlier interpretations of symbolic meanings. Nowhere in this series of sermons does Jacobus enter into an extravagant description of Christ's sufferings and the drama of the Crucifixion, nor does he contribute one iota from his imagination.[59] They are far less detailed in personal drama than even his chapter on the Passion in the *Legenda aurea*.[60] Obviously, these written sermons were not meant to be read aloud verbatim.

Vernacular preached sermons (whether written out or *reportatae*) were completely different. For example, the words of Jean Gerson, rector of the University of Paris and one of the foremost theologians of the early fifteenth century, could move crowds. His vernacular sermon on the Passion of Christ is a masterpiece of re-creation and active imagination. Thus, when Christ bid his mother goodbye on Maundy Thursday:[61]

Alas, what a parting that was. "Goodbye, my beautiful son," you, audience, might say. O sweet and most beautiful mother [who said]: "Goodbye, my only joy and comfort. I will never see you here again." Thus saying or perhaps keeping silent, only [expressing her feelings] in sighs, groans, and weeping (as I might religiously think), embrace your son . . . who is going to be killed. . . . You embrace him tenderly and lean your weeping face on his shoulder or on his chaste visage and then recover your strength. And you begin: "Alas, my son, also my father, my lord, and my glorious God . . . I beg you, I, your desolate mother . . . have mercy on this mother and stay for this evening here with us in Bethany, so that you avoid the fury of the traitorous Jews who wish to deliver you to death."

Martha, Mary Magdalene, and the apostles all cried at the leave-taking in Bethany. The preacher, not content with their overt gestures, wishes to plumb the hearts of the participants in the Passion drama: "But I would really like to know what you felt, O traitor, disloyal Judas . . . what was your heart, your look when you looked and saw such bitter complaints? O heartless heart . . . how did you dare appear that day; tell me, Judas, did you dare look at him?" And why, he asks, did Mary Magdalene, who knew of Judas's contacts among the priests, assume that those contacts were intended to mollify the priests and lessen their hostility to Christ? "O Mary Magdalene, you do not know how things really are. You are speaking to him who is the means of all the evil and mischief." And why, complains Gerson, do the Gospels, so irritatingly, tell us so little about what Mary felt and did during the Crucifixion? Did not the angel who comforted Christ in Gethsemane also comfort his mother?[62] When Christ could no longer carry his cross, did not his mother and the Magdalene offer to carry it for him?

You, devout Christian people, would indeed wish to know, I believe, where was the piteous and aching mother of Our Lord during this time of harsh need, of mortal and unjust sentencing, of injurious blasphemies and villainous deeds against her innocent and blessed son. And since I have no certain scripture, I will use credible conjectures as at the beginning, not presuming to assert [the veracity of the tale], but in order to move you to religious devotion.[63]

All this is imaginative preaching at its best, but interspersed with these vivid re-creations is some solid theological dogma, prayers, and Gospel texts. Gerson knew that some people argued that Christ was God and therefore did not suffer at all, and thus there is no need for Christians to mourn or pity him. This, said Gerson, is an illusion. Indeed, according to his divinity, Christ was immortal and impassible, but even so he was also man and had suffered, though voluntarily, the greatest pain any man had ever suffered: "If the pain of infernal punishment were not so terrible, why would justice inflict such suffering on the Son of God in order to deliver us from that punishment?"[64]

Gerson had not invented the imaginative re-creation. Two generations earlier, Bernardino of Siena had speculated in a similar manner:

I think that the Magdalene, seeing him depart from [Bethany] to Jerusalem, begged sweetly that he should not go for fear that he would be killed, and said to him: "How can I manage without you, my sweet comfort?" . . . And the Virgin Mary, I think . . . said: "O, my little son [figliuolo mio], don't go." Her emotions pushed her, and with great love she opposed his going, but her reason was content. Think of the prayers of Martha, Lazarus, and the other disciples, all begging him not to go to Jerusalem.[65]

Even charismatic preachers needed mnemonic aids to help their public retain the story. The twelve pains of Christ were a useful way to structure a sermon. The list was not necessarily the same everywhere, but the number, twelve, was a constant. Bernardino of Siena constructed the entire story of the Passion around the twelve pains, counting as the first pain the leave-taking at Bethany and ending with Christ's five wounds as the twelfth. Gerson first told the detailed narrative and then provided a succinct list. In contrast with Bernardino, his list is more thematic than narrative, stressing shame rather than physical pain or grief. Divestiture of clothing was one pain, nudity another, and mock royal clothing a third of his twelve pains. Was Christ naked on the cross, or did Mary cover his loins with a veil?[66] Pelbart of Themeswar, a later Hungarian Franciscan, began the list with the total of Christ's pains and ended with Christ's grief over his mother's pains.[67] In any case, listeners remembered that there were twelve pains during the Crucifixion:

> Take [the question of] how very painful was the Passion of Christ. I am afflicted, he says. He was afflicted by twelve separate pains. The first pain that Christ had was from his mother, from his disciple Mary Magdalene, from Martha and Lazarus and the others who were there. . . . The second pain that Jesus had was on Maundy Thursday. . . . [The Last Supper] . . . the third pain. It follows that after Christ's words it was already evening, and he left Jerusalem with his disciples. . . . [The agony in Gethsemane].[68]

Mnemonic numbering came up several times during Crucifixion sermons. Thus, during the flagellation, Christ received 5,865 wounds, and while on the cross, he received five.[69] Mary had seven swords stuck into her.[70] These ostensibly finite numbers served both as mnemonic aids and as an indicator of an infinity of suffering.

These details were born, not in the minds of fifteenth-century preachers, but in those of thirteenth-century monastic authors. Three anonymous texts, attributed to the Venerable Bede, to St. Anselm, and to St. Bernard, provided the basic narrative. Two, Pseudo-Bede and Pseudo-Bernard, are entitled meditations, while the third is a dialogue between Pseudo-Anselm and the Virgin, using her as a witness who recounts the Crucifixion.[71] Those meditations, meant for monks, gave the detailed picture of the Crucifixion that was destined to become common knowledge two centuries later.

Parallel to the meditations upon the Passion, the late thirteenth century saw the birth of a new genre, also destined to flesh out sermons eventually. Lives of Christ, written by Franciscans at first, appeared and quickly became popular. One of the notable early ones was Ubertino da Casale's (1259–1325) controversial *Arbor vitae crucifixae Jesu*.[72] As a leader of the Spiritual Franciscans, Ubertino's aim was to assert Christ's absolute poverty and the position of Francis as his heir, but most of his text was still a straightforward biographical re-creation of Christ's life and death, with an extensive section on the Passion.

The biographies added a new element. Christ's body was heir to the Holy Ghost and to a virgin woman. Women's bodies, according to several thirteenth-century preachers, were more tender, and hence more sensitive, than men's, and virgins were the most sensitive of all. Thus, though male, Christ partook of the pain sensitivity of virgin women, and he was the most tender and most virginal of all: "When something is more tender, thus it

suffers more severely. There was never a body as sensitive to suffering as the
Savior's body. The woman's body is tenderer than that of a man. Christ's
flesh was totally virginal, for he was conceived of the Holy Ghost and born
of a virgin. Thus Christ's passion was the sharpest of all, for he was tenderer
than all virgins."[73] This is one of the most interesting statements concerning Christ's gendered nature. Caroline Bynum has shown Christ as mother,
feeding his children.[74] This, however, is Christ the virgin, a Christ whose
entire humanity derives from a virgin woman and partakes nothing of human maleness. Humbert de Romans (1200–1277), master-general of the
Dominican order, and Bonaventure of Bagnoreggio, minister-general of the
Franciscans, preached the same idea roughly during the same midcentury
years. Such was the impact of Bonaventure's Christological writing that one
of the most popular biographies of Christ, the *Meditaciones vite Christi,*
was attributed to his pen.

When the Franciscan John of Caulibus, probably the real author of the
Meditaciones vite Christi,[75] reached the Crucifixion, he followed Christ
from his arrival at Gethsemane all the way to the removal of his body from
Calvary, re-creating and detailing each stage. He was also responsible for
adding several sources of pain to the Crucifixion, such as the stretching of
his arms and legs to fit the allotted spots on the cross.[76] As we shall see, the
main departure from tradition in the *Meditaciones* was the idea of Christ's
entire life as Passion.

The *Meditaciones* earned translation into Italian and Middle English
and great popularity under the false attribution to St. Bonaventure.[77] It
was followed by an equally popular and much translated work, Ludolph of
Saxony's *Vita Jesu Christi.* Ludolph (d. 1378), a Carthusian, wrote his biography shortly after John of Caulibus had written his. He was following the
Meditaciones as a genre of detailed biography, but his work was far more
comprehensive and sophisticated than that of his Franciscan predecessor.
Ludolph incorporated all the patristic and exegetical explanations of each
phase of Christ's life. All explanations and meditations, from Augustine to
Bernard, found a place in his work.[78] Though encyclopedic in its scope, the
text is anything but dry and factual. The emotional appeal rang out loud and
clear: "Cry, therefore, mourn, and grieve, my soul, let your eyes pour tears,
let the pupils of your eyes not keep silent. . . . You will mourn if you consider the tears of the women . . . the tears of the sufferer, of his mother."[79]
The author moves easily from impersonal narrative to direct speech and appeal to the reader. The scope of the Passion had grown as well: where John
had a few pages for the Passion, one-fourth of Ludolph's *Vita* concentrated
upon it. By the end of the fourteenth century, most of Christ's life had be-

come a prelude to the Crucifixion, but the entire biography had also gained in detail and depth. If, during the early Middle Ages, the Crucifixion was a minor detail in God's human biography, during the later Middle Ages the entire life became a prologue to the Crucifixion. The themes enunciated in these biographies appear also in individual visions of devout laypeople.

Ludolph's biography was actually written as a meditational text. Private meditations became popular as instructional reading material. This popularity reveals the imaginary landscape of the Passion in the minds of many devout Christians all over Europe. The meditations were often phrased in a language that would not bear translation into painting, sculpture, or theater. Who, for example, has ever seen in visual art a naked Christ whose loins have been quickly covered by his mother's torn veil? Or a blood-smeared, disheveled, unveiled Pietà? Or a Holy Family in which both mother and baby are crying bitterly following a painful circumcision, each wounded by the other's tears? Such things could be told, even written. Apparently, they could not be painted.

Late medieval meditations were based upon the late-eleventh-century tradition of John of Fécamp and Anselm of Canterbury.[80] This tradition, fully analyzed by Fulton, contained several elements that were crucial to the spirituality of later centuries. First, the role of the Virgin and her sufferings was exalted beyond any precedent. Even more important was the careful cataloging of Christ's torments, one after the other. Mostly, these meditations were not meant as exercises in piety but, to quote Fulton, were meant "to forge new tools with which to *feel*" (italics in original).[81] The ardent wish to unite with Christ and Mary's pain, to sense it in one's own body, appears in the prayers and meditations of both writers.

The early-thirteenth-century pseudonymous works supply details later included in Passion narratives. In the wake of Anselm's own writing, the pseudonymous meditations adopted direct speech for Christ and his companions, thus putting the interlocutor in the midst of the scene: "You might think, if the lady his mother were there, what she would have done, and say in your heart: `O my lady, how is it that you do not wonder where your beloved son is going? O lady, what an evil, bitter day tomorrow will be for you, when you hear and see such a cruel spectacle."[82] Pseudo-Anselm's meditation is a dialogue with the Virgin, and it is she who asserts that none of the evangelists had told the whole tale, especially where her role was concerned.[83] This position of a putative witness allowed the authors to add details, such as a loincloth for Christ: "Thus, all naked he was raised and stretched on the cross. But his most loving mother wrapped her head-veil around the shameful place."[84] The extraordinary level of pain that Christ had suffered because of his nature appeared here, too, though not in medical terminology: "first, because he was delicately raised, as the son of a virgin born of a royal line, for the noble suffer more when hurt than the ignoble."[85] This analysis, so different from the medical diagnosis, had far more appeal.[86] Christ's bleeding, too, began to assume copious proportions. When he was raised on the cross all his wounds opened and the Virgin's clothes were all drenched. Furthermore, he continued bleeding after death.[87] All these elements, as we have seen, recur in late medieval Passion sermons.

Meditations on the Passion are often visualizations interspersed with prayers, following the Passion step by step. The meditation pursued the daily liturgical *horarium*, with the seven monastic hours paralleling the seven stages of the Passion: "You were beaten at matins, accused at prime, proclaimed at terce, condemned at sext, and at none you died with crying and tears."[88] This division has been found in the writings of monks and hermits already in the twelfth and thirteenth centuries. Goscelin, a twelfth-century monk, recommended this discipline to Eve, a woman recluse and his ex-disciple: "Devote all hours to the sufferings of Christ. Adore him caught and jailed at midnight, whipped in the morning, brought to the cross at terce, while they called together 'let him be crucified,' thus crucifying him with their tongues. Hung on the cross at sext, dead at none, buried at vespers."[89]

A person meditating on the Passion ought to consider six things, said Ludolph of Saxony: imitation, compassion, wonder, exultation, resolution, and rest. These were the shorthand code words pointing to many devotional practices, from the inducement of emotion to actual sensations. By the fourteenth century, meditations upon Christ's Passion had long transcended the boundaries of monasteries. In fact, even Suso had written his meditations in vernacular German but still included in the *Little Book of Eternal Wisdom* the five offenses that scholastics had counted.[90] Domenico Cavalca's *Lo specchio della croce* was written in Italian and repeated the same motifs.[91]

Passion narratives transcended also the boundaries of the written word. When the English visionary Margery Kempe arrived at Rome in 1417, she sought out the house in which St. Bridget of Sweden had lived.[92] The illiterate, devout Englishwoman knew of the Swedish visionary of Rome. This episode illustrates that, while visions were unexpected gifts for the few, they were carefully recorded and often transmitted from one country to another. Though Margery's own text has survived in one copy only,[93] many others received a much wider publicity. While each vision was intrinsically personal, their translation, transmission, and wide distribution attest to their wide acceptance and popularity. They were no longer just a call for identification: they were the proof that it was possible to feel what Christ and Mary had felt by dwelling on all of the details in order.

Visions were sometimes granted in the wake of strenuous spiritual exercise. Mystics who had undergone religious training, such as Heinrich Suso and Richard Rolle, followed the traditional ways of meditating on the Passion.[94] But sometimes visions simply came as the result of a prayer or in the wake of a severe illness. They also could appear freely, like grace, an unearned and undeserved gift. But very often visions were closely connected with sensory pain. As Julian of Norwich (1342–ca. 1416) testified, pain diagnosed as bodily illness preceded her vision:

> Ande when I was thryttye wyntere alde and a halfe, god sente me a bode-lye syekenes in the whilke I laye thre dayes and thre nyghttes; and on the ferthe nyght I toke alle my rychttinges of haly kyrke, and wenyd nought tylle haue lyffede tylle daye. And aftyr this y langourede furthe two dayes and two nyghttes, and on the thyrde nyght I wenede afte tymes to hafe passede, and so wenyd thaye that were abowte me. Botte in this I was ryght sarye, and lothe thought for to dye, botte for nothinge that was in erthe that me lykede to lyeve fore, nor for nothynge that I was aferede fore, for I tristyd in god. . . . And I was answerde in my resone and be the felynges of my paynes that I schulde dye; and I asentyd fully with alle the wille of mye herte to be atte god ys wille. . . . Aftyr this my sight by ganne to fayle, and it was alle dyrke abowte me in the chaumbyr, and myrke as it hadde bene nyght. . . . The maste payne that I felyd was schortnes of wynde and faylynge of lyfe. Than wende I sothelye to have bene atte the poynte of dede. And in this sodeynlye alle my payne was awaye fro me, and I was alle hole, and namely in the overe partye of my bodye, as evere I was before or aftyr.[95]

As she told it, Julian had not at first wished to die, for her worship of God had not been fully accomplished, but she had accepted her fate. After being shriven and prepared for death, miraculously her own pain was taken from her. Then she suddenly felt a desire to achieve *compassio* with Christ, and what she received, to her astonished delight, was indeed a series of direct visions of the Crucifixion:

> I sawe the rede blode trekylle downe fro undyr the garlande, alle hate, freschlye, plentefully and lyvelye, right as me thought that it was that time that the garlonde of thornys was thyrstede on his blessede heede. Ryght so, both god and man, the same sufferde for me. I conseyvede

treulye and mighttyllye that itt was hym selfe that schewyd it me with owtyn any meenn.[96]

The desire for *compassio* meant that mystics wished not only to be on Calvary as witnesses but to feel what all participants, Christ as well as his followers, suffered then.[97] All visionaries insisted upon the uniqueness and inexpressibility of their experience. Angela of Foligno (ca. 1248–1309) wished to be *compartecipe* in Christ's pain by sensing it in her own soul.[98] She wanted to know of a pain that nobody else knew (and nobody had therefore ever written or preached about) and in her frustration appealed to the Virgin to reveal to her "something of that pain of your son of which I have no memory, for you saw the Passion more than any saint," for "I see what you saw with the eyes of the head and with the imagination." When her prayer was answered, she screamed, "Is there no saint who could tell me anything about this Passion *of which I hear no speech, not a single word, which my soul sees,* and it is such that I cannot say? So much pain!" (my italics).[99]

Margaretha Ebner also began her visionary life with illness.[100] As she gradually came to see her illnesses and pains as an integral part of her spiritual experience, the spiritual agony left her, though she kept bearing her sickness for God. Thereafter, her bouts of inexpressible pain coincided with her spiritual experiences. Her pain came upon her usually on Fridays, most often near Easter.[101]

During the following Lent . . . I grew very sick . . . as if I had seen His most painful sufferings with my own eyes. . . . Until that time I had never yet perceived true suffering in my whole life. My pain and the bitterness of my sorrow were so great that I thought nothing more painful could ever have happened to another human being, and I do not wish to exclude St. Mary Magdalene.[102]

The personalization of pain, juxtaposing the visionary with Mary Magdalene (but not with the Virgin), made it clear that indeed Margaretha felt as though she had been at the foot of the cross in person.

For the visionaries, seeing pain was akin to sensing it. In fact, it was indeed sensing. No wonder, then, that all Margaretha could tell of her experience was that it had taken place, no more. It had not come verbally, and she could not translate the vision (in both meanings of the word) into words. Similarly, Julian of Norwich insisted that "Swilke paynes I sawe that alle es to litelle that y can telle or saye, for itt maye nought be tolde."[103]

Visions often had effects on the bodies of the visionaries. I have already mentioned that Colette of Corbie's face looked battered and disjointed on Fridays, when she meditated upon the Passion.[104] Margery Kempe's visions of the Crucifixion caused her to burst into tears, twisting and turning so that she looked very much like a madwoman in a fit. Indeed, some people claimed the devil had gotten into her:

> Befor hir in hyr sowle sche saw hym veryly be contemplacyon, and that cawsyd hir to have compassyon. And whan thei cam up on to the Mownt of Calvarye, sche fel down that sche mygth not stondyn ne knelyn, but walwyd and wrestyd wyth hir body, spredyng hir armys abrode, and cryed wyth a lowde voys as thow hir her schulde a brostyn asundyr, for in the cite of hir sowle sche saw veryly and freschly how owyr Lord was crucifyed. Beforn hir face sche herd and saw in hir gostly sygth the mornyng of owyr Lady, of Sn John and Mary Mawdelyn, and of many other that lovyd owyr Lord.[105]

The records of ecstatic visions were of tremendous importance not only for the visionaries (who had had the experience, after all) but for their confessors and readers. Some, especially women visionaries, encountered skepticism and hostility, but many transmitted in words, to the best of their abilities, their immediate experience of ultimate pain in sharing the Passion. For readers who could not follow the same route, it was at least a step closer to what they wanted, if not the real thing.

Late Medieval Innovations: Lifelong Suffering

The wealth of pain expressions in identification with Christ and Mary increased significantly during the later Middle Ages. While the seeds of identification with Christ were born in the eleventh century, several elements especially seem to have grown, if not *ex nihilo*, at least from very modest roots, into remarkably weighty themes. In what follows, I shall concentrate upon one new motif: Christ's lifelong suffering. This was an innovation to a world long used to hearing of Christ and Mary's royal ancestry and to seeing a dignified Virgin leaning her cheek upon her hand in an age-old, restrained gesture of sorrow.

The idea that Christ's life was one long series of sufferings first appeared in the thirteenth century. Pseudo-Bernard's meditation is probably the first to bring up the subject: "Always think of him, . . . living there in extreme poverty and need, and coming back from there [i.e., Egypt] with the greatest effort . . . later subject to his parents, he who ruled over all creatures . . . then starving and thirsting in the desert, he who is the bread of life and the source of wisdom."[106]

Shortly thereafter, Bonaventure, too, insisted upon the lifelong Passion, perhaps because of his wish to create parallels between Christ and St. Francis, his hero. The lifelong Passion appears in a sermon to nuns and in his *Mystical Vine:* "From the day of his birth to that of his death he was constantly in pain and passions." "All of Christ's life was an example and a martyrdom . . . how poverty-ridden in his abstinence, how lavish in his vigils, how frequent his prayers, his face marked with labor and sweat, how diligent at going through towns and castles preaching and curing everwhere. Often he suffered hunger and thirst."[107] Later meditations stressed the same point. The Dominican Domenico Cavalca, in his *Lo specchio della croce*, began the tale of Christ's suffering at his birth:

> At birth, he had no place in a room, which was in a stable; thus, he was put in the manger between the ox and the ass. . . . Living, he had no home, no place of rest, nor any possessions. Dying, he had such a narrow bed that he could not lean his head. . . . At birth, he needed clothing, but the Virgin Mary was on the road and was so poor and ill-dressed that she had nothing with which to make it. . . . During his life, he was deprived of necessities . . . he suffered hunger. . . . Thus, we must believe that in all his life he suffered great deprivation.[108]

Visionaries, too, began thinking of Christ's life of suffering during the thirteenth century. Angela of Foligno, who had had no formal education but was closely connected to Franciscans, referred to the lifelong Passion of Christ in shorthand, while recounting her visions: "He began his life on the cross, he continued on the cross, he ended on the cross." "All his life he carried an invisible cross because of the ineffable and continuous pain that he bore."[109] Later visionaries even spoke with Christ about the subject. Margaretha Ebner's devotion was largely centered upon the child Christ. Searching for pain in his infancy, she came up with his circumcision, "the shedding of his all-powerful, holy blood."[110] In her visions, she conducted dialogues with the child Christ, asking him about his birth, his poverty, and his circumcision. Christ acknowledged that he had suffered from the cold on the night of his birth, that he had been poor, that Joseph had had to use his hose for swaddling the newborn, and that he had cried bitterly (as had his mother) and had bled profusely during his circumcision.[111]

Parallel to its entrance into visionary writing, the lifelong Passion became a standard topos in lives of Christ. Thus, the pain Christ suffered at his circumcision first appeared in the life of Christ written by John of Caulibus:

> For he very early began to suffer for us. . . . Suffer together with him, and cry with him, because today the infant cried hard. While it is right for us to rejoice greatly over our salvation in the midst of these solemnities, it is also right for us to suffer with him and to grieve deeply over his hardships and pains. You have heard how great affliction and want he experienced at his birth. Among other things consider the fact that, when his mother placed him in the manger, she placed his head on some small stone with perhaps just a little straw in between. . . . One would suppose that she would have more willingly placed there a lavish pillow if she had had it, but since she had nothing else she could put, with heartfelt regret she placed that stone there. You hear also that he shed his blood today; for his flesh was cut by his mother with a little stone knife. Is it not fitting to suffer along with him? Surely so, and for our own sake as well. The boy Jesus cried out today because of the pain which he felt in his flesh; for he had real flesh subject to pain just as other people.[112]

The baby Christ cried quite often, "to illustrate the misery of human nature and to hide himself behind his human nature, lest the devil recognize him."[113] John of Caulibus painted a touching picture of a teenage mother, heartbroken at her baby's crying, standing there crying too, and Jesus reaching up to touch her face, begging her not to cry. She professed herself unable to stop as long as he kept crying, and thus, pitying his mother, he choked his sobs on a hiccup and stopped crying.

Though the theological meaning of the circumcision as a prefiguration of the Crucifixion appears already in the twelfth century, the pain was a fourteenth-century innovation.[114] The great detailing of Christ's lifelong Passion, however, belonged to a more learned source. Ludolph of Saxony's *Vita Jesu Christi* followed John of Caulibus's work, and it is undoubtedly Ludolph's detailed and highly popular description that influenced later northern writers:

> if we wish to tell all that Christ had suffered in the world, no matter how much it is, especially since all of Christ's life on earth was a Passion. . . . Beginning at his Nativity, look how poor he was born, lacking both

home and clothes, born instead in a dirty stable, laid in a manger on
meager hay before brute animals, wrapped in dirty cloths; on the eighth
day he was circumcised, and already began to pour out his blood for us;
from there, he was taken, fleeing from Herod's persecution, to Egypt;
coming back, he was subjected to his parents during his entire childhood
and adolescence and was undoubtedly brought up in great poverty. Later,
having arrived at the time of his disclosure, look how he chose, at a time
of greatest cold, to be immersed when baptized in freezing water and
how at the time of his forty-day fast he was tortured, and how he suffered the devil's temptations, how many injuries and slanders he often
suffered from the Jews. . . . See how hard he worked, preaching every day
in the Temple, in synagogues, going from city to city, from land to land,
spending the nights often in prayer, curing the sick, exorcizing the possessed, raising the dead, feeding the hungry multitude; and on top of it,
he was subject to the laws of nature and exposed to hunger, thirst, and
other human weaknesses, albeit without sin.[115]

Jan van Ruusbroec (1293–1381) wrote his mystical treatise *Die geestelijke*
brulocht (*The Spiritual Espousals*) roughly in the same years as Ludolph
wrote his *Vita Jesu Christi*. It is unclear whether he was imitating Ludolph
or whether they were both following the same tradition. All the same, the
similarity is significant:

For he began to suffer early, as soon as he was born; that (suffering) consisted of poverty and cold. He was circumcised and shed his blood; he
was brought to safety in foreign lands; he served Lord Joseph and his
mother; he endured hunger and thirst, disgrace and scorn, the arrogant
words and deeds of the Jews; he fasted, he watched, and he was tempted
by the devil. He was subject to everyone. He went from country to country and from city to city to preach the gospel with great labor and with
great zeal.[116]

In other works, Ruusbroec paid little attention to the life and death of
Christ, which for him was merely the first coming. Two more comings,
vastly more important, were destined to follow. However, when he summarized this first coming, he accorded equal attention to the Passion of life
as to the Passion of death, considering both of equal importance.

From lives of Christ, the theme moved to sermons in the fifteenth century. In Gerson's sermon on the Passion, Christ's lifelong suffering gained
some notice: "He began his childhood in poverty, in pain, in tears, in hun-

ger, in thirst, in cold, in foreign travel to Egypt, in vigils, in temptations, in reproaching the wicked, in mortal persecution."[117] Gerson's context was that of the Passion, not the Nativity, and therefore he passed over the pain of life quickly.

Fifty years later, Gabriel Biel repeated Ludolph almost verbatim in one of his sermons, adding a few flourishes of his own. The Virgin's womb had been too tight for Christ. The first thing he had smelled was the offensive stench of the stables. Then he had had to undergo circumcision, which had also caused him pain. Herod's malice and the exile to Egypt were super-imposed on the baby's sufferings. Later, he grew up with hard work, absti-nence, vigils "of which the Scriptures only speak in general," and subjection to his mother and putative father. His home was poverty-stricken; destitu-tion, hunger, and thirst dogged him all his life. Once he had left home, he had had to face the hardships of the desert, temptations, endless wander-ing along the road, preaching, persecution, expulsion, and stoning. All this, before the agony in the garden and the Passion had even begun. Biel's list added little to what others had already said. Christ's death may have been what mattered to him, but Christ's life of pain was a central point.[118]

What is remarkable about this thread is that it takes every single ele-ment in Christ's life and weaves it into a pre-Passion Passion. Gestation was Passion; so was Nativity; exile, ministry, preaching, and miracles were all Passion. Even the authority of his parents and the frigid waters of the Jordan were an insult, a suffering, a burden. The minute enumeration of all of Christ's early pains is an echo of an earlier meditational practice that utilized every single suffering of Christ during the Passion. When Biel fol-lowed Christ's pains beyond the cradle to the womb, noting how every ele-ment added to his discomfort, he was working even farther backward from the Crucifixion.[119]

The theme of a lifelong Passion was only one of many woven into the tapestry of late medieval Christocentric piety. Many others, such as the sig-nificant increase in Mary's role in Christ's life and death (stressed by several authors) and the growth of the blood cult, have already been researched and written. What emerges from the above is that devotion to the Crucifixion in the later Middle Ages, and specifically to Christ's pain, was a dominant theme in contemporary religiosity.

Conclusion

As a certain melody will appear hesitantly at first in a concert and then reappear and grow until it insistently takes over the music, themes almost imperceptible in the twelfth century become central to late medieval experiencing of the Passion of Christ. Christ's wounded side, the instruments of the Passion, and the crown of thorns—these elements, surrounding the increasingly sorrowful stance and expression of the crucified and witnesses, privilege the element of physical pain in the Crucifixion. Added to the infliction and expression of pain is the contrast between the body's livid pallor and the flowing blood, stressing his human vulnerability and passibility. This was not the realm of pictorial art alone: all of these elements appear first in contemporary writings.[120] Visionaries saw them in their ecstasies, monks and nuns meditated upon them, and the laity heard about them in sermons and saw Passion plays.[121]

To what extent were the scholastic and devotional strands interconnected? It seems that the points of contact are few. Where scholars stressed Christ's perfectly balanced complexion as the source of his uniquely acute pain, devotional writings stressed his virginal female origins. Where scholars concentrated upon Christ's five offended senses, preachers spoke of Christ's compassion for his grieving mother. Generally speaking, devotional writings, along with other expressive arts, went much farther in re-creating the Crucifixion.[122]

CHAPTER EIGHT

Impassibility

In a world where pain was ubiquitous, and in a culture that glorified the sensation of pain, the idea that some people might be immune to pain was strange and unnatural. Was it a mark of diabolical powers, madness (as Hippocratic writings claimed), or sanctity? As with all extraordinary phenomena, any of these three explanations could fit a specific case. If impassibility existed at all, it was definitely unnatural. This chapter deals with two groups of people who felt no pain when suffering torture: martyrs and hardened criminals. The one link between the two is the fact that both were subjected to judicial torture, and both were capable of resisting it. Whether this miraculous ability resulted from greatness (or harshness) of spirit or from an immunity to pain is hard to tell. Furthermore, as discussed in chapter 5, the vocabulary of martyrology infused late medieval and early modern torture tractates.

The perception of torture as intended to break the spirit (while leaving the body relatively unharmed) permeated martyrological literature in late antiquity, providing a spiritual answer to the martyrs' ability to withstand torture. In the later Middle Ages, however, people who resisted torture were regarded, not as heroes, but merely as stubborn and hardened.

The first Christian authority to make impassibility a goal for the training of monks was Evagrius Ponticus. According to his treatise *Praktiké*, the first stage of monastic life consisted in trying to reach *apatheia* through transcending the passions and vanquishing the senses. Evagrius's ideas resemble those of the earlier Stoics and imply no miraculous freedom from pain. Rather, he advocated the cultivation of detachment from the senses and the passions. The entire first part of his treatise consists of a training program meant to help the monk reach *apatheia*. The earlier stage, *encrateia*, is a regime of continence and perseverance.[1] Thus, abstention from food and drink extinguish concupiscence.[2] Continence and *anachôrêsis* (monastic withdrawal) thus led to a mastery first of the body and subsequently of the passions of the soul. *Apatheia* included mastery over one's thoughts and dreams as well as one's physical drives. The ultimate victory over the passions and the senses would lead to the disappearance of physical natural qualities in monastic bodies.[3]

Nowhere, from start to finish, did Evagrius refer to physical pain or the ability to master or transcend it. The one to turn a monastic training program into a crude caricature was Evagrius's opponent Jerome. Jerome damned Evagrius's work (referring to it as *Peri apatheias*) by misrepresenting it as an argument for total insensibility, which, he contended, was beyond human capacity: "Evagrius of Ibera in Pontus, who sends letters to virgins and monks and among others to her whose name bears witness to the blackness of her perfidy [i.e., Melania], has published a book of maxims on apathy, or, as we should say, impassivity or imperturbability—a state in which the mind ceases to be agitated and, to speak simply, becomes either a stone or a god." The letter to Ctesiphon in which this paragraph appears is an all-out attack against anyone who dared disagree with Jerome on any matter of dogma. The fact that Evagrius had evolved a very careful training program for monks, trying to surmount their passions, made little difference when Jerome was on the warpath. Seemingly, he objected more to Evagrius's association with Melania and Rufinus than to his concept of impassibility. Nevertheless, the denial of human impassibility remained in place. Though Jerome did not mention martyrs anywhere in this context, the implication would have been clear: martyrs did suffer, and acutely so.[4]

Nevertheless, Jerome's attitude reflects Western medieval ideas about sensations in general and pain in particular. The idea of nonsensation sat awkwardly with notions of pain as expiation for human sin. Even early medieval monastic circles (to say nothing of later ones) did not encourage *apatheia*. To the contrary, they encouraged feelings and sensations with a stress upon expressivity in words and actions.[5] As an ideal, one might practice impassivity, controlling emotional expressivity, but the achievement of impassibility was not one of the goals of Western holiness. In conjunction with Jerome's crude equation of impassibility with the nonhuman—either the divine or simple matter—the mainstream of Western Christianity did not consider human insensitivity to pain a possibility. This attitude was so tacitly basic to Western envisioning of body and soul that it rarely needed stating.

Despite this down-to-earth general attitude, there remained tantalizing glimpses of impassibility at two ends of the human spectrum: among the

saints and among the sinners. How to interpret such super- or subhuman reactions was a great puzzle to those who dealt with the phenomenon. As most
people do when facing the incomprehensible, they opted for vagueness.

One of the earliest martyrdom narratives we have is that of Polycarp
(155/56). It comes to us via Eusebius, who was probably one of the most
influential authorities on the subject. Here martyrdom appears in a double
guise: heroism and impassibility. "Who could fail to admire their nobility
and endurance and love for their master?" A few lines later, however, he
seems to contradict himself: "Some reached such a pitch of noble endurance that not one of them let cry or groan escape him, showing to us all that
in the hours of their torture Christ's martyrs were absent from the flesh, or
rather that standing by their side their Lord conversed with them."[6] The
ambiguity continues in the narrative of Polycarp himself, where miraculous
insensibility appears side by side with endurance.[7]

Throughout the *Historia ecclesiastica,* Eusebius maintained the ambiguity we have just seen. Describing the martyrs of Palestine, he gives an
impressive but unclear account of a young Christian servant: "as if he were
without flesh and blood, he did not even appear to be sensible of his pains."
Another was tortured, "not as the flesh of a human being, but as stones and
wood, or any other lifeless object."[8] Elsewhere, miraculous impassibility
appears unquestionable. Eusebius met young Theodore of Antioch, who had
survived torture under Julian. "When we asked him whether he felt pain at
all, he said he barely felt it, for there was a young man standing next to him
who wiped his sweat away with a snow-white cloth soaked with cold water,
and thus he enjoyed himself and was sad when he was taken off the rack."[9]
Here the martyr himself testified to miraculous impassibility.

The cult of martyrs was inscribed in Christian communal memory and
identity during late antiquity, becoming an essential component of Christianity.[10] Writers and preachers throughout the Middle Ages referred to
Catherine of Alexandria, Vincent of Saragossa, or Lawrence of Rome and
assumed with a tolerable degree of certainty that their audience would automatically know the story.

The martyrs' acceptance of pain was as central as their heroism. The
predominant narrative invariably remained that of heroism and endurance,
highlighted by explicit gruesome details of torture. Martyrs were most often
depicted as welcoming and feeling pain. The tradition of Eusebius, though,
surfaced in later legendaries and sermons. Within martyrological literature,
late medieval authors contradicted themselves continually. The stories are
full of pain infliction, but pain itself is sometimes simultaneously affirmed
and denied in the same text. Furthermore, in the hierarchy of pain Christ's

suffering explicitly exceeded that of martyrs. Precisely because sensitivity to pain was the mark of the superior being, the pain of martyrs paled in comparison to Christ's.

The explicit statements concerning the martyrs' impassibility occur parenthetically within the context of Christ's Passion, contrasting it with the martyrs' actual impassibility. Thus, Domenico Cavalca spelled out the difference between Christ and the martyrs:

> even though Christ's soul was always blessed and saw God, nonetheless God miraculously left its sensitive part in a purely natural state, that is, without giving it any consolation or amelioration as he gave the martyrs, who joked about their pain and almost did not feel it. Thus, many [of them] walked on fire saying that it seemed to them that they were walking on rose petals. And it is known that many martyrs went to their martyrdom singing and joyous, as though they did not feel the pain and survived for many days in the harshest martyrdom.

Conversely, Christ was beset by fear and anguish at the beginning of his ordeal and survived only a few hours on the cross because of his intense pain.[11] John Bromyard made a similar comparison, arguing that the shining sun may warm a tree, but a man beaten under a shining sun still suffered just as much. God, inhabiting the martyrs, made them impassible (and Bromyard uses precisely this word) so that they suffered nothing, but God's light shed upon the Crucifixion did nothing to alleviate Christ's pains.[12]

The defiant attitude attributed to martyrs in their own stories was often construed as impassibility. They could jeer at their torturers because they truly felt no pain. However, when the martyrs themselves were the protagonists of the tale, they often claimed to be imitating Christ by suffering. Thus, martyrs identified with Christ in martyrdom narratives but were clearly distinguished from him in Crucifixion texts.

If we discard the Passion as any yardstick for human suffering, one must measure late medieval martyrdom narratives and the pain in them in comparison to the manner in which these stories were told earlier. The following analysis is largely based upon four martyrdom tales—Agnes, Agatha, Vincent, and Lawrence. All died as martyrs during the third- or fourth-century persecutions, and all their *acta* were repeated in different versions throughout the Middle Ages. All of them belong to the category of epic or semilegendary martyrs.[13] Their stories show them as being far beyond simple humanity. Though horribly tortured, they remained steadfast and sometimes even physically immaculate. Their heroic deaths were told in different narrative modes, with different emphases, from early Christianity to the fifteenth century and beyond. Here I have taken as a starting point Prudentius's *Peristephanon*,[14] comparing it with Jacobus de Voragine's work and later sermons.

Why follow the permutations of specific narratives across the ages? For anyone studying the history of pain in Western culture, martyrdom narratives are yardsticks of sensitivity. The same story, told in three different ways (always taking into account the type of narrative) might illuminate for us a landscape that is usually difficult to map. How important was the martyr's pain as part of her life or her death? How much of the telling was about pain, and how much about athletic contests? The shifts in emphasis across a millennium can tell us much about the nature of late medieval religiosity and its priorities.

Like all descriptions of behaviors, those of martyrs were carefully scripted. We have the standard ancient model of martyr behavior in the arena: arrogant, defiant, verbose, mocking.[15] This model alternated with the contemptuously silent model adopted by other martyrs. Either way, martyrs defied both authority and pain by either bearing pain bravely or ignoring it.

Apparently, both patterns—defiance and silence—were foreign to fifth-century everyday North African mores, for Augustine of Hippo found them extraordinary. How, marveled Augustine, could the martyr Vibia Perpetua (d. 203) have remained silent under torture in the arena? "Where was this woman, that she did not feel herself fighting that most savage of cows; that she asked when would what had already occurred [i.e., the fight in the arena] happen? Where was she? What did she see that she did not see this? What did she enjoy, that she did not feel this? By what love was she rapt, by what vision called away, by what potion intoxicated?"[16] Indeed, judging from Augustine's letters, the norms dictating the pain expressions for an ailing elderly bishop in fifth-century Africa were drastically different from those applying to third-century African women martyrs in the arena. In his own letters he complained vociferously of toothache and hemorrhoids, but Perpetua was silent, possibly drugged by a miraculous potion.

Given that most Western Christians after the third century were not required to die for their faith, the behavior of martyrs was transposed to sanctified narratives of Merovingian executions. The death of St. Leudegarius may well have been a calculated political execution, but it is remarkably similar to the deaths of the martyrs who people Prudentius's pages. A political opponent became a saint by the manner of his death: a slow, cruel agony born with impassive behavior.[17] The saint who sang psalms and prayed while being slowly chopped into pieces became a topos, repeated in the eleventh-century narrative of St. Emmeram's death in Bavaria.[18] No matter how hard to find martyrdom became, once encountered, its protagonists knew how to behave. Or rather, their biographers knew how they must have behaved. Their sensations are not part of the narrative.

Late medieval Christians were far more familiar with the late antique narratives (as retold by contemporary legendaries) than with heroic Franks. There are almost no detailed narratives of martyrish or even quasi-martyrish behavior in the later Middle Ages. The case of the persecuted Franciscans mentioned in chapter 2 shows how far the late antique model influenced the manner in which such new cases were told. Angelo Clareno, the Spiritual Franciscan leader, recorded the martyrdom of some *fraticelli*. Angelo wrote the history of the Franciscan order as a list of seven tribulations, beginning with the corruption of Brother Elias during Francis's absence in the East and ending with the death of Bernard Délicieux around 1320.[19] Part of the fifth tribulation took place in the kingdom of Naples around 1304, when a group of Spirituals was arrested and tortured by the local inquisitor, the Dominican Thomas of Aversa.

The torture session described does not conform in any way to any legal requirement of torture and is muddled enough to arouse doubt as to its veracity. One ostensibly negligible point does stand out, however. Thomas had first had a scaffold erected in Trevi but realized that torture was not a matter of spectacle, "because he saw that the bishop and leading men of the city would find such a spectacle with such people troubling to their eyes."[20] He therefore moved the entire procedure to the hill castle of Maginando, "a hidden place, fit for fell deeds," where the torture was performed in an enclosed place, a local house.[21] The methods described were genuine for the time and undoubtedly familiar to Angelo: strappado, a rope tightened around the skull, and the rack. Some of the Franciscans (one of them a priest) nearly died under torture, and two boys confessed to heresy—one under the influence of wine (though the narrative does not include the provision of beverages), the other under torture and threats of death. Even while confessing, the two destroyed their own credibility by yelling that, whatever the inquisitor wrote, the suspects were nevertheless all good Catholics. Thus, Thomas had obtained what he legally needed as proof—two full confessions. Subsequently, one Spiritual (also named Thomas) heard of the avowals and insisted that those who had confessed (apparently more than the two boys) were to recant. As we know, any suspect who confessed under torture had to verify his confession in court and could therefore still recant it.[22] Indeed, the following day they all resolutely recanted in the inquisitor's face. The inquisitor then prepared to take his revenge upon the stubborn

Brother Thomas, but the local castellan intervened.[23] At which point the inquisitor stopped his inquisition.

Angelo Clareno was not present at the occasion and wrote the account decades later. His description undoubtedly owes a great deal to familiarity with standard torture methods and with some of the subtleties of Romano-canonical law of proof. The rest of his account is culled, almost literally, from ancient martyrdom narratives. Thomas of Aversa is referred to as "this new Dacianus," in reference to the Roman emperor who had tortured St. Vincent to death. Like the original Dacianus in the ancient narrative, Thomas was subject to ungovernable fits of rage: he was "driven out of his mind with anger" and was "demented with fury," going so far as to personally work the pulley and later hit someone on the head for commending himself to Christ. All this, "although he was a learned man and of noble family."[24] At the peak of his fury the inquisitor had one of the boys raised naked on the rack and, personally shaking a lance at his breast, threatened to transfix him unless he confessed that all the suspects were heretics. The image of a naked boy stretched to breaking point and about to receive one more wound in the chest was a subtle but irresistible mnemonic pointer to the Crucifixion. The Spirituals and their supporters remained steadfast in their faith. As might be expected, Thomas of Aversa (who had also extorted money from all and sundry) died soon afterward, like all tyrants, in great pain and fear. He did admit his sins against the Spirituals, but this was not considered the saving grace of confession, as he had despaired of God's grace and was unquestionably headed for hell. This detailed mirror of martyrdom accords with the original tales also in all that concerns pain. The subjects were tired and hungry when they arrived at Maginando, but the frightful tortures inflicted on them did not affect their faith or their words. There is no record of screaming, begging, or any other reaction. The only sufferer whose pains are described in the text is the evil inquisitor on his deathbed.

The one great difference between this fourteenth-century narrative of torture and those of late antique martyrs is speech. Many early martyrs conducted a virulent verbal duel with their judges and audiences before and throughout their tortures. In contrast, none of the Franciscans' words are rendered in direct speech, and what Clareno does record is humble and pacific enough: they maintained that they were good Catholics. Caving under torture, some of them allowed the inquisitor to write another version, but in the end they recanted their confessions.

The deliberate framing of the persecution of Spiritual Franciscans in terms of early Christian martyrdom was a premeditated allusion to apocalyptic beliefs that saw St. Francis as a second Christ.[25] It was therefore necessary for his followers to imitate the followers of Christ, and for their enemies to imitate the enemies of early Christians. The history of courageous Christian behavior under persecution was destined to be retold time and again, every time with new martyrs, but every time with exactly the same modes of behavior assigned to both persecutors and persecuted.

To most late medieval Christians, however, martyrdom was a story of the ancient past.[26] The two main sources of martyrological knowledge for the laity were sermons and legendaries. Sermons *de sanctis* had been part of the Western Christian calendar for centuries, but legendaries were fairly rare until the thirteenth century. Compared with earlier martyrologies, they were infinitely more detailed and interesting. Legendaries compiled detailed lives of many saints—martyrs, virgins, and confessors.[27] Unlike other hagiographic documents, they were not simply mnemonic aids to liturgical practice. They contained stories, and these stories became a central source for preaching in the thirteenth century. The best known of these, the *Legenda aurea*, was first redacted by Jacobus of Voragine (1230–98) in 1267.[28] This compilation became a best-seller—translated into several vernacular languages, copied and recopied—and the basis of much subsequent sermon literature.[29]

The *Legenda aurea* was destined to have a protean history. Besides more than one thousand Latin manuscripts, it has survived in numerous vernacular translations. Each translation, however, changed the content as well. Thus, in Caxton's Middle English version one is apt to find English saints who had never made it into the original.[30] Thus, King Edward the martyr came to inhabit the *Golden Legend,* although his cult was a purely English affair. The *Legenda aurea* became the basis of many sermons (including those of Jacobus himself) and established an orthodox hagiography of the saints' lives.

The narratives of the third century and the thirteenth century form two contiguous links in a chain of transmission. Saints' passions had not vanished from writing and ritual during the intervening centuries; nor had Jacobus rescued them from oblivion. Throughout the Middle Ages there were martyrologies, sermons about martyrs, *vitae* of martyrs, and even plays like those of Hrosvitha of Gandersheim. Jacobus de Voragine, however, took little interest in the intermediate versions. He did not rely upon a continuous chain of transmission. Rather, he usually took his material—or so he claimed—directly from the original *acta* or *vita.* He rarely relied on intervening martyrologies, basing his writing upon the earliest sources he could find. Thus, late medieval audiences were fed Jacobus de Voragine's version of late antique saints—a version claiming its genealogy directly, so to speak, from the horse's mouth.[31]

The proliferation of saints' lives in drama, vernacular literature, iconography, and preaching undoubtedly created a closeness between audiences and favorite saints. Not all of them were martyrs, but martyrdom certainly made a better story. The death of a martyr was a mythological narrative, and its main thrust was to show not the power of human beings but the glory of God, who gave those humans the ability to withstand atrocious sufferings.

Most of the martyrological theater of horror is familiar through medieval and Renaissance paintings. Bartholomew being skinned, Sebastian transfixed with arrows, Lawrence roasted, Agatha undergoing breast removal, and Catherine on her wheel were all common artistic motifs. These, however, show the ideas of artists, not of the original narrators. One and all, they show the martyrs serenely accepting their tortures, as though feeling no pain. Judging from the late antique narrative, this was no innovation: late antique texts repeatedly describe martyrs as being miraculously above their tortures, aided by supernatural forces. Augustine spelled this out even more clearly than Prudentius: "If we consider the torturer's perturbation and the sufferer's calm, it is very easy to see who is under punishment and who is above it. . . . So great was the harshness of the pains inflicted on St. Vincent's members, and so great the confidence sounding in his words, that we might think one person was speaking while another was being tortured. And so indeed it was. His flesh suffered and his spirit spoke."[32] The late antique narrative does not show martyrs as serene and passive. Men or women, they were all aggressive, loquacious, challenging. Their torture did not break them, but it often did move them to expressions of sarcasm and disdain. The late antique martyr was not a victim but a victorious warrior.

This unmediated continuity makes the task of analysis easy, for the changes in martyrdom tales are not the result of evolving traditions; they are deliberate alterations. Though an analysis of four stories does not allow for sweeping generalizations, it does provide food for thought. There are adaptations that can be explained by sensitivity to the audience's experience and background; after all, one cannot present a thousand-year-old story without any new trappings to make it comprehensible and believable. At the same time, the atmosphere of the times, the sensitivity to suffering, and the concentration upon pain surface through a much more internalized narrative. While the late antique narrator of *acta* was careful to keep the observer's stance,[33] telling us what was done and spoken, his later successor tried on occasion also to interpret the deeds on more than one level. Finally, the late medieval story, dealing as it did with three-dimensional figures, was far more gendered.

By the later Middle Ages, martyrdom did not necessarily mean death by slow torture at the hands of pagans. It could come in the form of lingering, painful illness or self-inflicted ascetic practices. In fact, the real-life figures being burned at the stake were most often heretics or sodomites.[34] Nonetheless, just as Christ's Passion held a deep fascination for late medieval audiences, so did the passions of early Christians. Jacobus de Voragine assigned pride of place to early Christian martyrs. Almost two-thirds of the chapters devoted to saints focus on early Christianity.[35]

Jacobus was doing far more than merely conflating ancient sources. He was reshaping them in the manner of the thirteenth century; he continued with the enterprise, albeit in a slightly different genre, when he wrote his model sermons. His readaptation was the basis of much subsequent production of hagiographic sermons. In most cases, we have the antique source to compare with the thirteenth-century version and its successors and can see the difference. Pain loomed much larger in the version of Jacobus.

Let us take St. Augustine as an example. Though a crucially important saint, Augustine was martyr to nothing but hemorrhoids.[36] However, since he was included in the *Legenda aurea,* he had to suffer extravagantly and from something slightly less unsavory for late medieval sensibilities. Consequently, Jacobus gave preeminence to the toothache that attacked Augustine immediately after his conversion. Augustine did mention a toothache both in his *Soliloquies* and in his *Confessions,* relating that he could not speak from pain and had to write on a tablet to his familiars a request to join him in prayer for a cure.[37] Still, Jacobus included the insignificant case of the toothache in his biography of the saint.[38] Since Augustine had performed several posthumous miracles, this particular case was unnecessary for proving sanctity. It was inserted in order to paint Augustine as a sufferer, almost a martyr.

For each saint in his legendary, Jacobus provided a thumbnail sketch of the saint's identity and the meaning of his or her name. His martyrs were usually of noble extraction. According to both Jacobus and the Dominican preacher Leonardo of Udine (d. 1469), St. Lawrence's father was the duke of Hispania. After years of fruitless marriage, he promised God that he would devote his firstborn child to him. When the child was born "by a unique privilege of grace," the devil naturally took offense. He tried four times to kill the child, with the result that the parents, intimidated, deserted the afflicted boy. At this point, Pope Sixtus intervened, adopted the child, and brought him up as a Christian in Rome.[39] Though nobility might have argued enhanced pain sensitivity, Lawrence claimed during his martyrdom to feel nothing. Nevertheless, Jacobus lists him as a prime sufferer among martyrs, while still repeating his insensibility, quoting Ambrose to the effect that Lawrence was immune because he possessed the sense of refreshment of paradise.[40]

Another change in late medieval narratives is the role of women. In the late antique source, women martyrs were often as verbally aggressive as men. A millennium later, women martyrs became far less contentious. For late medieval preachers, Agatha was not a noblewoman who had chosen the humble status of Christ's servant but a virtuous bride of Christ. In the world of Jacobus, such a status was usually reserved to free, middle- or upper-class women. The exceptions to this meekness occur in the *South English Legendary*, where both male and female martyrs adhere more closely to ancient models.[41]

A similar gender difference can be detected in all the confrontations. While men became sharper in their speech, most women martyrs, like Agnes, became less aggressive.[42] One of the reasons for this relative taciturnity is not meekness but the deletion of theology from the stories. While Prudentius's heroes had to explain volubly what Christianity was about, Jacobus's had no such need. Speeches summarizing Christian belief, therefore, were deleted in most cases. In the case of Agnes, it left her rather short of words. She had been described in the original *acta* as wise beyond her years and had proven as much during her ordeal, but contentious females were not in the style of the thirteenth century.[43] In fact, even long-winded male martyrs such as Vincent and Lawrence had their speeches cut.

At the same time, the style of speech, especially that of male martyrs, became far rougher and more insulting. The late medieval Vincent taunted Dacianus in a style far less dignified than that of his late antique predecessor: "Oh happy me! The harder you try to frighten me, the more you begin to do me favors! Up, then, wretch, and indulge your malicious will to the full! You will see that I am stronger by God's virtue in being tortured than you are in torturing me!" "The way you talk, Dacianus! What you are saying proves me right and my torturers wrong!"[44] One can almost hear Vincent mockingly chide Dacianus for his foul language. Lawrence became equally taunting, insisting in the same breath that he felt nothing but that he had always thirsted for pain. The self-contradictory taunts and challenges smack of a culture of invective that disregarded dignity for the sake of a verbal victory. The martyrs insisted that they thirsted for pain, but they did not say that they are suffering, nor did they evince pain in their gestures.[45]

The gory details of torture changed little. The same semimythological late antique instruments, the rack (*eculeus*), the fiery metal bed (*craticula*), and leg shackles (*ergastulum*), recur in many stories unaltered, and for good reason. The iconography of each martyr was strictly tied to the instrument of his or her torture, and any changes would have resulted in total confusion. How would people recognize Catherine of Alexandria without her wheel or Margaret of Antioch without the dragon? There is, however, another reason as well: the unfamiliarity of late medieval audiences with public torture and painful executions. Painful public executions were a common sight in the fifth century. This practice was revived in the early modern period: painful public execution rituals had come to copy (sometimes quite deliberately) ancient rituals. However, during the thirteenth century, when Jacobus was writing, people were not likely to have seen many public executions other than the burning of heretics or the hanging of thieves.[46] Much of the great and wondrous spectacle of Vincent being tortured within an inch of his life and laughing at it required an exercise of imagination from thirteenth-century audiences, for it was not something they were likely to have seen. Judicial torture, as we have seen in chapter 2, was secretly conducted in enclosed, anonymous spaces with as few witnesses as possible. The one notable change is in the torture of Agnes. Taken to the stake in the original story, the fire that failed to harm her (and presumably did not even hurt) became far more interesting in the later tales. Starting with the "Gesta sancte Agnetis," the flames parted, leaving her unharmed, and later simply cooled off and were spontaneously extinguished. Jean de Mailly had the harmless fire turning around and burning the bloodthirsty mob.[47] Jacobus's own sermons had Agnes going through two fires, one of which went out and the other provided her with refreshment. This two-fire tradition appeared also in Leonardo of Udine's sermons.[48]

The clearest fire of all burned in the story of Lawrence. Lawrence was not burned on a stake but was roasted on a *craticula*, but later sermons made much of the fire heating the metal griddle. Jacobus insisted that—like gold—Lawrence was purified, melted, and shaped in the crucible's fire. The motif of fire goes back to Maximus of Turin and to Prudentius, who claimed that the fire in Lawrence's heart vanquished the external fire, annihilating his pain. Jacobus de Voragine had Lawrence burning with five internal fires and three external ones; he also constructed an entire sermon around the various fires that fueled Lawrence's martyrdom.[49] None of them caused the martyr any pain.

Why privilege fire over other execution methods? In fact, in the *Legenda aurea* the predominant forms of death are precisely those any urban late medieval crowd would recognize: beheading and burning. Hanging, the most common form of all, was too uncomfortably close to crucifixion and too ignoble, in late medieval terms, for the punishment of martyrs. But the executions that Jacobus dwelled upon were familiar and real to his audiences, not some outlandish ancient torture that nobody could really imagine.

Late medieval motifs also predominated when it came to the torture and execution of women. The sexual persecution so prevalent in late antique sources was attenuated, perhaps to avoid titillation but also with a clear agenda in mind. While the details of antiquity could not be obliterated, threatened rape and mutilated breasts were not the main gist of late medieval sermons and legends. Jacobus's series of sermons on Agatha are a case in point. The central theme was not femininity but *virtus*. He began by likening Agatha to the virtuous woman of the book of Proverbs, the *mulier fortis*. Femininity appeared only in his quotation from the Song of Songs: "we have a little sister, and she has no breasts."[50] This is an opening for a very philogynous sermon. Rather than use breastlessness for a pornographic view of women, Jacobus wrote a panegyric of love. What distinguished Agatha in this sermon was her ardent love and identification with Christ; she suffered for him, and he for her. The sermon is redolent of fragrant herbs, praise of virginity, and praise of womanhood in general. The wounding of her breast has no sexual connotations; to the contrary, it is reminiscent of the wound in Christ's side. For Jacobus, Agatha had carried the *imitatio Christi* to the point of almost total identification. This was indeed the highest praise he could offer her. Nothing in this, however, has any sexual connotations.

Even the story of Agnes, the most explicitly sexual, underwent some purging. In antiquity, Agnes was first shown as a prepubescent young girl, twelve years old.[51] Next, her entire torture was by way of attempted rape. Stripped naked and led to a brothel, her modesty was miraculously saved by an angel, who hid her nudity under hair and brilliant light. The angel also gave her a white robe to wear, and all those entering the brothel were immediately awestruck and respectful. The only one still presuming to try to attack her immediately fell dead. It was only after this, and performing a miracle, that she was sentenced to the flames and later died by the sword. There is nothing remotely similar in the tortures inflicted on men. With all their imaginative cruelty, somehow the authors of *acta* never suggested threats of male rape or castration (quite common in Roman and Hellenistic society) as coercive measures. The virility/*virtus* of martyrs (both male and female) was constantly stressed, but women martyrs were still women.[52]

But late medieval sermons on Agnes paid little attention to the brothel, expanding instead the motif of Christ as Agnes's preferred bridegroom. Jacobus himself wrote two sermons on the theme, one of them an epithalamium on the wedding of Christ and Agnes.[53] The anonymous sermon edited by Robert Taylor is rife with quotations from the Song of Songs, and later sermons preserved the motif of love and marriage.[54] The bride, rather than the virgin, stands at the center of these sermons. As in the case of Agatha, Jacobus described her as the ultimate married housewife, the virtuous woman from Proverbs.

Two thirteenth-century stereotypes stand behind these new interpretations. One is the biblical stereotype of the virtuous matron, which any late antique writer would hastily have repudiated for women martyrs. The virtuous woman is a head of her household, an example to other women living in the world, combining strength, wisdom, and dignity. It is a stereotype that sits ill with women who chose to defy their world and status by refusing to marry and were prepared to pay the price for it. Yet, Jacobus deliberately chose to describe both Agnes and Agatha in those terms: as virgins well and truly married to Christ. Far more startling is the second stereotype: the similarity between the newly transformed martyrs and some of the living holy women of the thirteenth century. The image of women consumed by their love for Christ, being his bride, marrying him, and imitating him by having a wound in their breast is unthinkable in any context earlier than the thirteenth century, but it is a recurring motif in women's mystical writings of the time.[55] Even more importantly, it is a recurring motif in the biographies of those women composed by contemporary monks. Indeed, the legend of Agnes was recited as nine long lessons in Clarissan liturgy for the entire week of her passion: "A sort of `holy week' for women, the ancient Office of St. Agnes of Rome began on January 21, the date commemorating Agnes's trial and the beginning of her passion, and closed on January 28, the celebrated date of her death."[56] Clare of Assisi was familiar with the text of the legend and used it often in her letters to Agnes of Prague. Whether as matrons or Beguines, women like Agnes and Agatha were people audiences could relate to. They were not exotic, superhuman creatures. And their flesh-and-blood character accorded with much of the attempt to reify religious subjects at the time, to make them, if not completely comprehensible, at least conceivable to the laity.

This attempt permeates much of the interpretation of male martyrs as well. The complex of metaphors built around Lawrence's death are an illustration of how a preacher could construct a *rapprochement* between the laity and the imagined past. The most memorable things about Lawrence are the griddle and his last words: "it is cooked, turn [it] over and eat." Already the earliest written sources mention both. Ambrose of Milan, Augustine, and Prudentius repeated the saying.[57] This macabre bit of martyr humor probably earned Lawrence his enduring memorability, for many other martyrs had also been placed upon *craticula*. Though the cooking remained the most memorable part, the last two words in all of the narratives insisted that Lawrence had offered his burned flesh as food. The standard interpretation was that Lawrence was a sacrificial animal. The earliest version of the *passio* had Lawrence describing himself as *"hostia Christi."*[58] The *Passio Polychronii* and subsequent sources cited Lawrence as saying: "I have brought myself as a sacrifice to God for a sweet smell."[59] The words are a paraphrase of Leviticus 7:9, dealing with edible sacrifices. In the fifteenth century, Leonardo of Udine expanded the idea, citing both the wholly burned holocaust and the cooked sacrifice of which the priest may partake, once again likening Lawrence to food sanctified by fire.[60] According to Jacobus de Voragine, Lawrence himself viewed the entire martyrdom as a banquet, with himself as the food.[61] Subsequently, Jacobus inverted the theme of food, claiming that Lawrence had felt nothing during his martyrdom because he was so sated (fattened!) and drunk with feasting.[62] So, while suffering martyrdom, Lawrence was being fatted and roasted at the same time, eating torture and being readied for others' consumption. Lawrence was a sacrifice, but whether an edible one or a holocaust is not clear. The story was originally told in antiquity to people who were familiar with animal sacrifices and knew the difference between holocausts and partially edible sacrifices. By the later Middle Ages it was being told to people who knew nothing about animal sacrifice. Thirteenth-century audiences might have been somewhat familiar with the burning of heretics and they well knew how little was left of the burned body. Who was eating Lawrence then? The literal explanation of his words was a provocative invitation to the pagans to practice cannibalism, and the shadow of this interpretation coexists with the sacrifice on the altar. In antiquity, it has the great value of shock, of accusing the Romans of the ultimate dehumanization of cannibalism—an accusation often leveled at early Christians.[63]

But food and cooking do not stand alone in this story. They are joined with treasure and gold. As the old sources told, Lawrence had first rescued the church's treasure (was it gold?) through the alchemy of charity. Though in the *Legenda aurea* Jacobus drew the name's etymology from the laurel wreath of the victor at the games, in his sermons he followed the older tradition: *Laurentius* derived from *aurum*.[64] The motif of gold was enhanced far beyond its antique source. Like gold, which does not tarnish, Lawrence was proved and purified in the crucible's fire. Like gold, he was pliable under the blows of martyrdom and did not break. The *Legenda aurea* also tells how Lawrence had posthumously saved Emperor Henry I's soul in Henry's trial before God by bringing a pot of gold that the dead emperor had donated to the church of Eichstätt.[65] Lawrence himself became gold, and holy; the mundane human body could be transmuted into something finer and holier.

Examining our four martyrs one by one, it is possible to see the changes in their stories. Of all four, Agatha's story changed the least. She did exclaim, in all versions, about the governor's cruelty when he had her breasts cut off, but there is no mention in either early or late sources of her pain, only of her awareness of her disfigurement. Vincent, too, remained the hardened soldier of God. He not only wished to suffer but also possessed constancy (*constantia sufferendi*) and, mostly, the fortitude of a rock (*fortitudinem lapidis*).[66] Nothing could move him from his purpose, not because he was insensitive to pain, but because, as his name indicated, he was a victor by definition.[67]

The clearest change over time comes in the story of Lawrence. At the beginning, Lawrence was depicted as an able administrator, a clever clergyman who could dispense miracles and money but with no heroic stature. From Carolingian times on, he was shown as impassible. As far back as Ado's martyrology (ninth century), Lawrence had been immune. Jacobus of Voragine stressed this point, quoting first the words of Decius, who claimed that Lawrence could block out all pain through magic, and adding the testimony of Romanus (about to be baptized and martyred too), who saw a beautiful young man wiping Lawrence's forehead. In addition, Jacobus claimed that this immunity stemmed from Lawrence's satiety with the food of sacrifice. Finally, Lawrence himself insisted that the coals only brought him comfort, not a sense of burning.[68] However, the same Jacobus, when summing up the chapter in the *Legenda aurea*, pronounced him second only to Stephen, the protomartyr in the ranks of the martyrs, by reason of his pain.[69] What Jacobus needed to make a martyr was not insensibility but sensibility.

A similar ambiguity emerges in the late medieval stories of Agnes. The main change that one finds in the late medieval stories concerns the shift in emphasis toward emotivity and sensation, though Jacobus attributed her victory "perhaps to impassibility."[70] Both Jacobus and Leonardo of Udine, who told of the two fires she had gone through, were assuming primarily that Agnes was indeed vulnerable to the pain of fire, or at least that one ought to think of her sensations and readiness for physical torture. The Agnes who emerged from late medieval sermons was not the stern, fearless, precocious girl immune to all feelings who appeared in the early *Gesta*. She was genuinely in love with her bridegroom, not merely counting the advantages of an alliance with Christ rather than with the prefect's son, as in the *Gesta*; she managed to suppress her fear, and she was sensitive to fire. In short, she was human and passible.

What emerges from these altered narratives is a perception of martyrs as seekers after self-sacrifice, as human beings with specific feelings and commitment. Lawrence described himself as a sacrifice and claimed to have always wished for martyrdom, Agatha spoke of her willing abnegation. Vincent (in the late medieval versions) stressed his own thirst for pain and, with a more didactic turn, the need for any athlete (God's or the arena's) to train his body for his day of glory, to be able to win the battle.[71] Agnes grew lyrical telling of her ardent love for Christ.

The evidence of pain is consistent with all the other human attributes of the erstwhile superpeople. They did suffer; they did not possess miraculous impassibility. Even when tradition pointed in another direction, the interpretation of late medieval authors veered toward the humanity of the martyrs and their passibility. The change in the narratives of martyrdom humanized the martyrs, making them far more understandable to the laity. Martyrs were human and individual and had individual human experiences. Knowing about pain was certainly one of them.

The humanization of martyrdom was connected to two different developments. First, passibility had become the hallmark of *imitatio Christi*. One could not admire and practice the cult of nonsufferers in the thirteenth century when living saints were practicing self-infliction of pain and meditation to imitate Christ's Passion. But even more importantly, judicial torture had come to be universal practice. Though people did not see what was done to criminal suspects, enough was known about the emerging legal practice for people to know that torture invariably caused intense, terrible pain, and that it took either a miracle or extraordinary force of character to withstand it. When preachers spoke of martyrs confronting torture, they spoke to people who knew what torture was. By contrast, telling them of miraculous insensibility, at a time when jurists claimed that insensibility resulted only from evil magic, was neither credible nor productive. The reality of torture reshaped heroes and heroines in a more human form.

Scholastics saw things differently. Though most of the writing on martyrs was didactic, scholastics were sometimes required to consider martyrs. When they did so, their ideas were hardly original. It was not a subject that merited much attention in scholastic circles. For late medieval reality, martyrdom was part of an epic past, not an issue of present problems. Other than Thomas Becket and Peter Martyr, it was hard to find martyrs in thoroughly Christian Europe. Furthermore, the subject of contemporary martyrdom was touchy, and best avoided, for—if one supported the Franciscan agenda—St. Francis could have been termed a martyr or even a second Christ. Consequently, Dominican and secular masters of theology tried to steer clear of contemporary implications. Unlike angels, devils, paradise, and hell—all topics of immense relevance—martyrdom had little impact upon theological problems that needed solving.

Scholars dealing with the subject were not merely indifferent. They were also swimming in an alien sea. Almost all of the sources they had about martyrs came from a realm of knowledge outside their usual hunting grounds. Rather than the philosophical and theological material they were used to dealing with, they had to turn to sermons, poems, and legendaries. The texts dealing with martyrs were literary, emotive, commemorative, and hortatory. Almost the only church father who spoke of the martyrs' pain was Hilary of Poitiers, who, while trying to prove the (heretical) impassibility of Christ, claimed that, if martyrs were beyond pain and fear, all the more so was Christ.[72] To this, Augustine trenchantly responded that martyrs were not comparable to Christ.[73] There was nobody who could instruct thirteenth-century scholastics as to which part of their souls, for example, the martyrs used when confronting pain. All scholastics did was stretch the concept of martyrdom as far as possible, in time as well as issues. Impassibility, as they conceived it, was not a quality pertaining to postlapsarian terrestrial life. Adam and Eve in paradise and the glorious resurrected bodies at the end of times enjoyed immunity from pain, but martyrs did not come into the discussion.[74]

How, then, did martyrs resist torture? According to thirteenth-century scholars, pain could not vanquish them because they used their reason, or the upper part of their souls, to ward off the onslaught of passions provoked by external attacks.[75] Alternatively, their souls were strong enough to feel and internalize the pain but behave as though they felt nothing. No wonder, therefore, that they classed martyrdom under the virtue of fortitude. In other words, what the martyrs had was the ability to withstand and hide pain—impassivity—rather than the ability not to feel it.

William of Auxerre (d. 1231) was probably the first to devote a serious section to martyrs in his treatise on fortitude.[76] His only basis was a letter of Bernard of Clairvaux that explains why the Maccabees were celebrated by the church as martyrs.[77] Bernard had extended martyrdom also to those who had fought their entire life for Christ but died peacefully, such as John the Evangelist, and to those who died unwillingly, such as the Holy Innocents. Contrary to Bernard, William rejected the martyrdom of those who had not died violently, despite their wish. There were five types of martyrs, said William of Auxerre. There were martyrs who had died for preaching the truth (e.g., John the Baptist), martyrs for the defense of divine law (the Maccabees), for defense of the faith (Stephen the protomartyr), for the redemption of humanity (Christ), and the Holy Innocents, for whose sacrifice there was simply no good reason.[78] This classification, with relevant modifications, was to be followed by future generations of scholastics dealing with the subject. Pain was no criterion at all in this scheme. The central criterion was a violent death, even if it was as senseless as that of the Holy Innocents. In sharp disjunction from all the issues that authors of legendaries entertained, scholastics concentrated upon the martyrs' deaths, ignoring all that preceded those deaths.

Though William of Auxerre placed martyrdom under a subheading of fortitude, which allowed him to speculate on the multiple meanings of *passio*, his main argument concerned the free will, which was definitely a contemporary issue. Unlike the usual philosophical meaning of "passion," which presupposed something being done to the subject, the *passio* of a martyr was an active expression of self and free will.[79] Therefore, saints' passions did not derive from the passions of the soul. As usual, scholastics tended to cut such Gordian knots by relying upon the multiple meanings of the term. Citing his teacher, Prévostin of Cremona (ca. 1150–1210, a noted jurist), William of Auxerre distinguished between passions (actions inflicted upon the subject) leading to moral corruption and passions (willing suffering) leading to moral betterment. Both types imply passivity, but of two different types. His examples of the first type of passion are a virgin's rape (*violenta corruptio virginitatis*) or bearing a penalty (*violenta penarum susceptio*); suffering those would corrupt the *patiens* in some way. The second, as in receiving a whipping for Christ's faith or dying for him (*passio mortis*), was morally useful. "We therefore say . . . that *patientia* has two uses, that is, to suffer what must be suffered and to reject what must be rejected."[80] The severity of the criminal's or the martyr's punishment was irrelevant; all that mattered was the free choice to die. The echoes of judicial arguments concerning free will and torture can be heard in William's words.

Thomas Aquinas, writing two generations later, also placed the discussion of martyrdom within the category of virtues and fortitude. His interest, however, was different. Like William of Auxerre before him, he proved that martyrdom was part of the cardinal virtue of fortitude, but his main

argument was that death, not only suffering, was necessary for the definition of martyrdom.[81] Though William had instanced only martyr categories
that fitted this requirement, his main argument had been will, not death.
Thomas lived in a different climate, and his main aim was to narrow, rather
than stretch, the scope of martyrdom. At a time when Europe was rife with
extreme ascetic manifestations of holy women and men, one needed to draw
boundaries, lest living saints become martyrs. Both in the *Summa theologiae* and in his disputed questions, Thomas spoke little of what martyrs underwent on the way to death and what they were supposed to withstand. In
clear contrast to legendaries, where death merely capped the achievement
of suffering and courage, Thomas dismissed all but the death as a requirement of martyrdom.

Thomas did, however, make one extremely important point concerning
the suffering of martyrs. While arguing whether martyrs possessed charity
as well as fortitude, Thomas asserted that having perfect charity was what
enabled certain martyrs to bear their sufferings more lightly. His examples,
tellingly enough, were Vincent and Lawrence, who had loudly proclaimed
that they felt no pain.[82] Charity, in the sense of spiritual love, was what enabled martyrs to withstand suffering.[83] Here, almost hidden by a mountain
of arid arguments, lies the single scholastic explanation for the power of
martyrs to transcend pain. All martyrs, by definition, possessed fortitude
and could impassively resist pain. Those who added charity to their virtues
possessed impassibility.

There is a wealth of contradictory opinions concerning the pain of martyrs in Thomas's work. When dealing with the human will, Thomas clearly
distinguished between the passions of Christ and of the martyrs. "If one
asks whether the same way of feeling [*modo sentiendum*] exists in the Passion and in the martyrdom of saints, we say that there is a difference between the passion of the head and of the members."[84] Clearly, he believed in
the possibility of human fortitude but not in human impassibility.[85]

Like William of Auxerre, Thomas placed a great deal of weight upon
the will to suffer. This, however, brought him into conflict with a group of
highly favored martyrs: the Holy Innocents, slaughtered by Herod's orders
in infancy. The best Thomas could come up with to justify their martyrdom
was that the infants had been granted the status of martyrs by divine grace.
Thomas did cite "some" who claimed that the infants had miraculously
attained free will prior to their death, but as the Bible said no such thing,
he rejected this explanation.[86] It is unclear whom Thomas was referring to
as the inventor of accelerated growth. He was aware of Bernard's work and

summed it up with his usual clarity (a clarity absent in Bernard's own letter): "Bernard distinguishes three types of martyrs: by will, not murder, as
John [the Evangelist]; by will and murder, as Stephen; by murder, not will,
as the Innocents."[87] All the same, Thomas did not agree that the mere thirst
for martyrdom sufficed, and the Holy Innocents were indeed a stumbling
block, which he removed by declaring it a unique phenomenon.

What emerges from the works of William and Thomas is a clear, if
somewhat impersonal, picture of what scholastics thought of the sufferings
of martyrs. A lifetime of asceticism and self-inflicted pain, as several controversial holy people of the time practiced, did not constitute martyrdom.
Being murdered by heretics after a normal, albeit celibate life as a papal
functionary (as in the case of Peter Martyr, a Dominican killed by Cathars
in 1252) did make one a martyr.[88] One required external infliction of pain
and death to qualify as a martyr. Furthermore, martyrs were passible, for
they had the virtues and the will to withstand the assault while feeling the
pain. Possessing perfect charity, however, could promote the martyr to a
state of near impassibility, granted by fortitude.

These were absolutely human virtues and had nothing to do with interpretations of Christ's Passion. A century later, John Duns Scotus did state
that it was only by divine grace that martyrs could retain their reason *in
maximis tormentis,* but his point was merely that Christ had needed no
such grace in his Passion.[89] Thus, grudgingly did scholastics add the possibility of martyrs' receiving divine grace.

The discomfort of scholars with the idea of the impassibility of martyrs
becomes clear when we view the context in which some of their opinions
were written. Other than William of Auxerre and Thomas Aquinas, martyrdom did not play a role in *summae.* Most of the opinions, in fact, were
enunciated in the context of highly political canonization proceedings. The
thirteenth century was not only the time of holy men and women. It was
the time of royal and episcopal canonizations; a historical martyr king could
come in handy, and a murdered archbishop turned martyr, like Thomas
Becket, was of immense importance. Martyrs, naturally, were in short supply, but where they could be found, royal power insisted that scholars grant
them their seal of approval. Like many ostensibly futile intellectual exercises, therefore, martyrdom was relegated largely to quodlibetal questions.
All the same, the futility remains entirely in the eyes of the modern be-
holder. While some scholars considered martyrdom a minor subject, martyrs
and their sensations could be powerful tools for analyzing and interpreting
the realities of the thirteenth, rather than the fourth, century.

By 1285, royal dynasties were seeking saints. The kings of France had St. Louis, but whom did the kings of England have? Other than Edward the Confessor (ca. 1003–66), a nonmartyr by the very definition of his epithet, English royalty was short of saints. Was Edward (ca. 962–978/79), the murdered Anglo-Saxon king, a martyr?[90] Edward, it must be remembered, was murdered for purely dynastic reasons by his brother, a Christian. The question was put to an English, Paris-trained, and Oxford-based Franciscan, Roger Marston. As might be expected, Marston gave a favorable answer to the question, supporting the local tradition.[91] To do so, he stretched the definition of martyrdom as far as it would go. According to Marston, not only those who had died for the faith were martyrs, but those who had died fighting for justice (like John the Baptist or Thomas Becket) also merited the title. In addition, those who had unsuccessfully aspired to martyrdom (like John the Evangelist or St. Martin) and those who had been unwillingly and unwittingly slaughtered (like the Holy Innocents—and, of course, like Edward, though Marston deliberately omitted his name) also became martyrs. Finally, Marston quoted Augustine's statement that all proper Christian life, if it followed the Gospel, was martyrdom.[92] Such a statement, given by a learned scholar, perhaps shows good political sense, but it shows very little sense of scholastic tradition. Furthermore, the criterion of a violent death, which had been central to martyrdom from its earliest times, vanished completely. If an aspirant to martyrdom who had lived a virtuous life counted as a martyr, why not a murdered king? Though Marston was hardly the first to grant the palm to the victim of a political assassination, his seal of approval for a king with nothing but his murder to recommend him does explain why other theologians avoided the topic as much as possible.

All that was left to scholastics was the comparative approach. Scholastics brought up martyrs and their pain time and again within the context of the Passion, only summarily to dismiss them. Christ's pain and the Virgin's pain were infinitely worse than anything suffered by Vincent or Lawrence (again!).[93] Once more, the implication of scholastic discourse on the subject was that these martyrs were not superhuman, and although they had suffered atrociously, their pain was nothing compared with that of Christ and the Virgin.

Martyrdom narratives were part of the formative framework of late medieval devotion. In sharp contrast to the Crucifixion story, the tale of martyrdom was not about feeling pain at all. It was a tale of courage, defiance, miraculous interventions, and happy deaths. Late medieval versions contained more inner dimensions and sensitivity than the heroic mold of fifth-century narrative would allow. Late medieval martyrs were far more impassive than impassible.

The tantalizing possibility that martyrs were immune to suffering by divine grace, although mentioned occasionally, was never discussed systematically. The laity, though, speculated that some people, by some means, could undergo torture and feel nothing because they could screen off the pain somehow. This idea, as we shall see, was promoted in the dark parallel of martyrdom: the torture of criminals.

The few trial protocols we have from the Middle Ages record occasional cases of endurance under torture. Thus, Berthaut Lestalon of Montlhéry, tried in a Paris court as a recidivist thief, was twice tortured but still refused to alter his confession. He was sentenced to ear cropping and banishment from Paris for his "harshness" (dureté).[94] Another suspect before the court survived four torture sessions without confessing to anything. His stubbornness earned him banishment from the kingdom of France for life.[95]

The fact that such cases existed is not altogether surprising, given the French system of torture. While in the south of Europe almost all justices resorted to the strappado, which dislocated shoulders and destroyed bodies, French torture was milder and sometimes even resistible. It consisted of stretching people on either the small or the big trestle and pouring water into their mouths until they agreed to confess. While anything but mild, this method did not kill the tortured and produced a few heroes whose harshness saved their lives. At the same time, no French jurist that I know of discussed the ever-recurrent myth of criminal impassibility, because resistance was possible.

Did Berthaut Lestalon and others like him suffer pain? Protocols do not answer such questions. The only thing we know is that, like the martyrs of old, they persevered in their confessions and changed nothing under torture. Unlike martyrs, late medieval resisters were labeled obstinate and ill-willed. A similar phenomenon—the ability to resist torture without breaking down—documented under contradictory circumstances, received two opposing interpretations.

Nevertheless, in both cases the borderline between human resilience and supernatural aid remained vague. In both cases, jurists at some point were forced to conclude that their suspects were not heroic but impassible. How this impassibility was achieved depended upon context. In the case of a martyr, it could unquestionably be attributed to divine intervention. In the case of a live criminal, there were other forces, almost equally powerful, that could produce the same effect.

Criminals who felt nothing while being tortured, we must stress, were just as mythical as impassible martyrs. Their myth is far more closely connected to their own time than to the time of the early Christian martyrs. Given that the impassibility of martyrs remained in the realm of ambiguity, it is not surprising that a parallel phenomenon among suspected criminals who were tortured remains even more nebulous. Clearly, if the phenomenon existed, it was limited to two specific groups: professional criminals and witches. The idea that some innocents might be miraculously rendered immune to pain remained in the realm of miracle tales. In those stories, a wrongly accused innocent who prayed to a saint might be spared all sensation of pain, but in juridic literature the assumption was that all those tortured were guilty. If one bears in mind Baldus's caution that *indicia* should be as clear as the sun before sending a suspect to torture, "so that only the confession is lacking," the assumption made sense. They had already decided upon guilt, but they lacked the ultimate proof to convict and punish the suspect.[96] With this conviction in mind, jurists could not possibly countenance the idea that subjects of torture were immune to pain thanks to divine grace.

To the best of my knowledge, there are no extant medieval protocols of cases of people who withstood the strappado, survived, and walked away free other than the statement of Bartolomeo Canholati, described in chapter 2. To the contrary, many jurists speak of the danger of killing suspects under repeated torture.[97] All the same, the myth of impassible or hardy criminals recurs throughout the juridic literature from the thirteenth to the sixteenth century. In almost every case the author claims to have encountered the phenomenon in person, but the evidence remains in the realm of anecdote and reminiscence.

Nevertheless, we have seen throughout that, in the hierarchy of being, those who suffered were superior to those who did not. Noble, pure people were more sensitive to pain than gross peasants, and the same held true for noble organs in the body, such as the eyes, which were far more sensitive than the plebeian toes. As a rule, "honorable" people were not subjected to torture. Hence, those who did undergo the sufferings of torture were automatically assumed to be less sensitive to pain. Was it possible for them to exploit their inferior nature to evade justice?

Furthermore, underlying the suspicion that present impassibility might derive from suspect sources were two base concepts that needed little articulation. First, impassibility could only be viewed with suspicion. If Christ had suffered, and all those who wished to imitate him made sure they suffered, then people who felt no pain could not possibly be saintly, or even just good. Immune criminals were doubly questionable, for they certainly had debts to pay, and they were not paying them even under torture.

Second, as of the late fourteenth century, and especially during the fifteenth century, the trend of suspecting supernatural phenomena of demonic provenance strengthened. The main issue concerned the visions of (female) saints, which, Jean Gerson argued, probably came from the devil, not from God.[98] In this near-dualistic atmosphere, in which evil could generate almost perfect simulacra of divine manifestations, impassibility could also be construed as demonic. "And this is a matter of doubt . . . so that one can distinguish between angelic revelations and demonic illusions." "We are to be like spiritual moneychangers or merchants. With skill and care we examine the precious and unfamiliar coin of divine revelation, in order to find out whether demons, who strive to corrupt and counterfeit any divine and good coin, smuggle in a fale and base coin instead of the true and legitimate one."[99] Indeed, one of the standard proofs in witchcraft trials was the infliction of pain, on the assumption that a witch would feel nothing. Witchcraft suspects, therefore, join the ranks of plain criminals in their nefarious search for impassability.

In the following, we shall first survey the evidence for criminal impassability, which is mostly hearsay, and then try to interpret the mental infrastructure that demanded the existence of such a phenomenon. I would like to argue that, whether criminal impassability had existed or not, jurists were bound to invent it and maintain the myth. The very logical underpinnings of torture as a mode of eliciting proof relied upon the assumption that not all suspects automatically succumbed, for in that case, confession under torture was no proof.

There is a certain reluctant respect in the juridic myths of the hardened criminals who withstand torture without batting an eyelid, the respect of one contestant for another. Those were the criminals who possessed *duritia*, and juridic texts are full of stories about them. Odofredus (d. 1265), the indefatigable raconteur who taught at Bologna around the middle of the thirteenth century, spoke of those who were so hardened that they slept during torture.[100] His context, of course, was Ulpian's observation that different people reacted differently to torture, some being weaker or more fearful than others. Two centuries later Franciscus Brunus testified to the same sort of *duritia*, claiming that some professional criminals merely presented the aspect of death while tortured, and when it was over, they opened their eyes.[101] One jurist even described a man who was willing to undergo strappado for a few coins.[102] The stories jurists told include the myths concerning criminals training themselves secretly in the forest, by inflicting torture upon each other, so that they might resist in a real situation; of others who knew the trick of keeping their shoulder joints so flexible that the strappado did not dislocate them; and those who knew the system well enough to realize that one session was all they would suffer unless new evidence was produced, which gave them the necessary endurance.[103] The explanation, therefore, lay in the Houdini-like capabilities of hardened criminals to withstand torture. In all of these stories, there was no supernatural element whatsoever.

This attitude changed in the sixteenth century. Just as martyrologists could explain the martyrs' endurance only by understanding it as a gift of God's grace, sixteenth-century jurists resorted to witchcraft to explain the same type of endurance among criminals. The metamorphosis of one miraculous drug is a case in point. The mysterious anesthetic stone from Memphis, called Memphytes or Mesites, had a perfectly respectable ancestry until it came into the possession of criminals. Dioscorides mentioned it in the first century as an anesthetic: ground and mixed with water, it provided total insensitivity to pain. In the thirteenth century, it was mentioned in the highly popular but somewhat suspect *Secretum*, falsely attributed to Albert the Great. At the time, such a book of practical magic did not count as witchcraft or necromancy, nor were its contents anything but mildly shocking. Three centuries later, however, the same stone was mentioned as one of the magical tools criminals resorted to in their search for insensitivity and silence.

The difference between the thirteenth century and the sixteenth did not lie only in the identification of endurance with silence and witchcraft. Unlike earlier jurists, who could view hardened criminals in a detached, somewhat-admiring manner, sixteenth-century jurists were thinking about witches—those subversive, acutely dangerous malefactors, worse than any criminal, who must be made to speak at all costs. Their ability to withstand torture had nothing admirable about it and was not a matter for anecdotes. These men and women had had no criminal training but might well be endowed with the *maleficium taciturnitatis*. The resistance of some witchcraft suspects supported the belief in the *maleficium taciturnitatis seu insensibilitatis*. A series of potions, scrolls, and incantations could help the tortured suspect remain silent without feeling any pain, a fact that jurists found most disturbing.[104] The very use of the term *maleficium* indicates the era in which the supernatural explanation surfaced. Earlier, the word had simply meant crime. Albertus Gandinus's thirteenth-century treatise on criminal law was naturally named *Tractatus de maleficiis*, though not a word in it refers to witchcraft. By the sixteenth century, *maleficium* had

come to mean witchcraft. Most of the stories about both natural and supernatural resistance derive from sixteenth-century jurists. Paulus Grillandus
gained most of his fame not for his juridic treatises but for his demonologi-
cal work.[105] In his view, a silent "patient" was automatically guilty, either
as a professional criminal or as a witch.

Like all his predecessors, Grillandus claimed to have encountered the
phenomenon himself. He begins with the naturally hardened:

> There are some who are so terrible and robust that they fear neither pain
> nor torture, as though somebody else was feeling it in his body. . . . Some
> of them [survive] by the strength of their body and arms, others by their
> lightness, for they lift a light weight; some, who can turn their arms
> from the back forward and over their heads through suppleness, so that it
> seems they feel only a light pain, or none. And I have seen others too.[106]

Thus far, all fits with previous descriptions. But then comes a section carrying a new tune:

> I found some others who, with the aid of sorcery and incantations of the
> evil art, are so strengthened physically, or levitate, or fall into a deep sleep
> after being lifted, so that they suffer absolutely no pain in their body.
> And this is called *maleficium taciturnitatis sive insensibilitatis.*[107]

At this point, Grillandus begins enumerating the specific means. One is
the Mesites stone. Next are a number of incantations. The first mentions
the three people who hung on crosses together—Christ, Dismas, and Ges-
tas. The second is a verse from Psalms, "my heart is stirred" (Ps. 45:1). A
third charm wishes that, just as Mary's milk was sweet to Christ, so should
the upcoming torture be sweet to the reciter's arms. The theme of Christ
hanging from the cross, his arms wrenched backward, recurs in the incantations of men or women about to be in a somewhat-similar, and equally
painful, physical position. The same theme recurs in the recommendation
to recite all the words Christ said from his capture until his death. Grillandus knew all this because he had encountered the phenomenon several
times in Pisa and in Rome. As soon as his suspect was raised on the rope,
he fell asleep as though he was on his bed, without any screaming. He did
murmur a few words before falling sleep, but afterward he was as insensible
as a marble statue.[108]

Similar means had been described a few decades earlier in the *Malleus
maleficarum.* Heinrich Kramer tells the story of some heretics in Regensburg

(a story already related by Caesarius of Heisterbach two centuries earlier) who refused to confess, were sent to the stake, and proved immune to the flames. Attempts to drown them also failed. But in the end faith triumphed over evidence, and miracles were no vindication. The bishop made his entire flock fast for three days, with the result that the charm was discovered in the armpit of one heretic. Once it was removed, they all proved quite combustible.[109]

Grillandus actually managed to capture such a charm, a small piece of parchment embedded in the recalcitrant suspect's hair, with the following text upon it: "†Iesus auem [sic] transiens† per medium illorum ibat.† os non comminuetis ex eo.†" Nevertheless, upon being raised again, the suspect resorted to a spoken charm and once more remained silent. The persistent inquisitor tried the *taxillum* (small dice put between the toes) with no result, "always impudent, he was strengthened in his denial" (*sed in sua negativa semper audacius convaluit*). The frustrated magistrate was forced to close the case, and he had encountered similar ones in which other judges were baulked by the silent suspect.

What was one to do in the face of such sorcery? Grillandus cited "some" who claimed that certain prayers would dissolve the enchantment. Some of the psalms served this end: "O Lord, open my lips, That my mouth may declare Your praise" (Ps. 51:15), was altered into "O Lord, open my lips, and my mouth shall tell the truth." The previously mentioned Psalm 45:1, with suitable alterations, was as efficient for the interrogator as for the tortured. Nevertheless, Grillandus was skeptical. He had copied these remedies from earlier authorities but admitted he had never tried them or heard of them being tried. This skepticism, following upon his utter credulity in the earlier paragraphs, might indicate that even a zealous witch-hunter like Grillandus was careful to distinguish between phenomena he had encountered (and interpreted as witchcraft) and things he had only read about in his textbooks. Obviously, he prized his own experience and that of his colleagues over the written words of Paris de Puteo (1413–93), whose tall stories about insensibility were a byword.[110]

What can one conclude from this mixture of legends and observation? It is indeed possible that some people could withstand torture, even the dreaded strappado. More importantly, one can try and burrow under the layers of urban legends and tall tales to find what beliefs existed at the time concerning impassibility. Perversely, impassibility was possible not because it was miraculous but because it had become evil. It might have had supernatural causes, but jurists were equally content to ascribe it to physical fortitude. Nevertheless, it carried supernatural overtones. All the incantations quote scripture or speak of Christ, the Crucifixion, and Mary. It is as though criminal impassibility were the obverse of Christ's utter passibility. Alternatively, it could be the illegitimate descendant of martyrological impassibility. This possibility is clear in the heretics' story cited by Heinrich Kramer. As we saw, it was an old tale, not something he had experienced, and the story is an exact inversion of the classical martyrdom of St. Agnes, who (when accused of murdering the prefect's son, who had assaulted her) convinced all and sundry of her innocence by being incombustible. If incombustibility was proof of innocence in the patently innocent martyrs, it was proof of guilt in the patently guilty heretics.

The existence or nonexistence of recalcitrant suspects who refused to confess after torture is not something we can determine. Nevertheless, they did exist in the minds of jurists like Grillandus. How had they come into being? As we have seen, until the fifteenth century the powers of silent criminals were purely human, not even innate. They could be acquired by practice. Thereafter, the silence assumed the ominous overtones of *maleficium taciturnitatis vel insensibilitatis*. Recalcitrance was magically and wrongly acquired. Furthermore, the magic did not endow the suspects with any special virtue. It worked by pure sedation, entirely separate of the human will. It required no more physical or spiritual characteristics than did surgical anesthesia.

Was this insensibility akin or identical to the impassibility once attributed to martyrs? No medieval author would have agreed to such a proposition, and I would argue that they were right. To begin with, Evagrius Ponticus had meant something totally different when he spoke of *apatheia*. Jerome, deriding him, deliberately misunderstood a discipline of the soul and control of the passions for complete insensibility, "like a stone or a god." Nevertheless, some of the tales of martyrs depict people who could sense the pleasure of divine consolation but not the simultaneous pain of torture. These martyrs were therefore not insensible but merely immune to pain. Others, like Perpetua, felt absolutely nothing and were not really conscious during the torture. These cases do indeed resemble the insensibility of the criminals. But by the later Middle Ages martyrs possessed fortitude (in the spiritual sense) or constancy enough to persevere in their testimony of faith, despite the torture. According to the narratives, they did not pray for impassibility. They prayed for victory in the arena, and a victory without an enemy to beat was a hollow one. In fact, as Vincent testified, he had strenuously wished to feel pain, not to be insensible.

Martyrs, therefore, presented an entire scale, from total insensibility to acute pain. Recalcitrant criminals presented only two explanations: physical resilience or witchcraft and total insensibility. No jurist ever argued that those "harsh" criminals who refused to confess had suffered as much as any human could and yet had resisted by virtue of their spirit. Such an option was not granted to people who were assumed, by virtue of their interrogation, already to be criminals. It would have been a virtue, and one did not attach virtues to such people.

The vanishing impassibility of martyrs and the growing impassibility of criminals, though, are contemporaneous. While preachers and scholars attempted to endow martyrs with fortitude to bear pain, not with miraculous immunity, the latter had been transferred to the opposite side: the criminals and witches. If it were necessary to find yet another proof of the valorization of pain during the later Middle Ages, it is here. Suffering on earth was granted to martyrs, denied to the wicked. Presumably, their roles were reversed in the afterlife, but in the meantime they could stand as metonymies of the realms of pain and painlessness.

CONCLUSION

L ike the music of the time, the sounds of pain emerging from the later Middle Ages are polyphonic. Unlike good polyphonic music, they do not harmonize. Still, we hear, not a cacophony, but the interaction of different social and cultural trends. It is customary when speaking of pain in the later Middle Ages to stress the visible and audible—the culture of devotion in all its manifestations. It is important to remember that this culture was not purely Christocentric but concentrated also upon martyrs and martyrdom. Consequently, thaumaturgic descriptions of pain also acquired a hitherto-unknown dimension of emotivity.

The same is not true for other realms of expressivity, however. If one examines the language and attitudes of physicians, there is little evidence of any growth of medical sensitivity before the sixteenth century. The vocabulary and attitudes that coalesced in the thirteenth century were fairly constant two centuries later. The only palpable change is the disappearance of the anesthetic sponge myth.

In contrast, vernacular and pastoral theology evolved an entire hierarchy of pain, beginning with human suffering on earth and culminating in hell. In between stood martyrs and Christ, who did suffer on earth, but whose suffering was greater than any usual human pain. These texts were not univocal. When speaking of martyrs, the texts stressed their unique pain, gradually erasing the superhuman impassible image promulgated in late antiquity and incorporating the martyrs' sensations into those of general humanity. The same was true of Christ's pains, though theologians took care to differentiate clearly between martyrs and Christ in the context of Christological writing. All the same, stressing the martyrs' actual suffering made them more similar to Christ than did attributing to them heroic invulnerability.

One might have expected scholastics, in the wake of devotional activity, to pay more attention to pain. Scholasticism, however, is not commensurate with medicine. While physicians carried on an unbroken tradition from antiquity, the tools and social structures of scholasticism coalesced only in the second half of the twelfth century. As we have seen, scholastics provided the theoretical basis for disquisitions upon the Crucifixion and were equally ready to discuss the course of humanity, from Eden to resurrection, through purgatory and hell. At the same time, they took little or no interest in the literature of martyrdom, which grew to unprecedented proportions during the later Middle Ages. While scholasticism was active and changing throughout the later Middle Ages, there appears to have been little evolution in the argumentation concerning the field of pain. Realists and nominalists, Averroists and their opponents, all treated pain within roughly the same categories, arriving at roughly similar conclusions. The one discernible change over time is the growing stress upon the interior apprehension of pain as the central factor in sensation. By the fourteenth century, nominalist scholars like John Duns Scotus arrived at the conclusion that all that was necessary for the apprehension of pain was the interior sensation, rather than an exterior trauma. The scholastic concept of internal apprehension of pain was also the cornerstone of devotional *compassio*—the total identification with another's pain, to the point of sensing it in one's own self. Inner apprehension was a concept accepted by physicians, too, when one organ sensed the pain of another.

Scholasticism played a central role in the coalescence of the culture of pain by its very structural framework of argumentation. The same methods of thought and argument were passed on to medicine and law—two fields that had existed in different forms before scholasticism. There is little doubt that the scholastic adversarial method also affected how the ill and the criminally suspect were questioned. While torture had existed long before the thirteenth century (indeed, it is not clear that it had ever vanished), the mantle of learned studies of Roman law endowed it with respectability and legality. Indeed, it has been claimed that the growth of Passion narratives received its impetus from the practice of torture. Torture became an integral part of the inquisitorial mode of trial, achieving a vast literature that almost invariably avoided any mention of pain but spelled out practices of pain infliction and reactions to it. Overall, torture literature is repetitious and static, showing few changes over time. But, whereas early torture treatises avoided almost all mention of the actual methods and degrees of torture, authors of the fifteenth and sixteenth centuries could occasionally be quite explicit on the subject. Torture may not have come out of the dungeon, but its particulars became far more familiar to the laity, both in the guise of martyrdom sermons and in the juridical literature.

The pervasiveness of ideas on pain is best illustrated in the case of torture. We have seen that torture borrowed procedures from religious confession and a vocabulary from martyrologies. In both cases, the borrowed framework was a camouflage for totally different contents and meanings. The notion of magical or pharmacological impassibility, too, was born in classical medicine and witchcraft, but the contents of early modern torture had turned the myth from one of heroism into one of a maleficent force. The single case of Bartolomeo Canholati conflates torture, medicine, witchcraft, and faith all in one. Thus, reality, hiding behind prescriptive writing, might well show a far more coherent view of the uses of pain.

The teleological view of pain embraced almost all disciplines and practices. All else stemmed from the functionality of pain, including the growing stress upon self-mortification, upon meditating on the Crucifixion, upon the martyrs' humanity and vulnerability to pain, the explicitness of torture treatises, and the systematization of types of pain among physicians. All these stemmed from the idea that pain, though harrowing to humans, was useful in the end.

Going from the aches and pains of terrestrial humans, through heroic martyrs, all the way to Christ's crucifixion, the variegated meanings of pain within late medieval Christian life and beliefs shifted according to time and conditions, giving opposite interpretations to similar sensations. Pain could be good or evil according to context. If Christ's agony was payment for human sin, then even a headache or gallstones could be seen as salvific. Conversely, if martyrs suffered because evil forces were trying to coerce them into idolatry, then one could view pain as an evil, sinister force, trying to break down one's constancy and faith. Present pain differed from historical pain; live pain differed from the pain of the dead; divine pain was unique in essence, resembling no human pain at all.

As ideas about the usefulness of pain gained prominence, the idea of human impassibility declined in prestige. Physicians began arguing against soothing as an equivalent to curing, insisting upon a cure of the disease rather than the attendant pain. Living saints were anxious not to be spared pain. This attitude made sense: Christ was anything but impassible, and the impassibility of martyrs had dissolved into fortitude. Eventually, the very idea of impassibility became tainted by association with crime and witchcraft.

The impact of those changes was more in volume than in pitch, if one is to return to the metaphor of music. Not surprisingly, norms of behavior began allowing people to report their pains, to complain about them, and to seek help. They had done so before as well, but Margery Kempe's wailing is much louder than that of Anselm of Canterbury. The advice (sometimes obligation) to a parturient woman to scream as loudly as possible belongs firmly in the fifteenth and sixteenth centuries, when the pain of childbirth became identified with the necessary and useful uterine contractions. Even in this case of undoubted childbirth pain, there was a purpose to the screaming.

Are we to assume then that late medieval society became more empathetic toward human pain? By no means. The logical conclusion deriving from the utility of pain was that the more it was inflicted, the better. What we consider cruelty, such as slow, painful executions (a phenomenon associated more with the sixteenth than with the fifteenth century), was often viewed as a force for betterment. Being a *patiens* was often seen as salutary. Though physicians never concurred in any such opinion, much of the medical practice of the time was imbued with the idea that health was reached through discipline, not indulgence. While there is a great distance between recommending a strict regime of life and torturing suspects, physicians and surgeons did not shrink from painful procedures when they considered them necessary.

If one were to draw a distinction between the late medieval past and the modern (or postmodern) present, it is this. Poets and novelists like Virginia Woolf and W. H. Auden have spoken of the utter isolation and solitude of the sufferer, and all modern thinkers have acknowledged this fact. The modern sufferer is trapped inside her pain, unable to share or express it. In contrast, in the later Middle Ages pain was definitely a social sensation. Even if apprehended internally, pain was shared, discussed, and transmitted through speech, art, and patterns of behavior. The late medieval sufferer was not alone; she was surrounded by the entire human population of sufferers, by a cosmic history of pain.

NOTES

INTRODUCTION

The chapter-opening epigraphs are taken from Augustine, *De libero arbitrio*, ed. W. M. Green, CCSL 29 (Turnhout, 1970), 3.23.69; Alexander of Hales, *Glossa in quatuor libri sententiarum Petri Lombardi*, BFSMA 14 (Quaracchi, 1954), 168–69; Alexander of Hales, *Glossa in quatuor libri sententiarum Petri Lombardi*, 159; Matthew of Acquasparta, *Quaestiones disputatae*, BFSMA 18 (Quaracchi, 1959), 114; Henry of Ghent, *Quotlibeta magistri Henrici Goethals a Gandavo* (Paris, 1518), fol. 459; John Duns Scotus, *Quaestiones in tertium librum sententiarum*, vol. 14 of *Opera omnia* (Paris, 1894); Galen, *Opera omnia*, ed. Carolus Gottlob Kühn, 20 vols. (Leipzig, 1821–33), 8:80; Avicenna, *Liber canonis Avicenne revisus et ab omni errore mendaque purgatus summaque cum diligentia impressus* (Venice, 1507; repr., Hildesheim, 1964), fol. 38r; U. Lindblom et al., "Pain Terms: A Current List with Definitions and Notes on Usage," *Pain* 24, supplement 1 (1986): S217.

1. Modern philosophers who have tried to define pain have not fared any better than historians. See Nikola Grahek, *Feeling Pain and Being in Pain*, 2nd ed. (Cambridge, MA, 2007); Murat Aydede, ed., *Pain: New Essays on Its Nature and the Methodology of Its Study* (Cambridge, MA, 2005).

2. Manuele Gragnolati, "Gluttony and the Anthropology of Pain in Dante's *Inferno* and *Purgatorio*," in *History in the Comic Mode: Medieval Communities and the Matter of Person*, ed. Rachel Fulton and Bruce W. Holsinger (New York, 2007), 238–50; Robert Mills, *Suspended Animation: Pain, Pleasure and Punishment in Medieval Culture* (London, 2005); Mitchell B. Merback, *The Thief, the Cross, and the Wheel: Pain and the Spectacle of Punishment in Medieval and Renaissance Europe* (Chicago, 1999).

SETTING THE STAGE

1. See Caroline W. Bynum, *The Resurrection of the Body in Western Christianity, 200–1336* (New York, 1995), 137–55.

2. Bernardo Bazàn et al., éds., *Les questions disputées et les questions quodlibétiques*

dans les facultés de théologie, de droit et de médecine, 2 vols., TSMA 44–45 (Turnhout, 1985), 2:50–85.

3. Ibid., 23–25; John F. Wippel, "Quodlibetal Questions," in ibid., 160–66.

4. *The Myroure of Oure Ladye, Containing A Divotional Treatise on Divine Service* . . . , ed. J. H. Blunt, Early English Text Society (London, 1873); Elizabeth Schirmer, "Reading Lessons at Syon Abbey: The *Myroure of Oure Ladye*, and the Mandates of Vernacular Theology," in *Voices in Dialogue: Reading Women in the Middle Ages*, ed. Linda Olson and Kathryn Kerby-Fulton (Notre Dame, IN, 2005), 345–76; Domenico Cavalca, *Lo specchio della croce: Testo originale e versione in italiano corrente*, ed. Tito Sante Centi (Bologna, 1992).

5. For the typology of preachers' manuals, see Marianne G. Briscoe, *Artes praedicandi*, TSMA 61 (Turnhout, 1992).

6. Michel Zink, *La prédication en langue romane avant 1300*, Nouvelle bibliothèque du Moyen Âge 4 (Paris, 1976); Jean Longère, *La prédication médiévale* (Paris, 1983); Stephen of Bourbon, *Tractatus de diversis materiis predicabilibus*, ed. Jacques Berlioz and Jean-Luc Eichenlaub, 2 vols., CCCM 124 (Turnhout, 2002–6); Humbert de Romans or Stephen of Bourbon, "De dono timoris/Tractatus de habundantia exemplorum," London, British Library, MS Arundel 107; Arnold of Liège, *An Alphabet of Tales: An English 15th-Century Translation of the "Alphabetum narrationum,"* ed. Mary M. Banks, Early English Text Society (London, 1904–5) (I have used the Latin original in London, British Library, MS Harley 268). Thomas de Cantimpré contributed a great deal to the exempla literature in his *De apibus*. Thomas of Cantimpré, *Miraculorum et exemplorum sui temporis libri duo [De apibus]* (Douai, 1605).

7. Claude Bremond, Jacques Le Goff, and Jean-Claude Schmitt, eds., *L'exemplum*, TSMA 40 (Turnhout, 1982).

8. Jacobus de Voragine, *Legenda aurea*, ed. Giovanni Paolo Maggioni, Millennio medievale 6, testi 3 (Florence, 1998); all references to the *Legenda aurea* are to this edition. Johann of Werden [attr.], *Sermones dormi secure vel dormi sine cura* (Strasbourg, 1485).

9. For all the genres of sermons, from manuals to live sermons, see Beverly Mayne Kienzle, *The Sermon*, TSMA 81–83 (Turnhout, 2000).

10. Thomas of Chobham, *Summa de arte praedicandi*, ed. Franco Morenzoni, CCCM 82 (Turnhout, 1988); John Bromyard, *Summa praedicantium* (Basel, 1480).

11. On sermons and their different types, see (from the copious literature) David L. D'Avray, "Method in the Study of Medieval Sermons," in *Modern Questions about Medieval Sermons*, ed. Nicole Bériou and David L. D'Avray (Spoleto, 1994), 3–30; Kienzle, *Sermon*.

12. For a general survey of visions, see Peter Dinzelbacher, *Revelationes*, TSMA 57 (Turnhout, 1991).

13. Michael R. McVaugh, *The Rational Surgery of the Middle Ages*, Micrologus' Library 15 (Florence, 2006).

14. Nancy G. Siraisi, *Taddeo Alderotti and His Pupils: Two Generations of Italian Medical Learning* (Princeton, NJ, 1981), 270–82.

15. Rudolf Dekker, ed., *Egodocuments and History: Autobiographical Writing in Its Social Context since the Middle Ages* (Hilversum, Netherlands, 2002).

PART I

1. E.g., Mary-Jo DelVecchio Good et al., eds., *Pain as Human Experience: An Anthropological Perspective* (Berkeley, CA, 1992); Jean E. Jackson, *"Camp Pain": Talking with Chronic Pain Patients* (Philadelphia, 2000).

2. Nemesius of Emesa, *De natura hominis: Traduction de Burgundio de Pise*, ed. G. Verbeke and J. R. Moncho, Corpus Latinum commentariorum in Aristotelem Graecorum, suppl. 1 (Leiden, 1975), 92–93, 103–4.

3. Augustine stressed this point, making it clear that body and soul were created together. Augustine, *De genesi ad litteram libri duodecim*, ed. Joseph Zycha, CSEL 28/1 (Vienna, 1894), 178, bk. 6, chap. 7.

4. On patristic interpretations of gendered creation, see Gillian Clark, "Adam's Engendering: Augustine on Gender and Creation," in *Gender and Christian Religion*, ed. R. N. Swanson, Studies in Church History 34 (Woodbridge, UK, 1998), 13–22; H. S. Benjamins, "Keeping Marriage out of Paradise: The Creation of Man and Woman in Patristic Literature," in *The Creation of Man and Woman*, ed. Gerard P. Luttikhuizen, Themes in Biblical Narrative: Jewish and Christian Traditions 3 (Leiden, 2000), 93–106. Eve's creation played a very small part in this strain of thought. For the few who did consider Eve, see Humbert de Romans, sermon 94, "Ad omnes mulieres," in Humbert de Romans, Gilbert of Tournai, and Stephen of Bourbon, *Prediche alle donne del secolo XIII*, trans. Carla Casagrande, ed. Maria Corti, Nuova corona 9 (Milan, 1978), 5–7, cited in Bede Jarrett, *Social Theories of the Middle Ages* (New York, 1966), 72. Bonaventura, "Opusculum VI de perfectione vitae ad sorores," in *Doctoris seraphici S. Bonaventurae opera omnia*, ed. Aloysius Lauer (Quaracchi, 1898), 8:121; English translation in *The Works of Bonaventure*, vol. 1, *Mystical Opuscula*, trans. José de Vinck (Paterson, NJ, 1960), 242.

5. "Sciendum est quod de octo partibus plasmatum fuit corpus Ade. Una pars erat de limo terre unde facta est caro eius et inde piger erit. Alia pars erat de mari unde factus est sanguis eius et inde erat uagus et profugus. Tertia pars erat de lapidibus terre unde sunt ossa eius et inde erat durus et auarus. Quarta pars erat de nubibus, inde facte sunt cogitaciones eius et inde factus est luxuriosus. Quinta pars erat de uento unde factus est anelitus et inde factus est leuis. Sexta pars erat de sole unde facti sunt oculi eius et inde erat bellus et preclarus. Septima pars est de luce mundi unde factus est gratus et inde habet scienciam. Octaua pars est de spiritu sancto unde facta est anima et inde sunt episcopi et sacerdotes et omnes sancti et electi dei. Et sciendum quod deus fecit et plasmauit Adam in eo loco in quo natus est Iesus scilicet in ciuitate Bedleem que est in medio mundi, et ibi de quatuor angulis terre corpus Ade factum est, deferentibus angelis de limo terre de partibus illis, uidelicet Micaele Gabriele Raphaele et Uriele. Et erat illa terra candida et munda sicut sol, et conspersa est illa terra de quatuor fluminibus id est Geon Phison Tigris et Euphrates, et factus est homo ad imaginem dei, et insufflauit in faciem eius spiraculum uite scilicet animam. Sicut enim a quatuor fluminibus conspersus sic a quatuor uentis accepit flatus." "The Life of Adam and Eve," chap. 55.1, ed. Wilfried Lechner-Schmidt, trans. B. Custis with the assistance of G. Anderson and R. Layton, http://www.iath.virginia.edu/anderson/vita/english/vita.lat.html#per2 (accessed 8 March 2009); based upon *"Vita Adae et Evae,"* ed. Wilhelm Meyer, *Abhandlungen der philosophisch-*

philologischen Classe der Königlich bayerischen Akademie der Wissenschaften 14 (1878): 185–250. For vernacular versions, see Yves Lepage, "Les versions françaises médiévales du récit apocryphe de la formation d'Adam," *Romania* 100, no. 2 (1979): 145–64.

6. Though later philosophical and scientific trends identified man (*homo*, not Adam) as a composite of the four basic elements (earth, water, air, and fire), they did not carry this perception into the story of creation. See R. Allers, "Microcosmus: From Anaximandros to Paracelsus," *Traditio* 2 (1944): 319–407.

7. In this case we have no alternate creation of Eve. The text begins with the expulsion from paradise and ends with some explanations as to Adam's nature.

8. There are, according to Anderson, seventy-three extant Latin manuscripts of the *Life of Adam and Eve*, and Wilhelm Meyer consulted only the German manuscripts for his edition. For Latin versions, see Gary A. Anderson and Michael E. Stone, "An Electronic Edition of the 'Life of Adam and Eve,'" http://jefferson.village.virginia.edu/anderson/iath.report.html (accessed 8 March 2009). Although the manuscript research of the Latin branch is still very incomplete, I have not found any direct quotations of the text in late medieval sermons and theological works.

9. Bynum, *Resurrection of the Body*, 59–94.

10. Gragnolati, "Gluttony and the Anthropology of Pain," 242–44.

11. Hieronymus, *Epistolae*, ed. Isidore Hilfberg, CSEL 56/1 (Vienna, 1996), 246.

12. In the sermons of Jacobus de Voragine, St. Vincent is described as possessing *fortitudo lapidis*. Jacobus de Voragine, *Registrum in sermones de sanctis* (Lyons, 1520), sermon 69.

13. Danielle Jacquart and Claude Thomasset, *Sexualité et savoir médical au Moyen Âge* (Paris, 1985), 67–120.

14. See Naama Cohen-HaNegbi, "Accidents of the Soul: Emotions and Their Treatment in Medicine and Confession, 12th–15th Centuries, Spain and Italy" (Ph.D. diss., Hebrew University of Jerusalem, forthcoming).

15. Feter H. Niebyl, "The Non-naturals," *Bulletin of the History of Medicine* 45 (1971): 486–92.

16. Hildegard of Bingen, *Causae et curae*, ed. P. Kaiser (Leipzig, 1903), 43–44. See also Danielle Jacquart, "Hildegard et la physiologie de son temps," in *Hildegard of Bingen: The Context of Her Thought and Art*, ed. C. S. F. Burnett and Peter Dronke (London, 1998), 121–34; Victoria Sweet, "Hildegard of Bingen and the Greening of Medieval Medicine," *Bulletin of the History of Medicine* 73 (1999): 381–403.

17. Nancy G. Siraisi, *Medieval and Early Renaissance Medicine: An Introduction to Knowledge and Practice* (Chicago, 1990), 1–17; Jacquart and Thomasset, *Sexualité et savoir médical*, 68–73; Joan Cadden, *Meanings of Sex Difference in the Middle Ages: Medicine, Science, and Culture* (Cambridge, 1993).

CHAPTER ONE

1. "An ad Cybebes ibo lucum pineum?/puer sed obstat gallus ob libidinem/per triste uulnus perque sectum dedecus/ab inpudicae tutus amplexu deae, /per multa Matri sacra plorandus spado." Prudentius, *Peristefanon*, in *Carmina*, ed. Maurice Patrick Cunning-

ham, CCSL 126 (Turnhout, 1966), 337, bk. 10, ll. 196–200. For the epigraph I have used the English translation in Prudentius, *The Poems*, trans. Sister M. Clement Eagan, 2 vols. (Washington, DC, 1962–65), 2:199.

2. Peter Brown, *The Body and Society: Men, Women, and Sexual Renunciation in Early Christianity* (New York, 1988), 213–40.

3. Judith Perkins, *The Suffering Self: Pain and Narrative Representation in the Early Christian Era* (London, 1995), esp. 200–214.

4. *Vita vel passio Haimhrammi episcopi et martyris Ratisbonensis*, in *Passiones vitaeque sanctorum aevi Merovingici*, ed. Bruno Krusch, MGH, SSRM 4 (Hannover, 1902), 2:452–524.

5. Gregory of Tours, *Historiarum libri X*, ed. Bruno Krusch and Wilhelm Levison, MGH SSRM 1/1 (Hannover, 1961; repr., Hannover, 1993), 380–83, bk. 8, chap. 15.

6. Giles Constable, "Attitudes towards Self-Inflicted Suffering in the Middle Ages," in *Culture and Spirituality in Medieval Europe*, by Giles Constable (Aldershot, UK, 1996); Piroska Nagy, "Les larmes du Christ dans l'exégèse médiévale," *Médiévales* 27 (1994): 37–49.

7. Heinrich Suso, *Der Mystikers Heinrish Seuse O. Pr. deutsche Schriften*, ed. Nikolaus Keller (Regensburg, 1926), 18–19. Though he bled copiously, he was so aflame with love that he felt no pain.

8. See Catherine Vincent, "Discipline du corps et de l'esprit chez les flagellants au Moyen Âge," *Revue historique* 302 (2000): 593–614; Daniel Bornstein, *The Bianchi of 1399: Popular Devotion in Late Medieval Italy* (Ithaca, NY, 1993).

9. Richard Kieckhefer, *Unquiet Souls: Fourteenth-Century Saints and Their Religious Milieu* (Chicago, 1984), 89–95.

10. Giles Constable, "The Ideal of the Imitation of Christ," in *Three Studies in Medieval Religious and Social Thought*, by Giles Constable (Cambridge, 1995), 209–48.

11. Peter Brown, "The Rise and Function of the Holy Man in Late Antiquity," *Journal of Roman Studies* 61 (1971): 80–101.

12. Caroline W. Bynum, *Wonderful Blood: Theology and Practice in Late Medieval Northern Germany and Beyond* (Philadelphia, 2007).

13. Oddly enough, there is no practice of imitating martyrs. Presumably, martyrdom was within human reach and could be achieved without divine aid. Furthermore, martyrdom entailed the infliction of pain by others, not by one's own hand, and no such common practice is found outside flagellant processions.

14. "Et pono diversas species unguentorum, quo ex pluribus ea, quae potissimum sponsae uberibus congruant, eligamus. Est unguentum contritionis, et est unguentum devotionis, est et pietatis. Primum pungitivum, dolorem faciens; secundum temperativum, dolorem leniens; tertium sanativum, etiam morbum expellens." Bernard of Clairvaux, "Sermon 10," in *Sancti Bernardi opera*, vol. 1, *Sermones super Cantica canticorum*, 1–35, ed. Jean Leclercq, C. H. Talbot, and H. M. Rochais (Rome, 1957), 50.

15. William of Auvergne, *De sacramento poenitentiae*, in *Opera omnia*, 2 vols. (Paris, 1674), 1:464a. See also Carla Casagrande, "Guglielmo d'Auvergne e il buon uso delle passioni nella penitenza," in *Autour de Guillaume d'Auvergne (d. 1249)*, ed. Franco Morenzoni and Jean-Yves Tilliette (Turnhout, 2005), 189–201.

16. Pelbart of Themeswar, *Pomerium sermonum quadragesimalium tripartitus* (Hagenau, 1509), Quadragesimale I, dominica tertia, De penitentia, sermon 21, "De contritionis intenso dolore cum fletus ablutione." Cf. Piroska Nagy, *Le don de larmes au Moyen Âge: Un instrument spirituel en quête d'institution (V*ᵉ*–XIII*ᵉ *siècle)* (Paris, 2000), 25–40.

17. "Prima veritas quod dolor sensualis in contrito homine non requiritur quod sit intensior in omnibus dolorum aliorum comparatione." Pelbart of Themeswar, *Pomerium sermonum quadragesimalium tripartitus*, sermon 21.

18. For the significance of this legislation, see Katherine L. Jansen, *The Making of the Magdalen: Preaching and Popular Devotion in the Later Middle Ages* (Princeton, NJ, 2000), 199–200; Thomas Tentler, *Sin and Confession on the Eve of the Reformation* (Princeton, NJ, 1977), 16.

19. E.g., Thomas of Cantimpré, *Miraculorum et exemplorum sui temporis*, 306–7; Stephen of Bourbon, *Tractatus*, 1:69–70, 1:192, 2:232–33.

20. See Peter Abelard, *Sententie magistri Petri Abaelardi*, ed. David Luscombe, in *Petri Abaelardi opera theologica*, ed. Eligius M. Buytaert, CCCM 14 (Turnhout, 2006), 145; Stephen of Bourbon, *Tractatus*, 3:4.

21. Stephen of Bourbon, *Tractatus*, 3:60–62.

22. *Fratri Alberti magni ordinis predicatorum quondam episcopi Ratisponensis. In nomine sancte et individue trinitatis Amen. Incipit prohemium de arte bene moriendi* (Naples, 1476), particula quarta: "debet plorare, non oculis carnalibus sed lacrimis cordis, scilicet vera penitentia."

23. Bromyard, *Summa praedicantium*, s.v. "penitentia."

24. Stephen of Bourbon, *Tractatus*, 2:179–261.

25. Bromyard, *Summa praedicantium*, s.v. "penitentia," art. 5: "qui non inveniuntur cum quo non poterunt garrulare" [*sic*].

26. Stephen of Bourbon, *Tractatus*, 2:108–10, bk. 3, pt. 4.

27. Jansen, *Making of the Magdalen*, 207, 209. See also Jacobus de Voragine, *Sermones quadragesimales*, ed. Giovanni Paolo Maggioni (Florence, 2005), 295.

28. Nicole Bériou, *L'avènement des maîtres de la parole: La prédication à Paris au XIII*ᵉ *siècle*, 2 vols., Collection des études augustiniennes, Moyen Âge et temps modernes 31 (Paris, 1998), 1:465–73; Jean-Th. Welter, ed., *La tabula exemplorum secundum ordinem alphabeti, recueil d'exempla compilé en France à la fin du XIII*ᵉ *siècle* (Paris, 1926), 79.

29. Jacobus de Voragine, *Registrum in sermones de sanctis*, "Dominica xxii post festum trinitatis sermo primus."

30. Attributed in early printed editions variously to Albert the Great, Domenico Capranica, and Matthew of Cracow.

31. "Secunda temptatio est desperatio, qua est contra spem et confidentiam quam homo habere debet in deo. Cum enim infirmus doloribus cruciatur corpore, tunc diabolus dolorem dolori superaddit. . . . Proinde ad confidentiam veram: quam precipue infirmus in deum habere, debet in agone inducere cum debet dispositio Cristi in cruce. Tertia temptatio est inpatientia que est contra caritatem. Nam moriturus maxime dolor accidit corporis: hi precipue qui non morte naturali que rata est, sicut manifeste docet experientia, sed frequenter ex accidentibus, puta febre vel apostemate: aut alia infirmitate gravi et

afflictiva atque longa dissoluuntur . . . ut plerumque ex nimio dolore et in patientia amentes et insensati videntur." *Fratri Alberti magni ordinis predicatorum quondam episcopi Ratisponensis. In nomine sancte et individue trinitatis Amen.*

32. "Dolor nonnisi in naturis bonis . . . sed cum ad melius cogitur, utilis dolor est; cum ad deterius, inutilis. In animo ergo dolorem voluntas resistens potestati majori: in corpore dolorem facit sensus resistens corpori potentiori. . . . Item in corpore melius est vulnus cum dolore, quam putredo sine dolore, quae specialiter corruptio dicitur." Augustine, "De natura boni contra Manichaeos," PL 42:556–57.

33. "Ea vero, quae sunt doloris, sicut scis, mortificant et extinguunt concupiscentias voluptatum, desideriaque carnalia, ac secularia, ipsasque voluptates mortificant et abradunt hominibus. Iam autem nosti ex aliis quam noxiae sint hominibus voluptates huiusmodi et desideria, quia videlicet captivant, inebriant, debilitant, dissolvunt, excaecant, atque dementant in omne genus insaniae animas humanas, seu homines. Dolor igitur, qui omnia haec extinguit, et abradit ab eisdem, quam salutaris sit, apparet ex his, et quia revera medicina est, instar absynthij, vermes huiusmodi mortificans, et est velut lixivia abominanda huiusmodi inquinamenta diluens; propter haec igitur duo, videlicet mortificationem istam et ablutionem a vitiis, nominata videtur aqua tribulationis in sermonibus prophetarum. Sciendum etiam tibi est, quod ipsam avaritiam, atque superbiam radicitus exterminat cum seminibus earum, et quemadmodum ignis lateres, et omnia alia vasa fictilia firmat, atque fortificat, et obduratione quodammodo armat; non solum contra aquam, sed etiam contra se; lateres enim excocti nec ignem timent, nec aquam, sic dolor praesentium tribulationum animas humanas armat atque fortificat, et velut armaturam quandam eis patientiam operatur et praestat." William of Auvergne, "De anima," in *Opera omnia*, pt. 1/3, chap. 5, 1:764a. See also ibid., 766b: "quis enim non videat delectabilia corporalia inflammant desideriis animas, et irretiunt atque captivant voluptatibus, similiter ut quaedam tristabilia contristant easdem? Quot enim molestias desideriorum, quot et quantos dolores, cruciatus turpium amorum speciosae mulieres ingerant animabus stultorum et interdum animabus etiam sapientium, quis non videat?"

34. William avoids an older tradition, which likens man to gold that is purified in fire. See Alcuin, "Epistolae," PL 100:451, letter 180: "Aurum examinatur in fornace, tu purior splendescat ex flammis (Prov. 27, 21); et homo in dolore corporis excoquitur, ut purior exsiliat anima de ergastulo carceris sui. Placeat tibi castigatio paterna." The simile does recur in martyrological literature.

35. Using absinthe as a metaphor for a cleanser of souls appears also in the works of other thirteenth-century theologians. See Jacobus de Voragine, *Sermones quadragesimales*, 152–53.

36. The term *aqua tribulationis* is nowhere in the Bible. It is, however, the standard exegetical interpretation of the Flood. See *Biblia Latina cum glossa ordinaria* (Strassburg, 1480/81; repr., Turnhout, 1992), ad Gen. 7, fol. 38°. Cf. Rupert of Deutz, "Commentariorum in genesim liber quartus," PL 167:346; Philippe de Harveng, "De institutione clericorum tractatus sex," PL 203:852.

37. William of Auvergne, *Opera omnia*, 1:764a–767a.

38. "Si vero volueris utilitates dolorum invenire, et numerare, quomodo dolor et aqua tribulationis vocatur et ignis in sanctis, authenticisque sermonibus, considera actus et

operationes ignis naturalis, et invenies similitudinem et proportionem earum operationes et utilitates spirituales." Ibid., 766a.

39. On Avicenna's influence upon William, see Alan E. Bernstein, "Esoteric Theology: William of Auvergne on the Fires of Hell and Purgatory," *Speculum* 57 (1982): 529–31; Alan E. Bernstein, "Theology between Heresy and Folklore: William of Auvergne on Punishment after Death," *Studies in Medieval and Renaissance History* 5 (1982): 5–44.

40. "Harum igitur quaestionum prima est, an curet creator benedictus et sublimis universa et singula, et de universis et singulis. Secunda, qualiter curet de malis, quae iustis, et sanctis hominibus accidunt in hac vita . . . qualiter et qua utilitate vel usu sustineat hic florere malos, florere inquam potentijs, divitijs, et delitijs. Similiter qua utilitate, vel fructu sustineat bonos affligi hic, et etiam opprimi in malis, et ipsos malis dominari bonis, et multiplici tyrannide, atque violentia graffari in eos." William of Auvergne, *Opera omnia*, 1:754a.

41. This is a deliberate inversion of the legal definition of torture, which often included "*tormentum est torquere mentem.*" Mario Sbriccoli, "'Tormentum id est torquere mentem': Processo inquisitorio e interrogatorio per tortura nell'Italia communale," in *La parola all'accusato*, ed. Jean-Claude Maire Vigueur and Agostino Paravicini Bagliani (Palermo, 1991), 17–32.

42. "Libenter etiam debemus suscipere tribulationes propter multiplicem virtutum quam habent. Prima virtus est quod mentem sanant, . . . Tribulatio vero corporis est velut tortura animam sanans. Tortura videtur esse vulnus vel infirmitas, cum tamen sit sanitas. Sic tribulatio infirmitas videtur, cum tamen sit sanitas mentis. . . . Tribulatio est medicina Altissimi. . . . Ideo qui infirmus est mente, debet gaudere quando datur sibi tribulatio, tanquam spem habens de salute, cum tantum medicus intromittat se de ipso. Secundo, tribulationes debita nostra solvunt, et est magna valde misericordia Dei, quod pro poenis futuris recipit tribulationes praesentes. Talis enim est, ac si ille, cui debentur marcae auri vel argenti, reciperet pro eis fabas vel lapillos, quibus facta est computatio. Plus enim faba una est respectu marcae argenti, quam tribulatio praesens respectu poenae futurae. . . . Tertio, tribulatio signum est divini amoris. . . . Quarto, tribulatio erudit hominem. . . . Quinto, tribulatio odium praesentis vitae inducit." William of Auvergne, "Sermo secundus dominicae in sexagesima," in *Opera omnia*, 2:36b.

43. Jean Gerson, "La médecine de l'âme," in *Oeuvres complètes*, ed. Palémon Glorieux (Paris, Tournai, and Rome, 1968), 7/2:404–7.

44. Johannes Herolt, *Sermones discipuli de tempore et de sanctis una cum promptuario exemplorum* (n.p., [1503?]), sermon 128, "De infirmitatibus."

45. "Nil etenim refert a quibus rebus patiantur, sed quantum patiantur; quia vis doloris non in tormento sed in sensu patientis consistit. Quid enim prodesset etiamsi elementorum foris cruciantium materia abesset, et patientium tamen dolor intus propterea non minor esset? Ut quid ignem ac flammam times, nisi quia uri times? Sed si vulnera et plagae non dolerent, quis arma aut tela timeret? Vide ergo quod omnia haec a quibus dolor esse potest non timentur nisi propter ipsum dolorem. Tolle sensum doloris, non est quod timeas." Hugh of Saint Victor, "De sacramentis Christiane fidei," PL 176:585–86. I have taken the English translation from Hugh of Saint Victor, *On the Sacraments of the Christian Faith*, trans. Roy Deferrari (Cambridge, MA, 1951), 424.

46. Augustine, *Confessionum libri tredecim*, ed. Lucas Verheijen, CCSL 27 (Turnhout, 1981), 162–70, bk. 10.

47. Genesis 34:25: "quando gravissimus vulnerum dolor est."

48. "Primo itaque die considerationis recurrit ad memoriam amputata licentia amata consuetudinis, et absque dubio dolor efficitur, dolor utique gravis. . . . Secundo die considerationis seconde invenit se animus per detrimenta corporis pervenisse ad damna mentis, et fit utique dolor quanto justitior, tanto fortassis et gravior. Tertio die considerationis tertiae deprehendit se gravia pertulisse de sententia propria, sed graviora expectare debere de sententia divina." Richard of Saint Victor, "Benjamin minor," PL 196:40–41, chap. 55. Richard's interpretation is entirely original. The *Glossa ordinaria* to the Bible has no comment to make on the three days of pain. For "Benjamin minor," see Ineke van 't Spijker, *Fictions of the Inner Life: Religious Literature and Formation of the Self in the Eleventh and Twelfth Centuries* (Turnhout, 2004), 136–44, esp. 141.

49. William of Ockham did consider protracted sensation after the injury also a factor, but a sensory one. See William of Ockham, *Quodlibeta septem*, ed. Joseph C. Wey, Opera philosophica et theologica 9 (St. Bonaventure, NY, 1980), 269, quodlibet 3, q. 17, art. 2.

50. It is interesting to compare Richard's attitude toward the psychological and shaming effects of circumcision to Abelard's description of his castration. He, too, avoids the mention of pain and concentrates on shame.

51. William of Auvergne, "De moribus," in *Opera omnia*, 1:192–259. Partially translated in Bernstein, "Theology between Heresy and Folklore," 27.

52. William of Auvergne, *Opera omnia*, 1:211a; Bernstein, "Theology between Heresy and Folklore," 29.

53. "Ego sum ianitor et custos cordis humani . . . ego sum ianitor gladium ex utraque parte acutum, sive bipennem divine sententiae . . . ego sum tortor, non ad mortificandum, sed potius ad vitam." William of Auvergne, *Opera omnia*, 1:195b–196a.

54. For a similar use of a good torturer, see below, chap. 2, and Gratian, *Decretum*, vol. 1 of *Corpus iuris canonici*, ed. Emil Friedberg (Leipzig, 1881), C. 5, q. 5, c. 4.

55. The term *auditores* is problematic. It might also have meant participants in the mass who were not yet entitled to the Eucharist, but in the context of Thomas's work "listeners" or "audience" is the proper rendition.

56. See Morenzoni's summary of Thomas's biography in Thomas of Chobham, *Summa*, xxxi–xxxvi.

57. Ibid., 32–53. For an excellent survey of preaching, see Lester K. Little, "Les techniques de la confession et la confession comme technique," in *Faire croire: Modalités de la diffusion et de la réception des messages religieux du XIIe au XVe siècle*, Collection de l'École française de Rome 51 (Rome, 1981), 87–99.

58. "Et si talis cogitatio aliquem ad bonum convertit ex imaginatione timoris illarum penarum . . . maxime hoc convertere ad bonum deberet." Bromyard, *Summa praedicantium*, s.v. "pena," art. 7.19.

59. "Inquisitio que fit ad eruendam veritatem per tormenta et corporis dolorem." There are several variations of this definition, but they have little meaning. Albertus Gandinus, *Tractatus de maleficiis*, vol. 2 of *Albertus Gandinus und das Strafrecht der Scholastik*, ed. Hermann Kantorowicz (Berlin and Leipzig, 1926), 156–57.

60. "Sed nec in isto ex forma malorum iudicandorum agitis erga nos, quod ceteris negantibus tormenta adhibetis ad confitendum, solis christianis ad negandum, cum, si malum esset, nos quidem negaremus, uos uero confiteri tormentis compelleretis. Neque enim ideo non putaretis requirenda quaestionibus scelera, quia certi essetis admitti ea rex nominis confessione, qui hodie de confesso homicida, scientes homicidium quid sit, nihilominus ordinem exquiritis admissi. Quod peruersius est, cum praesumatis de sceleribus nostris ex nominis confessione, cogitis tormentis de confessione decedere, ut negantes nomen pariter utique negemus et scelera, de quibus ex confessione nominis praesumpseratis. . . . Vociferatur homo: 'christianus sum.' Quod est, dicit; tu uis audire quod non est. Veritatis extorquendae praesides de nobis solis mendacium audire laboratis! 'hoc sum,' inquit, 'quod quaeris an sim. Quid me torques in peruersum! confiteor, et torques: quid faceres, si negarem?' plane aliis negantibus non facile fidem accommodatis: nobis, si negauerimus, statim creditis." Quintus Septimius Florens Tertullianus, "Apologeticum," in Opera, ed. Elygius Dekkers, CCSL 1–2 (Turnhout, 1954), 1:89.

61. This misuse of the law of evidence was rectified by Diocletian, who issued an edict depriving Christians of their Roman citizenship, thus making them liable to torture under almost any circumstances. See Joyce E. Salisbury, The Blood of Martyrs: Unintended Consequences of Ancient Violence (London, 2004), 24–25.

62. Lucy Grig, "Torture and Truth in Late Antique Martyrology," Early Medieval Europe 11 (2002): 332–34.

63. Angelo Clareno, Liber chronicarum, sive tribulationum ordinis minorum, trans. Marino Bigaroni, ed. Giovanni Boccali, Pubblicazioni della Biblioteca francescana, chiesa nuova 8 (Assisi, 1998), 618.

64. Esther Cohen, The Crossroads of Justice: Law and Culture in Late Medieval France, Brill's Studies in Intellectual History 36 (Leiden, 1993), 148–49.

65. Bronislaw Geremek, La potence ou la pitié: L'Europe et les pauvres du Moyen Âge à nos jours, trans. Joanna Arnold-Moricet (Paris, 1987), 159–262.

66. The use of male gender here is deliberate; very few women were executed during the later Middle Ages. See Cohen, Crossroads of Justice, 94.

67. Lindsay Bryan, "Marriage and Morals in the Fourteenth Century: The Evidence of Bishop Hamo's Register," English Historical Review 121 (2006): 481, 485.

68. Cohen, Crossroads of Justice, 181–95.

69. See Michel Foucault, Discipline and Punish: The Birth of the Prison, trans. Alan Sheridan (London, 1977), 9–11, for a totally atypical execution.

70. Cohen, Crossroads of Justice, 146–61.

71. Wolfgang Schild, "Das Strafrecht als Phänomen der Geistesgeschichte," in Justiz in alter Zeit, ed. Christoph Hinckeldey (Rothenburg o.d.T., 1984), 7–58.

72. See below, chap. 2.

73. Isabelle Guérin, La vie rurale en Sologne aux XIV et XV siècles (Paris, 1960), 295–96.

74. Stephen of Bourbon, Tractatus, 1:150–51; John Gobi, Scala coeli, ed. Marie-Anne Polo de Beaulieu (Paris, 1991), no. 905, where the time spans are different. Also cited by Herolt, Sermones discipuli, sermon 128, who gives the alternatives of one day in purgatory and thirty years in sickness.

75. Stephen of Bourbon, *Tractatus*, 1:143–47; Thomas of Chobham, *Summa*, 32–35.

76. Jacques Le Goff, *La naissance du purgatoire* (Paris, 1981).

77. "Augustinus, in libro De ciuitate Dei: Octo genera penarum in legibus describit Tullius: dampnum, uincula, uerbera, talionem, ignominiam, exilium, mortem." Stephen of Bourbon, *Tractatus*, 1:146.

78. Ibid., 140–92; Thomas of Chobham, *Summa*, 32–38.

79. Jacobus de Voragine, *Registrum in sermones de tempore* (Lyons, 1520), "Dominica XIII post festum trinitatis sermo tertius."

80. Jacobus de Voragine, *Registrum in sermones de sanctis*, "Dominica xxii post festum trinitatis sermo primus"; Jacobus de Voragine, *Sermones quadragesimales*, 153.

81. Roberto Caracciolo, *Prediche de frate Roberto vulgare* (Milan, 1515), 13v–14r.

82. C. M. Van der Zanden, *Étude sur le "Purgatoire de saint Patrice"* (Paris, 1927), 4–26; *Le purgatoire de saint Patrice*, ed. J. Vising (Gothenburg, 1916).

83. Giovanni Mattiotti, *Santa Francesca Romana: Edizione critica dei trattati latini di Giovanni Mattiotti*, ed. Alessandra Bartolomei Romagnoli, Storia e attualità 14 (Vatican City, 1994), 877–78.

84. Bromyard, *Summa praedicantium*, s.v. "mors," arts. 20–21; Thomas of Chobham, *Summa*, 51–52.

85. Gobi, *Scala coeli*, no. 626.

86. Jo Ann McNamara, "The Need to Give: Suffering and Female Sanctity in the Middle Ages," in *Images of Sainthood in Medieval Europe*, ed. Renate Blumenfeld-Kosinski and Timea Szell (Ithaca, NY, 1991), 212–21; Stephen of Bourbon, *Tractatus*, 1:175–76.

87. Constantine the African, "De morborum cognitione et curatione," in *Opera* (Basel, 1539), bk. 7, chap. 14.

88. It would be interesting to compare the amount of intellectual effort expended in the search for the alchemical process of converting base matter into gold with the effort not expended in the search for effective anesthesia.

CHAPTER TWO

1. John Langbein, *Torture and the Law of Proof* (Chicago, 1977); Edward Peters, *Torture*, expanded ed. (Philadelphia, 1996).

2. Langbein, *Torture and the Law of Proof*, 3–11.

3. See below, n. 19.

4. The idea that early medieval legal systems operated purely upon a system of belief was first embraced by Henry Charles Lea, in his *Superstition and Force* (Philadelphia, 1870), and was not exploded until the publication of Wendy Davies and Paul Fouracre, eds., *The Settlement of Disputes in Early Medieval Europe* (Cambridge, 1986).

5. Carlo Ginzburg, "Clues: Roots of an Evidential Paradigm," in *Clues, Myths, and the Historical Method*, by Carlo Ginzburg, trans. John Tedeschi and Anne Tedeschi (Baltimore, MD, 1989), 96–126.

6. Peter Brown, "Society and the Supernatural: A Medieval Change," *Daedalus* 104 (1975): 133–51.

7. The Romans did not invent the system. For Greek precedents, see Page duBois, *Torture and Truth* (London, 1991); Yan Thomas, ed., *Du châtiment dans la cité: Supplices corporels et peine de mort dans le monde antique* (Rome, 1984).

8. Compare the theory of torture as summarized in Lisa Silverman, *Tortured Subjects: Pain, Truth, and the Body in Early Modern France* (Chicago, 2001), 51–70.

9. "Quaestionem intellegere debemus tormenta et corporis dolorem ad eruendam veritatem." *Dig.* 47.10.15.41. All references and translations are from *Corpus iuris civilis*, ed. Paul Krueger, Theodore Mommsen, and Rudolph Scholl, trans. Alan Watson, 3 vols. (Berlin, 1884–95; repr., Philadelphia, 1985).

10. *Dig.* 48.18.7.

11. *Dig.* 48.18.10pr., 48.18.15.1.

12. *Dig.* 48.18.18pr.

13. *The Theodosian Code and Novels and the Sirmondian Constitutions*, ed. Theodore Mommsen, trans. Pharr Clyde (Princeton, NJ, 1952), 9.5.1, 9.7.4, 9.16.4. See also David Hunt, "Christianising the Roman Empire: The Evidence of the Code," in *The Theodosian Code*, ed. Jill Harries and I. N. Wood (Ithaca, NY, 1993), 143–58.

14. *Cod.* 9.8, 3.26, 9.8, 4.27, 9.18, 7.28; *Dig.* 49.1, etc.

15. "Quaestioni fidem non semper nec tamen numquam habendam constitutionibus declaratur: etenim res est fragilis et periculosa et quae veritatem vallat. nam plerique patientia sive duritia tormentorum ita tormenta contemnunt, ut exprimi eis veritas nullo modo possit: alii tanta sunt inpatientia, ut quodvis mentiri quam pati tormenta velint: ita fit, ut etiam vario modo fateantur, ut non tantum se, verum etiam alios criminentur." *Dig.* 48.18.1.23.

16. "Quaestiones neque semper in omni causa et persona desiderari debere arbitror, et, cum capitalia et atrociora maleficia non aliter explorari et investigari possunt quam per servorum quaestiones, efficacissimas eas esse ad requirendam veritatem existimo et habendas censeo." *Dig.* 48.18.8pr.

17. Patrick Geary, "Judicial Violence and Torture in the Carolingian Empire," in *Law and the Illicit in Medieval Europe*, ed. Ruth Mazo Karras, Joel Kaye, and Ann E. Matter (Philadelphia, 2008), 79–88.

18. Charles Donahue Jr., "Proof by Witnesses in the Church Courts of Medieval England: An Imperfect Reception of the Learned Law," in *On the Laws and Customs of England: Essays in Honor of Samuel E. Thorne*, ed. Morris S. Arnold (Chapel Hill, NC, 1981), 128: "When the Bolognese glossators began writing, the standard methods of proof in the secular courts were ordeal, battle, and compurgation."

19. Rebecca V. Colman, "Reason and Unreason in Early Medieval Law," *Journal of Interdisciplinary History* 4 (1974): 571–91; Brown, "Society and the Supernatural"; Paul Hyams, "Trial by Ordeal: The Key to Proof in the Early Common Law," in *On the Laws and Customs of England: Essays in Honor of Samuel E. Thorne*, edited by Morris S. Arnold (Chapel Hill, NC, 1981), 90–126; Robert Bartlett, *Trial by Fire and Water: The Medieval Judicial Ordeal* (Oxford, 1986); Stephen D. White, "Proposing the Ordeal and Avoiding It: Strategy and Power in Western French Litigation, 1050 to 1110," in *Cultures of Power: Lordship, Status, and Process in Twelfth-Century Europe*, ed. Thomas N. Bisson (Philadelphia, 1995), 89–123.

20. See the articles in Davies and Fouracre, *Settlement of Disputes in Early Medieval Europe*.

21. Raoul C. Van Caeneghem, "The Law of Evidence in the Twelfth Century," in *Proceedings of the Second International Congress of Medieval Canon Law* (Rome, 1965), 297–310.

22. Richard M. Fraher, "IV Lateran's Revolution in Criminal Procedure: The Birth of *Inquisitio*, the End of Ordeals, and Innocent III's Vision of Ecclesiastical Politics," in *Studia in honorem eminentissimi cardinalis Alphonsi M. Stickler*, ed. J. Rosalius and L. Castillo, Studia et textus historiae iuris canonici 7 (Rome, 1992), 108–10. The Fourth Lateran Council (1215) did not forbid ordeals; it merely forbade any clerical participation in them.

23. Bartlett, *Trial by Fire and Water*, 17n11; Gregory of Tours, *Liber in gloria martyrum*, ed. Bruno Krusch, MGH, SSRM 1 (Hannover, 1885), 542–43. For an English translation, see *Glory of the Martyrs*, trans. Raymond Van Dam (Liverpool, 1988), 104–5.

24. Hyams, "Trial by Ordeal," 93, citing a miracle from the life of St. Swithin, mentions that the slave who had undergone the hot-iron ordeal had felt "immediate, searing pain." This is the only example of which I know.

25. Jacques Berlioz, "Les ordalies dans les exempla de la confession (XIIIe–XIVe siècles)," in *L'aveu: Antiquité et Moyen Âge; Actes de la table ronde organisée par l'École française de Rome, Rome, 28–30 mars 1984* (Rome, 1986), 323–28.

26. Peters, *Torture*, 48.

27. Ibid., 40–73; Richard M. Fraher, "The Theoretical Justification for the New Criminal Law of the High Middle Ages: 'Rei Publicae Interest, Ne Crimina Remaneant Impunita,'" *University of Illinois Law Review* (1984): 577–95.

28. Esther Cohen, "Inquiring Once More after the Inquisitorial Process," in *Die Entstehung des öffentlichen Strafrechts: Beiträge zu einer Bestandaufnahme*, ed. Dietmar Willoweit (Cologne, 1999), 41–65.

29. Fraher, "IV Lateran's Revolution," 110.

30. Stephan Kuttner, *Kanonistische Schuldlehre von Gratian bis auf die Dekretalen Gregors IX*, Studi e testi 64 (Vatican City, 1935); Stephan Kuttner, "The Revival of Jurisprudence," in *Renaissance and Renewal in the Twelfth Century*, ed. Larry Benson and Giles Constable (Oxford, 1982), 299–338.

31. Peters, *Torture*, 43. See also Van Caeneghem, "Law of Evidence."

32. Jacques Chiffoleau, "Sur la pratique et la conjoncture de l'aveu judiciaire en France du XIIIe au XVe siècle," in *L'aveu: Antiquité et Moyen Âge; Actes de la table ronde organisée par l'École française de Rome, Rome, 28–30 mars 1984* (Rome, 1986), 341–43.

33. "Nam ferri candentis vel aquae ferventis examinatione confessionem extorqueri a quolibet sacri non censent canones." Ivo of Chartres, "Decretum," bk. 9, c. 27 (PL 161:599). Gratian, *Decretum*, C. 2, q. 5, c. 20. It is clear from Gratian's context that he had read the letter as referring to ordeals. See also Petrus Browe, *De ordaliies*, 2 vols. (Rome, 1933), 1:14.

34. "Viri honeste viventes et qui gratia vel amicitia vel pecunia corrumpi non possunt, solo iure iurando ad testimonium recipiantur. Vilissimi vero homines et qui facile corrumpuntur, non solo sacramento recipiantur, sed tortoribus subiciantur, id est ad iudicium ignis vel aque ferventis." *Tübingen Lawbook*, chap. 53, quoted in Piero Fiorelli,

La tortura giudiziaria nel diritto comune, 2 vols. (Milan, 1953–54), 1:117. For the date and place of origin of the *Tübingen Lawbook*, see Peter Weimar, "Zur Entstehung des sogenannten Tübinger Rechtsbuchs und der Exceptiones legum romanarum des Petrus," in *Studien zur europäischen Rechtsgeschichte*, ed. Walter Wilhelm (Frankfurt a.M., 1972), 1–24; James A. Brundage, *The Medieval Origins of the Legal Profession: Canonists, Civilians, and Courts* (Chicago, 2008), 91.

35. Fiorelli, *Tortura giudiziaria nel diritto comune*, 1:84–85.

36. For attempts to avoid ordeal, see Hyams, "Trial by Ordeal," 93–94.

37. *Decretales dni. Papae Gregorii IX suae integritati una cum glossis restitutae*, in *Corpus juris canonici emendatum et notis illustratum*, Gregorii XIII. pont. max. iussu editum, pt. 3 (Rome, 1582), 1835–51, bk. 5, tit. 34–35; I have used the *editio princeps* of the *Decretales* rather than Friedberg's edition in order to examine the glosses as well. Yvonne Bongert, *Recherches sur les cours laïques du Xe au XIIIe siècle* (Paris, 1948), 206; Fiorelli, *Tortura giudiziaria nel diritto comune*, 1:232–33; Fraher, "IV Lateran's Revolution," 105–7; Winfried Trusen, "Der Inquisitionsprozeß: Seine historischen Grundlagen und frühen Formen," *Zeitschrift der Savigny-Stiftung, kanonistische Abteilung* 105 (1988): 168–230; Karl B. Shoemaker, "Criminal Procedure in Medieval European Law: A Comparison between English and Roman-Canonical Developments after the IV Lateran Council," *Zeitschrift der Savigny-Stiftung, kanonistische Abteilung* 116 (1999): 174–202.

38. PL 171:277; see the next section.

39. Hyams, "Trial by Ordeal," 105.

40. See below, chap. 8.

41. The Latin term *reus* can mean either "suspect" or "criminal."

42. "Reos tormentis afficere, vel suppliciis veritatem extorquere, censura curiae est, non Ecclesiae disciplina. Unde et ab ejus animadversione abstinere debuisti, quem pecuniam tuam furto suspicaris asportasse. Neque enim carnifex es, sed sacrifex." Hildebert of Lavardin, "Epistolae," PL 171:277 (letter 52).

43. Edward Peters, "Destruction of the Flesh—Salvation of the Spirit: The Paradoxes of Torture in Medieval Christian Society," in *The Devil, Heresy, and Witchcraft in the Middle Ages: Essays in Honor of Jeffrey B. Russell*, edited by Alberto Ferreiro (Leiden, 1998), 131–35; Sbriccoli, "Tormentum id est torquere mentem."

44. Augustine, *De ciuitate Dei*, bk. 19, chap. 6, quoted in Peters, "Destruction of the Flesh," 133n3.

45. "Aliquando, misericordes, et in ipso dubio, nolunt homini pro incerta pecunia, certa inferre supplicia. Ad hanc etiam misericordiam vos etiam provocare nos et exhortari decet. Melius enim, si habet, amittis, quam, si non habet, excrucias, aut occidis. . . . Nolentes reddere quos novimus et male abstulisse, et unde reddant habere, arguimus, increpamus, detestamur, quosdam clam, quosdam palam, sicut diversitas personarum diversam videtur posse recipere medicinam, nec in aliorum perniciem ad majorem insaniam concitari. . . . Aliquando etiam, si res magis curanda non impedit, sacri altaris communione privamus." Augustine, *Epistulae*, ed. A. Goldbacher, CSEL 44 (Vienna, 1904), letter 153, 420–21.

46. Fiorelli, *Tortura giudiziaria nel diritto comune*, 1:76–77.

47. R. I. Moore, *The Formation of a Persecuting Society: Power and Deviance in Western Europe, 950–1250* (New York, 1987), 11.

48. "A mane ergo usque ad vesperum tortus, deciesque suspensus, decies depositus, cum jam se deficere videret, judex etiam juraret, quod si se ulterius suspendi permitteret, jam deinceps vivens non deponeretur." Herman of Tournai, "De miraculis sancta Maria Laudunensis et de gestis venerabilis Bartholomaei episcopi et S. Nortberti libri tres," PL 156:1014. The event took place between Bartholomew's assumption of the bishopric of Laon (1113) and Anselm of Laon's death (1117).

49. "Illi, qui aut in fide catholica, aut inimicitia suspecti sunt, ad pulsationem episcoporum non admittantur. Nec illi, qui aliorum sponte crimina confitentur. Et ideo replicanda sollicite est ueritas, quam sponte prolata in illis habere uox non potest. Hanc diuersis cruciatibus e latebris suis religiosus tortor exigere debet, ut dum penis corpora subiciuntur, que gesta sunt fideliter et ueraciter exquirantur." Gratian, *Decretum,* C. 5, q. 5, c. 4.

50. Gratian was not completely consistent on this point. While discussing regular criminal procedure, he did admit that those who had confessed to a secret (rather than a notorious) crime while coerced by torture had the right to appeal their condemnation. Gratian, *Decretum,* C. 2, q. 6, c. 41, §§ 12–13. The implication is that the breaking of the will might not necessarily lead to the truth.

51. *Decretales,* 758, bk. 2, tit. 21, c. 1.

52. John H. Arnold, *Inquisition and Power: Catharism and the Confessing Subject in Medieval Languedoc* (Philadelphia, 2001).

53. Henry A. Kelly, "Inquisition and the Prosecution of Heresy: Misconceptions and Abuses," *Church History* 58 (1989): 444–45.

54. Mary C. Mansfield, *The Humiliation of Sinners: Public Penance in Thirteenth-Century France* (Ithaca, NY, 1995).

55. For the theology of penitence and confession, see Paul Anciaux, *La théologie du sacrement de pénitence au XIIe siècle,* Universitas Catholica Lovaniensis dissertationes, ser. 2, 41 (Louvain and Gembloux, 1949); Nicole Bériou, "La confession dans les écrits théologiques et pastoraux du XIIIe siècle: Médication de l'âme ou démarche judiciaire?" in *L'aveu: Antiquité et Moyen Âge; Actes de la table ronde organisée par l'École française de Rome, Rome, 28–30 mars 1984* (Rome, 1986), 261–82. For the practice of confession, see Alexander Murray, "Confession before 1215," *Transactions of the Royal Historical Society,* 6th ser., 3 (1993): 51–81.

56. For example, the *Liber feodorum,* covering rents from 1198 to 1293, was compiled in 1302; Philippe de Beaumanoir wrote his *Coutumes du Beauvaisis* in 1283; Albertus Gandinus completed the final version of his Roman-canonical treatise on crime, *Tractatus de maleficiis,* in 1299, quoting a somewhat earlier *Tractatus de tormentis.* Other treatises of both Roman-canonical and customary law belong at the earliest in the second half of the thirteenth century.

57. Berlioz, "Ordalies," 338.

58. Gerald of Wales, *Descriptio Kambriae,* ed. James F. Dimock, Rolls Series 21/6 (repr., London, 1964), 215–16; Mansfield, *Humiliation of Sinners,* 66–67.

59. Peter Abelard, "Abelard's Letter of Consolation to a Friend," ed. J. T. Muckle, *Mediaeval Studies* 12 (1950): 195–202; Betty Radice, ed., *The Letters of Abelard and Heloise,* Penguin Classics (Harmondsworth, UK, 1974); Michael T. Clanchy, *Abelard: A Medieval Life* (Oxford, 1997), 173–203.

60. Anciaux, *Théologie du sacrement de pénitence*, 164–230.

61. Mayke De Jong, "Power and Humility in Carolingian Society: The Public Penance of Louis the Pious," *Early Medieval Europe* 1 (1992): 29–52; Cohen, *Crossroads of Justice*, 177–80.

62. For shame as an integral part of confession, see Anciaux, *Théologie du sacrement de pénitence*, 252. Shame came to occupy a more central place in the theology of confession during the thirteenth century. See Pierre-Marie Gy, "Les définitions de la confession après le quatrième concile du Latran," in *L'aveu: Antiquité et Moyen Âge; Actes de la table ronde organisée par l'École française de Rome, Rome, 28–30 mars 1984* (Rome, 1986), 291, citing Alexander of Hales, "confessio peccati pudorem habet, et ipsa erubescentia est gravis poena."

63. Cohen, *Crossroads of Justice*, 181–201.

64. Léon Dacheux, *Un réformateur catholique de la fin du XVe siècle: Jean Geiler de Kaysersberg, prédicateur à la cathédrale de Strasbourg, 1478–1510* (Paris and Strasbourg, 1876), 45–49.

65. Walter Ullmann, "Reflections on Medieval Torture," *Juridical Review* 56 (1944): 123–37; Walter Ullmann, "Some Medieval Principles of Criminal Procedure," in *Jurisprudence in the Middle Ages*, by Walter Ullmann (London, 1980).

66. E.g., "De generali consuetudine Italie quotidie servamus contrarium, et specialiter in furtis, quia magis frequentatur." Albertus Gandinus, *Tractatus de maleficiis*, 164. "Adeo quidem hoc verum est, quod plene convictus non indigeat tormentis, quia superfluum est tunc adhibere tormenta . . . licet de consuetudine torquentur, ut appellare non possint." Baldus de Ubaldis, *Consiliorum sive responsorum . . .* (Venice, 1580), 5.61.1.

67. Whether laboratory experiments are any more truth revealing than judicial torture remains to be proven. One is led to speculate upon the great number of extremely painful experiments on animals conducted in the name of "truth" and "knowledge."

68. North of the Alps the situation was different; most university law school graduates in northern France went into royal administration. See E. M. Meijers, "L'Université d'Orléans au XIIIe siècle," in *Études d'histoire du droit*, ed. R. Feenstra and H. F. W. D. Vischer (Leiden, 1976), 3:3–148.

69. The overwhelmingly Italian origin of torture treatises is remarkable. A possible reason is the different level of professionalization of law in different countries. While medieval Italian communes often employed trained jurists as either advisers or judges, this was rarely the case north of the Alps. Thus, only in 1499 did King Louis XII formally order that all incoming magistrates of the Parlement of Paris be subject to an examination prior to their admission; J. H. Shennan, *The Parlement of Paris* (Ithaca, NY, 1968), 136. A university degree (not necessarily in law) was not required until the sixteenth century.

70. Fiorelli, *Tortura giudiziaria nel diritto comune*, 1:133–85.

71. Albertus Gandinus, *Tractatus de maleficiis*, 155–77. See also Martino Semeraro, "Osservazioni in margine al '*Tractatus de tormentis*': Attribuzione e circolazione dell'opera sulla base di alcuni manoscritti," *Initium: Revista catalana d'història del dret* 4 (1999): 479–86, who conjectures that, indeed, Gandinus might have been the original author, not the plagiarist.

72. Guido de Suzaria [attr.], "Tractatus de tormentis sive de indicijs et tortura," in *Decimum volumen tractatuum e variis iuris interpretibus collectorum* (Lyons, 1599), fol. 85r; Albertus Gandinus, *Tractatus de maleficiis*, 155–56. By the last question the author meant merely the effects upon the judicial procedure, not upon the suspect.

73. Guido de Suzaria, "Tractatus de tormentis," fol. 87v.

74. Franciscus Brunus, *Tractatus de indicijs et tortura* (Siena, n.d., 1480s), fol. 222r.

75. "[I]nquisitio que fit ad eruendam veritatem per tormenta et corporis dolorem." There are several variations of this definition, but they have little meaning. Albertus Gandinus, *Tractatus de maleficiis*, 156–57.

76. Ibid., 158.

77. This passage, with variations, appears in almost all treatises. Once more, it is the development of a Roman maxim.

78. Albertus Gandinus, *Tractatus de maleficiis*, 159: "nam plerique, dum torquentur, perire solent."

79. Bartolus of Sassoferrato, *Repetitio super materia quaestionum sive torturarum*, vol. 10 of *Omnia quae extant opera . . .* (Venice, 1615), 253, art. 34. For the requirement of multiple *indicia*, see Richard M. Fraher, "Conviction according to Conscience: The Medieval Jurists' Debate concerning Judicial Discretion and the Law of Proof," *Law and History Review* 7 (1989): 39–40, 51–54.

80. Franciscus Brunus, *Tractatus de indicijs et tortura*, fol. 222v; Albertus Gandinus, *Tractatus de maleficiis*, 162–64.

81. Albertus Gandinus, *Tractatus de maleficiis*, 165–66.

82. Bernard of Parma, gloss to *Decretales*, 481–82, bk. 1, tit. 40, c. 3: "hanc (que cadet in constantem) etiam sepe ex ipsius qui patitur magnanimitate vel pusillanimitate metimur, quia in magnanimo levis, in meticuloso violenta invenitur." Quoted in Kuttner, *Kanonistische Schuldlehre*, 311. The fear needed to intimidate a woman was lesser, claimed Bernard (*Decretales*, 1429, gloss to bk. 4, tit. 1, c. 14).

83. *Cod.* 2.19.4, 7, 2.4.3 ("non quemlibet timorem, sed maioris malitatis"); *Dig.* 4.2.3–7.

84. Kuttner, *Kanonistische Schuldlehre*, 309. In the sixteenth century, Paulus Grillandus mentions that, although some derived the term *tortura* from *terrendo* (frightening), this etymology was faulty. Paulus Grillandus, *Tractatus de hereticis: Et sortilegijs omnifariam coitu eorumque penis item de questionibus et torturae ac de relaxatione carceratorum Domini Pauli Grillandi Castilionei ultima hac impressione summa cura castigatus: Adaitis ubilibet summariijs: Prepositosque perutili: Repertorio speciales sententias aptissime continente* (Lyons, 1545), fol. 28r.

85. *ST*, Supplementum, q. 47, art. 2; quoted in Johannes Fried, "Wille, Freiwilligkeit und Geständnis um 1300," *Historisches Jahrbuch* 105 (1985): 422.

86. Fried, "Wille, Freiwilligkeit und Geständnis um 1300," 421–22.

87. Bonifacius de Vitalinis, "Tractatus maleficij cum additionibus & apostillis D. Hieronymi Chuchalon Hispani," in *Tractatus diversi super maleficiis, nempe Do. Alberti de Gandino, Do. Bonifacii de Vitalini, Do. Pauli Grillandi, Do. Baldi de Periglis, Do. Jacobi de Arena* (Lyons, 1555), 453. The printed text says *fumum*, but this might be a misprint for *funem* (rope, strappado), which is what Franciscus Brunus (*Tractatus de indicijs et tortura*, fol. 225v) said.

88. Franciscus Brunus, *Tractatus de indicijs et tortura*, fols. 226v, 229v; Baldus de Ubaldis, *Consiliorum sive responsorum*, 5.479.1; Albertus Gandinus, *Tractatus de maleficiis*, 167–68.

89. Albertus Gandinus, *Tractatus de maleficiis*, 168; Franciscus Brunus, *Tractatus de indicijs et tortura*, fol. 223r.

90. Paulus Grillandus, "De questionibus & tortura tractatus," in *Tractatus diversi super maleficiis, nempe Do. Alberti de Gandino, Do. Bonifacii de Vitalini, Do. Pauli Grillandi, Do. Baldi de Periglis, Do. Jacobi de Arena* (Lyons, 1555), 668: "ita ut nihil aliud deficiat quam sola elevatio. . . . Et ista proprie non dicitur tortura; quia vere corpus non torquetur, nec sentit dolorem; sed potius est quidam mentis timor."

91. For a summary of the cautions concerning torture, see Ullmann, "Reflections on Medieval Torture."

92. Baldus de Ubaldis, *Consiliorum sive responsorum*, 3.364.4; Fraher, "Conviction according to Conscience."

93. Baldus de Ubaldis, *Consiliorum sive responsorum*, 3.364.6, 5.427.10.

94. Most present-day legal historians are agreed that the *ius commune* was indeed an effective influence upon legislation and legal procedures throughout Europe. See Kenneth Pennington, "Learned Law, *Droit Savant, Gelehrtes Recht:* The Tyranny of a Concept," *Rivista internazionale di diritto comune* 5 (1994): 197–209. Given the near-total absence of criminal protocols for the Middle Ages, it is impossible to prove that the *ius commune* permeated actual criminal proceedings.

95. Bonifacius de Vitalinis, "Tractatus maleficij," 456–57.

96. "Et licet sit tutius et minus suspectum, quod testes adhibeantur confessionem et perseverat [*sic*], ut dictum est; tamen bene stabitur actis factis coram iudice per notarium in secreto et sine testibus . . . et ita de consuetine generali observatur quae vicem legis obtinet." Ibid., 457.

97. Grillandus, "De questionibus & tortura tractatus," 670.

98. Ariel Glucklich, *Sacred Pain: Hurting the Body for the Sake of the Soul* (Oxford, 2001).

99. Bonifacius de Vitalinis, "Tractatus maleficij," 456. The *stanghetta* involved encasing the suspect's legs in wooden rods and constricting them.

100. Franciscus Brunus, *Tractatus de indicijs et tortura*, fols. 225v–26ro; Fiorelli, *Tortura giudiziaria nel diritto comune*, 1:197–98.

101. "Non permittunt unquam dictum reum dormire nec quiescere, in tantum quod ad tardius in duabus noctibus et uno die reus omnia confitebitur, promissa sibi quiete. . . . Ideo teneas menti hoc genus tormenti, quia est maximae potentiae et non affligit corpus, adeo quod nunquam ex eo iudex teneretur in sindicatu." Quoted in Fiorelli, *Tortura giudiziaria nel diritto comune*, 1:200–201n64.

102. Grillandus, "De questionibus & tortura tractatus," 668–74; Grillandus, *Tractatus de hereticis*, fols. 97vo–100vo.

103. Here Grillandus quoted Baldus de Ubaldis's lectures on the *Codex*, in which Baldus wrote about appearance in court, not torture. It is important to note that both Baldus and Grillandus made the medieval medical distinction between fever as a symptom and the various illnesses known as fever at the time—quartan, tertian, and hectic fevers.

104. "Sed hic in levi tortura fieri non potest, quod corpus non torqueatur nec patiatur aliqualem dolorem: licet sit levis dolor, dolor est, et infertur iniuria dignitati, vel innocentiae ipsius rei." Grillandus, "De questionibus & tortura tractatus," 670.

105. "Et istud est saevissimum genus tormenti. Et dicunt doc[tores] qui scripserunt de hac materia quod tunc corpus ipsius rei dilaniatur, membraque et ossa quodammodo dissolvuntur, et evelluntur a corpore. Et hac dicitur gravior poena quam utriusque manus abscissio." Ibid., 671.

106. *Dig.* 48.18.7. The phrase "tortus salvus innocentie vel supplicio conservetur" recurred in the writings of several medieval jurists, with small changes: the *Digest* spoke of a slave (*ut servus salvus sit vel innocentiae vel supplicio*); medieval jurists spoke of *tortus* rather than *servus*. Guido de Suzaria, "Tractatus de tormentis," fol. 85r; Albertus Gandinus, *Tractatus de maleficiis*, 156. The implication was, of course, that people were tortured only in cases of capital crimes; there was no possibility of being absolved from torture for any option of a punishment less than death.

107. Ullmann, "Reflections on Medieval Torture," 133.

108. "Et ibi in prima tracta cordae cum nihil confiteretur, fecit eum secundo levari sursum, et deorsum mergi, et cum adhuc etiam nihil confiteretur, fecit idem fieri tertia vice absque eo, quod credere deberet, quod dictus tortus esset sic de levi moriturus, qui tamen impatiens doloris in dicta tertia tormentatione diem clausit extremum. Et ideo credentibus torquentibus quod dictus tortus expiraverit, adhuc dederunt sibi parum de aqua pro experientia vitae; tamen re vera expiraverat omnino." Baldus de Ubaldis, *Consiliorum sive responsorum*, 5.61.1. The case, like many other *consilia*, is probably a putative one, but people did die under torture, especially that of strappado.

109. Bartolus of Sassoferrato, *Repetitio*, 255, art. 30.

110. Franciscus Brunus, *Tractatus de indiciis et tortura*, fol. 226r.

111. Bartolomaeus Caepolla, *Consilia criminalia* (Brescia, 1490), *consilium* 61; Bonifacius de Vitalinis, "Tractatus maleficij," 451–52.

112. This case was published by Hermann Kantorowicz in his *Albertus Gandinus und das Strafrecht der Scholastik* (Berlin and Leipzig, 1907), 1:202, Urk. 20: "Super septimo libello dato dicto d. Ghalvano per Iohanem Ioanini quo petiit, ipsum d. Ghalvanum puniri, quia eidem Iohani intullit minas tormentorum, ducendo eum sub tondolo . . . quod predictus d. Ghalvanus per syndicos in lib. centum bon. condempnetur, quia plene probatum [est] quod dicto Iohani minas intullit tormentorum et eidem in ea parte dicto Iohani non servavit statutum de tondolo et tormento, ut tenebatur, et maxime quia constat ipsum Ioanem esse privilegiatum et de societatibus populi."

113. For the full text of the statute, see Hermann Kantorowicz, "Studien zum altitalienischen Strafprozeß," in *Rechtshistorische Schriften*, ed. Helmut Coing and Gerhard Immel (Karlsruhe, 1970), 327–28, first published in *Zeitschrift für die gesamte Strafrechtswissenschaft* 44 (1924): 97–130. For the difference between various types of lawyer, see Brundage, *Medieval Origins of the Legal Profession*, 282.

114. *Aconitum napellus*, found mostly in Friuli and the Dolomites. Like most aconites, it is poisonous.

115. Konrad Eubel, "Vom Zaubereiunwesen anfangs des 14. Jahrhunderts," *Historisches Jahrbuch* 18 (1897): 612. I thank Dr. John Arnold for bringing this episode to my attention.

116. Ibid., 609–25.

117. Ibid., 619.

118. We can assume that the deposition was truthful. Had Bartolomeo broken down and confessed his pro-papal sympathies and activities, he would not have emerged alive from the dungeon to tell the tale.

119. "Circa merita processus honorabilis viri Tanini de Porta civis et mercatoris Viennensis appellantis in hac causa et procuratoris fiscalis curie communis dicte civitatis Vienne appellati. . . . Ex alio etiam capite male fuit tractus in causam ipse de Porta coram iudice communi Viennensi, que de iure communi antequam in criminalibus possit procedi sine privato denunciatore per viam inquisitionis requiritur quod precedat de tali pretenso crimine *fama seu infamia publica a fidedignis super inquirendis; non solum semel sed pluries sit tanta fama quod generet scandalum tale quod sine periculo tolerari non possit* [my italics]. . . . Et si iudex aliter procedat ad inquisitionem processus est ipso iure nullus. . . . Maxime ubi reus inquisitus dicit se non infamatur, prout fecit dictus de porta coram dicto iudice communi Vienne. Tunc enim iudex primo cognoscere debet de asserta infamia, et si hoc pretermittat gravat partem: et potest ipsa pars gravata a tali iudice appellare tanquam gravatus." Gui Pape, *Consilia domini Guidonis Pape cum repertorio* . . . (Lyons, 1533), fols. 126r, 127v, *consilium* 89, arts. 1, 7.

120. Nicolas de Tudeschis [Panormitanus], *Consilia, quaestiones et tractatus Panormitani* (Lyons, 1534), fol. 46v, *consilium* 92. See also James A. Brundage, "The Rise of Professional Canonists and Development of the *Ius Commune*," *Zeitschrift der Savigny-Stiftung, kanonistische Abteilung* 112 (1995): 26–63.

121. Daniel Baraz, *Medieval Cruelty: Changing Perceptions, Late Antiquity to the Early Modern Period* (Ithaca, NY, 2003), 27, 166.

122. Heinrich Kramer [Institoris], *Malleus maleficarum*, ed. and trans. Christopher S. Mackay, 2 vols. (Cambridge, 2006), 1:15–28.

123. Ibid., 557–717.

124. Ibid., 578–81, 584–96, 608–12.

125. Ibid., 605–8, 597.

126. Ibid., 616: "questionent eum moderate utpote sine sanguinis effusione, scientes quod questiones sunt fallaces et sepius, ut tactum est, inefficaces."

127. Ibid., 618–19: "Quod si nec sic poterit ad terrorem vel etiam ad veritatem induci, tunc per secunda aut tercia die questionanda—ad continuandum tormenta non ad iterandum, quia iterari non debent nisi nova supervenissent indicia."

128. Ibid., 620–21.

129. Jean Améry, *At the Mind's Limits: Contemplations by a Survivor on Auschwitz and Its Realities*, trans. Sidney Rosenfeld and Stella P. Rosenfeld (Bloomington, IN, 1980), 33, 36.

CHAPTER THREE

1. Contrary to the usual narrative of modern science, taxonomy is as old as Aristotle at least and was practiced throughout scholastic disciplines from the thirteenth century onward. See Scott Atran, *Cognitive Foundations of Natural History: Towards an Anthropology of Science* (Cambridge, 1990).

2. I have not explored the chain of transmission from late antique and Byzantine medicine, to Jewish and Arab medicine, and thence to late medieval medicine. There may well have been authors writing about pain before Avicenna, but I doubt their work had much direct influence upon most medical authorities in the West.

3. Peregrine Horden, "Pain in Hippocratic Medicine," in *Religion, Health and Suffering*, ed. John R. Hinnells and Roy Porter (London, 1999), 295–315.

4. Rosa María Moreno Rodríguez and Luis García-Ballester, "El dolor en la teoría y práctica médicas de Galeno," *Dynamis* 2 (1982): 3–24.

5. Galen, *Opera omnia*, ed. Carolus Gottlob Kühn, 20 vols. (Leipzig, 1821–33), 8:80: "primas doloris species duas esse, repentinam temperamenti alterationem et continuitatis solutionem." Note that the Latin translation of Galen referred to the Greek *krasis* as *temperamentum*. The term *complexio* for this concept was accepted only in the eleventh century; see Danielle Jacquart, "De crasis à complexio: Note sur le vocabulaire du tempérament en latin médiéval," in *La science médicale occidentale entre deux renaissances (XIIe s.–XVe s.)*, by Danielle Jacquart (Aldershot, UK, 1997).

6. Concerning Gerard of Cremona, see Luis García-Ballester, *La búsqueda de la salud: Sanadores y enfermos en la España medieval* (Barcelona, 2001), passim.

7. On the six naturals and the nonnaturals, see Niebyl, "Non-naturals."

8. "Quoniam dolor est una ex dispositionibus non naturalibus que corpori animalis accidunt: in causis eius sermonem faciemus universalem." Avicenna, *Liber canonis Avicenne revisus et ab omni errore mendaque purgatus summaque cum diligentia impressus* (Venice, 1507; repr., Hildesheim, 1964), fol. 38r. English translation in Avicenna, *The Canon of Medicine (al-Qanun fi'l-tibb)*, trans. O. Cameron Gruner et al., ed. Seyyed Hossein Nasr, Great Books of the Islamic World (Chicago, 1999), 246.

9. See below, chap. 5.

10. I have borrowed the translation of Luis García-Ballester for "malitia complexionis diversa," "complexión patológica desequilibrada," in the introduction to Arnau de Villanova, *Commentum super tractatum Galieni de malicia complexionis diverse*, ed. Luis García-Ballester and Eustaquio Sánchez Salor, Arnaldi de Villanova opera medica omnia 15 (Barcelona, 1985), 76–77.

11. "Dicimus igitur quod dolor est sensibilitas rei contrarie. Omnes vero doloris cause in duobus comprehenduntur generibus, scilicet genere mutationis complexionis cito facte et est malitia complexionis diverse, et genere solutionis continuitatis." Avicenna, *Liber canonis*, fol. 38r. I have changed Gruner's use of the term "temperament" to "complexion," according to Gerard of Cremona's usage.

12. Siraisi, *Taddeo Alderotti*, 224–26; Arnau de Villanova, *Tractatus de consideracionibus operis medicine sive de flebotomia*, ed. Luke Demaitre and Pedro Gil-Sotres, Arnaldi de Villanova opera medica omnia 4 (Barcelona, 1988), 218–19; Bernard de Gordon, *Lilio de medicina*, ed. Brian Dutton and María Nieves Sánchez (Madrid, 1993), 1:184; Bernard de Gordon, *Lilium medicinae: Tractatus nimirum septem foliis sive particulis, accuratissimam omnium morborum, tam uniuersalium, quam particularium, curationem complectens*, ed. Peter Uffenbach (Frankfurt, 1617), 71; Henri de Mondeville, *Die Chirurgie des Heinrich von Mondeville*, ed. Julius Leopold Pagel (Berlin, 1892), 395.

13. Luke Demaitre, "Medieval Notions of Cancer: Malignancy and Metaphor," *Bulletin of the History of Medicine* 72 (1998): 611, quoting Guy de Chauliac, *Guigonis de Caulhiaco inventarium sive chirurgia magna*, ed. Michael R. McVaugh, 2 vols., Studies in Ancient Medicine 14 (Leiden, 1997), 1:57.

14. Moreno Rodríguez and García-Ballester, "El dolor"; Galen, *Opera*, 8:70–71; Aristotle, *De anima*, trans. J. A. Smith, Works of Aristotle (Oxford, 1931), 2.11.3.422a–424a; Aristotle, *De sensu et sensibili*, trans. J. I. Beare, Works of Aristotle (Oxford, 1931), 3.436a. See Cynthia Freeland, "Aristotle on the Sense of Touch," in *Essays on Aristotle's "De anima*," ed. Martha C. Nussbaum and Amélie O. Rorty (Oxford, 1992), 228–34; Siraisi, *Taddeo Alderotti*, 223–26.

15. For a thorough discussion of all positions concerning the location of pain, see Per-Gunnar Ottosson, *Scholastic Medicine and Philosophy: A Study of Commentaries on Galen's "Tegni" (ca. 1300–1450)* (Naples, 1984), 239–46.

16. Gilbertus Anglicus, *Healing and Society in Medieval England: A Middle English Translation of the Pharmaceutical Writings of Gilbertus Anglicus*, ed. Faye M. Getz (Madison, WI, 1991), xviii.

17. Paul Diepgen, "Aus der Geschichte des Schmerzes und der Schmerzbehandlung," *Medizinische Mitteilungen* 8 (1936): 218–25.

18. This view was contradicted by the steady publication of early medieval medical manuscripts during the early decades of the twentieth century. See Henry E. Sigerist, *Studien und Texte zur frühmittelalterlichen Rezeptliteratur*, ed. Karl Sudhoff, Studien zur Geschichte der Medizin 13 (Leipzig, 1923; repr., Vaduz, 1977).

19. Roselyne Rey, *The History of Pain*, trans. Louise Elliott Wallace, J. A. Cadden, and S. W. Cadden (Cambridge, MA, 1995), 44–49.

20. Had anyone used only Homer or Virgil as sources for medicine in antiquity, their work would have been dismissed as inconsequential.

21. Johan Huizinga, *The Autumn of the Middle Ages*, trans. Rodney J. Payton and Ulrich Mammitzsch (Chicago, 1996), chap. 1; Norbert Elias, *The Civilizing Process*, trans. Edmund Jephcott, 2 vols. (Oxford, 1994), 1:191–205; Robert Muchembled, *L'invention de l'homme moderne: Culture et sensibilités en France du XVe au XVIIIe siècle* (Paris, 1994).

22. Daniel de Moulin, "A Historical-Phenomenological Study of Bodily Pain in Western Man," *Bulletin of the History of Medicine* 48 (1974): 540–70.

23. Michael R. McVaugh and Luis García-Ballester, "Therapeutic Method in the Later Middle Ages: Arnau de Vilanova on Medical Contingency," *Caduceus* 11 (1995): 73–86.

24. Gilbertus Anglicus, *Healing and Society*, xxii; Percival Horton-Smith Hartley and Harold Richard Aldridge, *Johannes de Mirfeld of St. Bartholomew's, Smithfield: His Life and Works* (Cambridge, 1936), 50.

25. John of Mirfield, *Surgery [Breviarium Bartholomaei, Part IX]*, trans. J. B. Colton (New York, 1969), 217.

26. Avicenna, *Liber canonis*, fol. 43v; Avicenna, *Canon of Medicine*, 282.

27. Constantine the African, "De morborum cognitione et curatione," 157, bk. 7, chap. 14; Avicenna, *Liber canonis*, fol. 39r; Avicenna, *Canon of Medicine*, 251.

28. William de Saliceto, *Chirurgia*, trans. P. Pifteau (Toulouse, 1898), 325–31; Guy de Chauliac, *Chirurgia*, 1:169–70, 2:146; Bernard de Gordon, *Lilio de medicina*, 1:185, 188; Bernard de Gordon, *Lilium medicinae*, 71–76, 196–218.

29. Michele Savonarola, *De gotta la preseruatione e cura per lo preclaro medico m. Michele Sauonarola ordinata: E intitulata allo illustre Marchese di Ferrara S. Nicolo da Este*, ed. Georgius Vegius (Pavia, 1505), canto 4. I am indebted to Chiara Crisciani for drawing my attention to this text and providing me with a photocopy.

30. Jean de St. Amand, *Die Concordanciae des Johannes de sancto Amando: Nach einer Berliner und zwei Erfurter Handschriften*, ed. Julius Pagel (Berlin, 1894).

31. Mondino de Liuzzi, *Practica de accidentibus*, ed. Giuseppe Caturegli, Scientia veterum: Collana di studi di storia della medicina 107 (Pisa, 1967), 25–26; Arnau de Villanova, *Tractatus*, 218; Petrus Hispanus, *Thesaurus pauperum*, in *Obras médicas de Pedro Hispano*, ed. Maria Helena Da Rocha Pereira (Coimbra, 1973), 115–33; Fernando Salmón, "Academic Discourse and Pain in Medical Scholasticism (Thirteenth–Fourteenth Centuries)," in *Medicine and Medical Ethics in Medieval and Early Modern Spain: An Intercultural Approach*, ed. Samuel S. Kottek and Luis García-Ballester (Jerusalem, 1996), 136–53; Fernando Salmón, "Pain and the Medieval Physician," *American Pain Society Bulletin* 10, no. 3 (2000).

32. Jacques Despars, "Summula Jacobi de Partibus per ordinem alphabeti singulorum remediorum singulis morbis conferentium," in *Supplementum in secundum librum compendii secretorum medicinae Ioannis Mesues medici celeberrimi*, by Francesco de Piedmont (Venice, 1531).

33. Guy de Chauliac, *Chirurgia*, 1:436.

34. These ingredients are no more than a sample. They are taken from Paul Meyer, "Recettes médicales en français publiées d'après le manuscrit 23 d'Évreux," *Romania* 18 (1889): 573, 575, 576; Paul Meyer, "Recettes médicales en français publiées d'après le manuscrit BN Lat. 8654ᴮ," *Romania* 37 (1908): 371; Paul Meyer, "Recettes médicales en provençal d'après le manuscrit R. 14.30 de Trinity College (Cambridge)," *Romania* 32 (1903): 273, 276–78, 284; Maria Sofia Corradini Bozzi, ed., *Ricettari medico-farmaceutici medievali nella Francia meridionale*, Studi della Accademia toscana di scienze e lettere 159 (Florence, 1997), passim; Guy de Chauliac, *Chirurgia*, 1:434–46; "Recettes de mede-cine (XVᶜ siècle)," Paris, Bibliothèque nationale de France, Nouvelles acquisitions latines 152; Jehan Sauvage de Picquigny, "La nouvelle physique attraite de plusieurs autheurs par . . . secrets de medecine pour traiter maladies du corps humain," Paris, Bibliothèque de l'Arsenal, MS 3174, passim; Claude de Tovar, "Contamination, interférences et tenta-tives de systematisation dans la tradition manuscrite des recéptaires medicaux français: Le recéptaire de Jean Sauvage," *Revue d'histoire des textes* 3–4 (1973–74): 115–91, 239–88; John Arderne, *Treatises of Fistula in Ano, Haemorrhoids and Clysters, from an Early Fifteenth-Century Manuscript Translation*, trans. D'Arcy Power, Early English Text Soci-ety (London, 1910), 88–89, 100–101; John Arderne, *De arte phisicali et de cirurgia (1412)*, trans. D'Arcy Power, Research Studies in Medical History of the Wellcome Historical Medical Museum 1 (London, 1922), 27, 38, 48–50; *Boec van medicinen in Dietsche: Een Middelnederlandse compilatie van medisch-farmaceutische literatuur*, ed. W. F. Daems, Janus, Suppléments 7 (Leiden, 1967), 185–86, 194, 294; Constance B. Hieatt and Robin

'F. Jones, eds., *La novele cirurgerie* (London, 1990); Gilbertus Anglicus, *Healing and Society*, xxxv–xxxvii, 1–6, 32–41, 64–68.

35. Mondino de Liuzzi, *Practica de accidentibus*, 20–21.

36. Helen King, "The Early Anodynes: Pain in the Ancient World," in *The History of the Management of Pain*, ed. Ronald D. Mann (Carnforth, Lancashire, 1988), 52–53; John M. Riddle, *Dioscorides on Pharmacy and Medicine* (Austin, TX, 1985), 67–69.

37. Siraisi, *Taddeo Alderotti*, 291–92.

38. Guy de Chauliac, *Chirurgia*; Sauvage de Picquigny, "Nouvelle physique," MS 3174, fol. 25r; Arderne, *De arte phisicali*, 27; Arderne, *Treatises*, 103–4.

39. E.g., Arderne, *Treatises*, 89–90; *Boec van medicinen*, 186.

40. See, e.g., Theodoricus Borgognoni, *Surgery*, trans. E. Campbell and J. B. Colton, 2 vols. (New York, 1955), 1:149.

41. McVaugh, *Rational Surgery*, 107–9; "Recettes de medecine," Nouvelles acquisitions latines 152, fol. 1v: "Calidoma trita et corta ac capiti emplastrata tollit dolorem frontis . . . fronti applicata dolorem ex frigiditate tollit."

42. Arderne, *Treatises*, 102–4; Henry E. Handerson, *Gilbertus Anglicus: Medicine of the Thirteenth Century* (Cleveland, OH, 1918), 27, 36; Faye M. Getz, *Medicine in the English Middle Ages* (Princeton, NJ, 1998), 49–53.

43. "Recettes de medecine," Nouvelles acquisitions latines 152, fol. 11r; Tony Hunt, *Popular Medicine in Thirteenth-Century England: Introduction and Texts* (Wolfeboro, NH, 1990), 88.

44. "Recettes de medecine," Nouvelles acquisitions latines 152, fol. 10v; Hunt, *Popular Medicine*, 28, 81–82; Oswald Cockayne, *Leechdoms, Wortcunning, and Starcraft of Early England, Being a Collection of Documents . . . Illustrating the History of Science in This Country before the Norman Conquest*, 3 vols., Rolls Series 35 (London, 1864; repr., Nendeln, 1965), 3:65.

45. Michael R. McVaugh, "*Incantationes* in Late Medieval Surgery," in *Ratio et Superstitio: Essays in Honor of Graziella Federici Vescovini*, edited by Giancarlo Marchetti, Orsola Rignani, and Valeria Sorge, Fédération internationale des Instituts d'études médiévales: Textes et études du Moyen Âge 24 (Louvain-la-Neuve, 2003), 331. This statement, if one is to take the Gospels as its source, is partially true. The wound on Christ's side, inflicted after his death, is mentioned only in the Gospel of John (19:34). As Christ was dead, it could not have caused pain. Nevertheless, it did flow with water and blood.

46. Getz, *Medicine in the English Middle Ages*, 41.

47. Sigerist, *Studien und Texte zur frühmittelalterlichen Rezeptliteratur*.

48. Ibid., 25, 33, 37.

49. Dietlinde Goltz, *Mittelalterliche Pharmazie und Medizin, dargestellt an Geschichte und Inhalt des "Antidotarium Nicolai," mit einem Nachdruck der Druckfassung von 1471*, ed. Wolfgang-Hagen Hein, Veröffentlichungen der Internationalen Gesellschaft für Geschichte der Pharmazie e. V., neue Folge, 44 (Stuttgart, 1976). I have used the facsimile in Goltz's work as my text and have compared it with Fontanella's edition of a vernacular translation: Lucia Fontanella, *Un volgarizzamento tardo duecentesco fiorentino dell' "Antidotarium Nicolai": Montréal, McGill University, Osler Library* 7628, Pluteus testi 3 (Alessandria, 2000), v–xvii. For the dating of the *Antidotarium*, see

Gundolf Keil, "Zur Datierung des 'Antidotarium Nicolai,'" *Sudhoffs Archiv: Zeitschrift für Wissenschaftsgeschichte* 62 (1978): 190–96.

50. Goltz, *Antidotarium Nicolai*, s.v. "Unguentum agrippa."

51. Ibid., s.v. "Tyriaca magna Galieni, Theodoriton yperiston."

52. Ibid., s.v. "Litontripon."

53. Ibid., 149. The author's conclusion is that painkillers were as important then as now; if, she says, one excludes from the total of 142 medicines those compounds that are meant only as ingredients for other medications, more than half of all remaining prescriptions are analgesics.

54. Pseudo–Yāh'annā Ibn Māsawaih, "Grabadin, id est compendii secretorum medicamentorum liber secundum, qua propria remedia ad singularum partium corporis morbos docentur," in *Johannes Mesuae medici clarissimi opera* (Venice, 1531). The Arab original has never been found; concerning the *Grabadin*, see Danielle Jacquart, "L'enseignement de la médecine: Quelques termes fondamentaux," in *La science médicale occidentale entre deux renaissances (XIIᵉ s.–XVᵉ s.)*, by Danielle Jacquart (Aldershot, UK, 1997).

55. John M. Riddle, "Theory and Practice in Medieval Medicine," *Viator* 5 (1974): 179–83.

56. Hunt, *Popular Medicine*; Tovar, "Contamination"; "Recettes de medecine," Nouvelles acquisitions latines 152; Corradini Bozzi, *Ricettari*; *Boec van medicinen*; Francis B. Brévart, "Between Medicine, Magic, and Religion: Wonder Drugs in German Medico-Pharmaceutical Treatises of the Thirteenth to Sixteenth Centuries," *Speculum* 83 (2008): 1–57.

57. E.g., Sauvage de Picquigny, "Nouvelle physique," MS 3174, fol. 59vo: "Pour savoir si feme est fole de corps ou pucelle. . . . Pronostique pour espier si la feme est mechyne ou non. . . . Pronostique pour savoir de quel enfant feme soit enceinte. . . . Pronostique de mort. Prenez du sang ou de larme au malade et let de feme norrice denfant masle et mesle ensemble si se iougnent ensemble il mourra et si non il vivra. Idem oignez les piez du malade des le talon iusque lortail de lart et le remaignent de lart gettez a un chien se li maladez doit eschaper il le mangera et si non il ne tastera." These subjects are highly reminiscent of the literature of secrets rather than medicine: see Charles-Victor Langlois, *La connaissance de la nature et du monde d'après des écrits français à l'usage des laïcs* (Paris, 1927); William Eamon, *Science and the Secrets of Nature: Books of Secrets in Medieval and Early Modern Culture* (Princeton, NJ, 1996).

58. Ernst Wickersheimer, "Bénédiction des remèdes au Moyen Âge," *Lychnos* (1952): 96–101. The subject still requires much research.

59. Avicenna, *Liber canonis*, bk. 5; Arnau de Villanova, "Antidotarium," in *Opera omnia*, forthcoming. I am grateful to Michael McVaugh for allowing me to see the draft of the forthcoming edition of Arnau's *Antidotarium* in the Opera medica omnia series. Guy de Chauliac, *Chirurgia*, 1:434–36.

60. McVaugh, *Rational Surgery*.

61. Ibid., 13–52.

62. See above, n. 34.

63. For other botched phlebotomies, see Getz, *Medicine in the English Middle Ages*, 13.

64. Arnau de Villanova, *Commentum*, esp. 176. Arnau repeated the same opinion in a *consilium*, where he added a stringent warning against quacks. See n. 71 below. Arnau

de Villanova, *Doctrina Galieni de interioribus secundum stilum Latinorum*, ed. Richard J. Durling, Arnaldi de Villanova opera medica omnia 15 (Barcelona, 1985), 314–15. This text is more an elaboration of Galen than a commentary.

65. Arnau de Villanova, *Tractatus*, 218–24.

66. Avicenna, *Liber canonis*, fol. 39r; Avicenna, *Canon of Medicine*, 251.

67. Danielle Jacquart, "Le regard d'un medecin sur son temps: Jacques Despars (1380?–1458)," *Bibliothèque de l'École des chartes* 138 (1980): 60; Danielle Jacquart, *La médecine médiévale dans le cadre parisien: XIVᵉ–XVᵉ siècle*, Penser la médecine (Paris, 1998), 125n17, 517.

68. Mondino de Liuzzi, *Practica de accidentibus*, 19.

69. Ibid., 20.

70. E.g., concerning earache, "Secundo dolor vel est pungitivus vel pruritivus vel gravativus vel extensivus vel commixtus ex istis"; concerning stomach pains, "dolor pungitivus vel mordicativus vel ulcerativus." Cristoforo Barzizza, *Introductorium practicae medicinae* (Pavia, 1494), fols. 84r, 141v.

71. Arnau de Villanova, *Arnaldi Villanovani philosophi et medici summi opera omnia* (Basel, 1585), col. 1494.

72. Laurent Joubert, *The Second Part of the Popular Errors*, trans. Gregory David de Rocher (Tuscaloosa, AL, 1995), 78–81.

73. Jole Agrimi and Chiara Crisciani, *Les consilia médicaux*, trans. Caroline Viola, TSMA 69 (Turnhout, 1994).

74. Bartolomeo Montagnana, *Consilia magistri Bartolomei Montagnane* (Venice, 1525); "Consilia magistri Bartolomei Montagnane," Rome, Biblioteca apostolica Vaticana, MS Vat. Lat. 2471, fols. 49v–52v, 199r.

75. "Consilia magistri Bartolomei Montagnane," MS Vat. Lat. 2471, fols. 157v–175r, 178v, 250r.

76. Savonarola, *De gotta*, canto 4; Baverio Maghinardo de Bonetti, *Praestantissimi medici et philosophi clarissimi D. Ioannis Bauerij de Imola consiliorum de re medica sive morborum curationibus liber* (Strasbourg, 1542), fols. 21r–33v, 135r.

77. E.g., Bartolomeo Montagnana, *Consilia*, consilium 129; "Consilia magistri Bartolomei Montagnane," MS Vat. Lat. 2471, fol. 199r; Marcus Gatinarius, *De curis egritudinum particularium novi Almansoris practica uberrima* (Venice, 1521); Arnau de Villanova, *Opera omnia*, 1491–98. Practically all *consilia* begin by recommending a moderate lifestyle, as do medical textbooks, e.g., Alonso de Chirino, *El menor daño de la medicina*, ed. María Teresa Herrera (Salamanca, 1973); Arnau de Villanova, *Regimen sanitatis ad regem Aragonum*, ed. Luis García-Ballester, Michael R. McVaugh, and Pedro Gil-Sotres, Arnaldi de Villanova opera medica omnia 10/1 (Barcelona, 1996).

78. Guy de Chauliac, *Chirurgia*, 1:404–6.

79. *The Trotula: A Medieval Compendium of Women's Medicine*, ed. Monica H. Green (Philadelphia, 2001), 99–103.

80. Michele Savonarola, *Ad mulieres Ferrarienses de regimine pregnantium et noviter natorum usque ad septennium*, published as *Il trattato ginecologico-pediatrico in volgare di Michele Savonarola*, ed. Luigi Belloni (Milan, 1952), 110–11.

81. *Trotula*, 100; Pseudo–Arnau de Villanova, *Breviarium practicae medicinae* (Venice, 1494), bk. 3, chap. 4.

82. "Quod omnino vitupero et omnibus vere fidelibus talia diabolica necnon medicamina similia fugienda esse censeo." Pseudo–Arnau de Villanova, *Breviarium practicae medicinae*, bk. 3, chap. 4. I am indebted to Naama Cohen-HaNegbi for this reference.

83. Marianne Elsakkers, "In Pain You Shall Bear Children (Gen 3:16): Medieval Prayers for a Safe Delivery," in *Women and Miracle Stories: A Multidisciplinary Exploration*, ed. Anne-Marie Korte (Leiden, 2001), 179–209; Hunt, *Popular Medicine*, 90.

84. Vincent of Beauvais, *Speculum historiale* (Douai, 1624; repr., Graz, 1965), 252, 258, bk. 7, chaps. 85, 99.

85. For childbirth charms that promise a successful but not necessarily painless delivery, see Don C. Skemer, *Binding Words: Textual Amulets in the Middle Ages* (University Park, PA, 2006), 235–78.

86. McVaugh, *Rational Surgery*.

87. Theodoricus Borgognoni, *Surgery*, 2:119–31; Guy de Chauliac, *Chirurgia*, 1:169, 2:146.

88. Theodoricus Borgognoni, *Surgery*, 2:147–51.

89. Guy de Chauliac, *Chirurgia*, 1:403.

90. E.g., Mondino de Liuzzi, *Practica de accidentibus*, 19, 25; Arnau de Villanova, *Opera omnia*; Ugo Benzi, *Consilia medica* (Venice, 1523), passim.

91. Bartolomeo Montagnana, *Consilia*, fols. 50r, 52v: "propter quod ultimate concluditur quod non est mirabile si huic viro aliquin supervenit destitutio virium corporis. Imo propter nocumentum stomachi vehementer colligati cerebro cordi et vehementer nocentur olim membrorum principalium operationes vitalis et animalis motiva sensitiva et naturalis vegetativa; que sunt fere omnes corporis humani virtutes a plurimis sapientium lipothomie et pro parte cordi."

92. Guy de Chauliac, *Chirurgia*, 1:391.

93. For the ideology of phlebotomy, see Pedro Gil-Sotres, "Sangre y patología en la medicina bajomedieval: El substrato material de la flebotomía," *Asclepio* 38 (1986): 73–104; Pedro Gil-Sotres, "Derivation and Revulsion: The Theory and Practice of Medieval Phlebotomy," in *Practical Medicine from Salerno to the Black Death*, ed. Luis García-Ballester et al. (Cambridge, 1994), 110–55; Roger French, "Astrology in Medical Practice," in *Practical Medicine from Salerno to the Black Death*, ed. Luis García-Ballester et al. (Cambridge, 1994), 30–59. On the history of medieval phlebotomy, see Linda E. Voigts and Michael R. McVaugh, eds., "A Latin Technical Phlebotomy and Its Middle English Translation," *Transactions of the American Philosophical Society* 74, no. 2 (1984): 1–7.

94. Constantine the African, "De morborum cognitione et curatione," 157–58, bk. 7, chap. 14; Avicenna, *Liber canonis*, fol. 39r; Avicenna, *Canon of Medicine*, 251.

95. Petrus Hispanus, "Libro della flebotomia," London, Wellcome Library, MS 617, fols. 48v–49r; "Anonymi practica medicinae," Paris, Bibliothèque nationale de France, Nouvelles acquisitions latines 733, fols. 22v, 23v; "Traités de medecine," Paris, Bibliothèque de l'Arsenal, MS 1024, fol. 204v; Voigts and McVaugh, "Latin Technical Phlebotomy," 42–50.

96. Arnau de Villanova, *Opera omnia*, 1491–98, 1501–6; "Consilia magistri Bartolomei Montagnane," MS Vat. Lat. 2471, fols. 26r–26v; Gil-Sotres, "Derivation and Revulsion," 133–40.

97. Joubert, *Second Part of the Popular Errors*, 78–81.

98. Arnau de Villanova, *Tractatus*, 218; Savonarola, *De gotta*, canto 4.

99. Berlioz, "Ordalies," 338.

100. Guy de Chauliac, *Chirurgia*, 1:414, 443: "cito facta sit et cito transeat illata impressio," "nisi esset in casu in quo paciens propter eius pusillanimitatem non esset ausus attendere ignem, aut in casu in quo vellemus facere cauteria ad evacuandum et derivandum; tun enim ruptorium propter dolorem et escarram grossum quam dimittit, debilitando locum, maiorem provocat fluxum." Cf. Henri de Mondeville, *Chirurgie*, 541–47.

101. Guy de Chauliac, *Chirurgia*, 2:357–58.

102. Ibid., 1:415; Henri de Mondeville, *Chirurgie*, 363.

103. Guy de Chauliac, *Chirurgia*, 1:415.

104. Arnau de Villanova, *Commentum*, 176.

105. Arnau de Villanova, *Regimen*, 466–67.

106. The term *cancrum* in medieval Latin could refer to any type of tumor or growth. Martin de Saint-Gilles warned that cauterizing a cancerous lesion was "moult perilleuse chose"; quoted in Demaitre, "Medieval Notions of Cancer," n. 103.

107. Guy de Chauliac, *Chirurgia*, 1:415.

108. Duns Scotus, *Questiones*, 568.

109. Guy de Chauliac, *Chirurgia*, 1:306: "Et membro separato cauterizetur sanum cum ferro ignito ad hoc apto aut cum oleo ferventi . . . et ligetur." McVaugh mentions in his notes to Chauliac (2:251) that he could not trace this attribution to its source.

110. Ibid., 307: "quia honestius est medico quod cadat per se quam si incideretur. Semper enim quando inciditur remanet rancor et cogitacio in paciente quod posset remanere."

111. John of Salisbury, *Policraticus*, ed. K. S. B. Keats-Rohan, CCCM 118 (Turnhout, 1993), 115–20, bk. 3, chap. 13.

112. See Fourth Lateran Council (1215), canon 3.

113. In a bitter diatribe against physicians in general, Roger Bacon, who was not a physician, accused them of killing their patients with opium. Roger Bacon, "De erroribus medicorum," in *Essays on the History of Medicine Presented to Karl Sudhoff*, trans. E. T. Wittington, ed. Charles Singer and Henry E. Sigerist (Oxford, 1924), 142. Guy de Chauliac, *Chirurgia*, 1:305–8.

114. Guy de Chauliac, *Chirurgia*, 1:307 ("de membris superfluis amputandis"), 1:436 ("de antidotis localibus apostematum").

115. Ambroise Paré, *Oeuvres complètes* (Paris, 1628; repr., Geneva, 1970), 3:547–51.

116. McVaugh, *Rational Surgery*, 108–10.

117. Isidore of Seville, *Etymologiarum sive originum libri XX*, ed. W. M. Lindsay, 2 vols. (Oxford, 1911), 30, bk. 17, chap. 9.

118. For the three manuscripts and the recipes, see Daniel de Moulin, *De heelkunde in de vroege Middeleeuwen* (Leiden, 1964), 120–25; Willem F. Daems, "Spongia somnifera: Philologische und pharmakologische Probleme," *Beiträge zur Geschichte der Pharmazie* 22 (1970): 25–26.

119. Goltz, *Antidotarium Nicolai*, s.v. "spongia somnifera." The recipe includes opium, henbane, seeds of green mulberries, lettuce, poppy, and ivy.

120. Gilbertus Anglicus, *Healing and Society*, xxxvii; Arderne, *Treatises*, 101.

121. Though a text once attributed to Arnau de Villanova contains an antidotary with an entire chapter on opiates and their uses, nothing is known of the author. *Antidotarium* in Arnau de Villanova, *Opera omnia*, 336–494, chap. 21, cols. 442–63: de opiatis.

122. Guy de Chauliac, *Chirurgia*, 1:307 ("de membris superfluis amputandis"), 1:436 ("de antidotis localibus apostematum").

123. Marguerite L. Baur, "Recherches sur l'histoire de l'anesthésie avant 1846," *Janus* 31 (1927): 24–39, 63–90, 124–37, 170–82.

124. Peter Murray Jones, *Medieval Medical Miniatures* (London, 1984), 65; Loren Mackinney, *Medical Illustrations in Medieval Manuscripts* (Berkeley, CA, 1965), 208 (fig. 81B), 229 (fig. 51, cautery), 237 (fig. 68), 244 (fig. 81C); Robert S. Gottfried, *Doctors and Medicine in Medieval England, 1340–1530* (Princeton, NJ, 1986), 237.

125. McVaugh, *Rational Surgery*, 110.

126. Jocelyn of Furness, "The Life of Saint Kentigern," ed. and trans. Cynthia Whiddon Green (M.A. thesis, University of Houston, 1998), http://www.gypsyfire.com/Translation.htm (accessed 9 March 2009). Jocelyn, however, was not citing any specific case; he was merely trying to explain how a virtuous unmarried princess, the saint's mother, had somehow gotten pregnant without in any way infringing upon the uniqueness of the Virgin and without sinning. She had prayed to the Virgin, begging that she might imitate her by getting pregnant, and indeed her womb was blessed. The author did not know how this had happened. His way of avoiding an embarrassing acknowledgment is to say that much can happen to people while they are unconscious under medication.

127. Arderne, *Treatises*, 101.

128. Linda E. Voigts and Robert P. Hudson, "'A Drynke That Men Callen Dwale to Make a Man to Slepe Whyle Men Kerven Him': A Surgical Anesthetic from Late Medieval England," in *Health, Disease, and Healing in Medieval Culture*, ed. Sheila Campbell, Bert Hall, and David Klausner (London, 1992), 34–35.

129. Guy de Chauliac, *Chirurgia*, 1:306: "Et modum est quod involuatur membrum a parte sana et a parte corrupta cum ligamentis, et teneatur firmiter per ministros."

130. David Kunzle, "The Art of Pulling Teeth in the Seventeenth and Nineteenth Centuries: From Public Martyrdom to Private Nightmare and Political Struggle?" in *Fragments for a History of the Human Body*, ed. Michel Feher, Ramona Naddaff, and Nadia Tazi (New York, 1989), 3:29–89.

CHAPTER FOUR

1. Mark Zborowski, *People in Pain* (San Francisco, 1969), 18–48. For criticism of Zborowski and his method, see Arthur Kleinman et al., "Pain as a Human Experience: An Introduction," in *Pain as Human Experience: An Anthropological Perspective*, edited by Mary-Jo DelVecchio Good et al. (Berkeley, CA, 1992), 1–28.

2. Barbara Newman, "Possessed by the Spirit: Devout Women, Demoniacs, and the Apostolic Life in the Thirteenth Century," *Speculum* 73 (1998): 733–70; Uhlinka Rublack, "Pregnancy, Childbirth and the Female Body in Early Modern Germany," *Past and Present* 150 (1996): 84–110; Elisheva Baumgarten, *Mothers and Children: Jewish Family Life in Medieval Europe* (Princeton, NJ, 2004), 43–52.

3. The art of letter writing did not coalesce in rigid forms until the twelfth century and became paramount only during the first half of the thirteenth century. See Alain Boureau, "The Letter-Writing Norm, a Mediaeval Invention," in *Correspondence: Models of Letter-Writing from the Middle Ages to the Nineteenth Century,* ed. Roger Chartier, Alain Boureau, and Cécile Dauphin (London, 1997), 36–52.

4. "Secundum spiritum quantum Domino placet atque ipse uires praebere dignatur, recte sumus, corpore autem, ego in lecto sum, nec ambulare enim nec stare nec sedere possum rhagadis uel exochadis dolore et tumore." Augustine, letter 38, in *Sancti Aurelii Augustini epistulae,* ed. K. D. Daur, CCSL 31 (Turnhout, 2004), 156–57.

5. Symmachus, "Epistolae," PL 18:323.

6. "Multum enim iam tempus est, quod surgere de lecto non ualeo. Nam modo podagrae dolor cruciat, modo nescio quis in toto corpore cum dolore se ignis expandit. Et fit plerumque ut uno in me tempore ardor cum dolore confligat et corpus in me animus que deficiat. Quantis autem aliis necessitatibus extra haec quae retuli infirmitatis afficiar, enumerare non ualeo. Sed breuiter dico quia sic me infectio noxii humoris inhibit, ut uiuere mihi poena sit, sed mortem desideranter exspectem, quam gemitibus meis solam esse credo posse remedium." Gregory the Great, *Registrum epistolarum,* ed. Dag Norberg, CCSL 140 (Turnhout, 1982), 889–90. See also 500, 898.

7. Michel de Montaigne, *Essais,* ed. Maurice Rat, 2 vols. (Paris, 1962), 2:172–76.

8. Einhard, "Epistolae," PL 104:525–26.

9. "Nam et nimia ventris solutio et renium dolor sic in me alternando sibi succedunt, ut nulla dies fuerit, postquam de Aquis promoui, quin hac vel illa infirmitate laborarem. Sunt pariter haec et alia quae mihi ex illo morbo, in quo anno praeterito jacui, contigerant, dextri videlicet femoris continuus torpor ac splenis pene intolerabilis dolor. His passionibus affectus, valde tristem ac pene omni jucunditate carentem duco vitam." Ibid., 526.

10. Gerbert of Aurillac, "Epistolae alia Gerberti," PL 139:259.

11. Letter to Christian, archbishop of Mainz (1179), in Hildegard of Bingen, *Epistolarium,* ed. L. Van Acker, 3 vols., CCCM 91 (Turnhout, 1991–2001), 1:67. English translation in *The Letters of Hildegard of Bingen,* trans. Joseph L. Baird and Radd K. Ehrman, 3 vols. (New York, 1994–2004), 1:67.

12. Richard W. Southern, *Saint Anselm and His Biographer: A Study of Monastic Life and Thought, 1059–c. 1130* (Cambridge, 1966), 67–76; Giles Gasper, "'A Doctor in the House'? The Context for Anselm of Canterbury's Interest in Medicine with Reference to a Probable Case of Malaria," *Journal of Medieval History* 30 (2004): 245–61.

13. Anselm of Canterbury, *The Letters of Saint Anselm of Canterbury,* ed. and trans. Walter Frölich, 3 vols. (Kalamazoo, MI, 1990–94), 1:320–21.

14. Ibid., 140.

15. Petrarch referred briefly to his ailments in *Le familiari,* ed. V. Rossi and U. Bosco, 4 vols. (Florence, 1933–42), 1:47–48. Most of what he wrote on pain is in *De remediis utriusque fortune.* See *A Dialogue between Reason and Adversity: A Late Middle English Version of Petrarch's "De remediis,"* ed. F. N. M. Diekstra (Assen, 1968), 2–41; Karl A. E. Enenkel, "Pain as Persuasion: The Petrarch Master Interpreting Petrarch's *De remediis,*" in *The Sense of Suffering: Constructions of Physical Pain in Early Modern Culture,* ed. Jan Frans van Dijkhuizen and Karl A. E. Enenkel (Leiden, 2009), 91–164.

16. "The maste payne that I felyd was schortnes of wynde and faylynge of lyfe." *A Book of Showings to the Anchoress Julian of Norwich*, ed. Edmund Colledge and James Walsh (Toronto, 1978), 209; Angela of Foligno, *Il libro della beata Angela da Foligno*, ed. Ludger Thier and Abele Calufetti (Grottaferrata, 1985), 724–37.

17. Kieckhefer, *Unquiet Souls*.

18. Suso, *Deutsche Schriften*, 18–19. English translation in *The Exemplar: Life and Writings of Blessed Henry Suso, O.P.*, trans. M. Ann Edward, 2 vols. (Dubuque, IA, 1962), 1:13–14; Raymond of Capua, "Vita sanctae Catharinae Senensis," *AASS*, 3 April, 901–2. See also Caroline W. Bynum, *Holy Feast and Holy Fast: The Religious Significance of Food to Medieval Women* (Berkeley, CA, 1987), 212, 274, for several other cases.

19. Thomas of Cantimpré, "Vita Christinae Mirabilis," AASS, 5 July, 650–56. English translation in *The Life of Christina Mirabilis*, trans. and ed. Margot H. King (Toronto, 1986; repr., Toronto, 1989). For recent writing about Christina, see Anke E. Passenier, "The Life of Christina Mirabilis: Miracles and the Construction of Marginality," in *Women and Miracle Stories: A Multidisciplinary Exploration*, ed. Anne-Marie Korte (Leiden, 2001), 145–78; Robert Sweetman, "Christine of Saint-Trond's Preaching Apostolate: Thomas of Cantimpré's Hagiographical Method Revisited," *Vox Benedictina* 9 (1992): 67–97; Newman, "Possessed by the Spirit," 763–68, and the bibliography there; Barbara Newman, "Devout Women and Demoniacs in the World of Thomas of Cantimpré," in *New Trends in Feminine Spirituality: The Holy Women of Liège and Their Impact*, ed. Juliette Dor, Lesley Johnson, and Jocelyn Wogan-Browne (Turnhout, 1999), 35–60.

20. Thomas of Cantimpré, "Vita Christinae Mirabilis," 654–55; both Passenier, "Christina Mirabilis," and Sweetman, "Christine of Saint-Trond's Preaching Apostolate," claim that Thomas of Cantimpré deliberately constructed her life as an apostolate and a mission. There is little doubt that all we know of Christina is due to her biographers. The fact that they did not attempt to "civilize" her behavior indicates that, far from being bizarre or an indication of demonic possession, this was acceptable behavior for a holy woman.

21. "Pro his et hujusmodi sorores ejus, et amici erubescentes non modice, eo quod eam homines plenam daemonibus reputarent, nequissimum quemdam et fortissimum virum conveniunt, qui accepta mercede eam insequeretur ac caperet, et vinculis ferreis manciparet." Thomas of Cantimpré, "Vita Christinae Mirabilis," 653; English translation from Thomas of Cantimpré, *Life of Christina Mirabilis*, 19.

22. For an overview of Douceline and her life, see Philippine de Porcellet, *The Life of Saint Douceline, a Beguine of Provence*, trans. Kathleen Garay and Madeleine Jeay, Library of Medieval Women (Cambridge, 2001), 1–24. For a detailed treatment of St. Douceline, see Daniel E. Bornstein, "Violenza al corpo di una santa: Fra agiografia e pornografia; A proposito di Douceline di Digne," *Quaderni medievali* 39 (1995): 31–46.

23. Philippine de Porcellet, *La vie de sainte Douceline, fondatrice des Béguines de Marseille, composée au treizième siècle en langue provençale*, ed. J.-H. Albanès (Marseille, 1879), 73–81; Philippine de Porcellet, *Life of Saint Douceline*, 49–52.

24. Philippine de Porcellet, *Vie de sainte Douceline*, 93.

25. Placido T. Lugano, ed., *I pocessi inediti per Francesca Bussa dei Ponziani (Santa Francesca Romana)*, 1440–1453, Studi e testi 120 (Vatican City, 1945), 29, 61–61.

26. Elisabeth Lopez, *Culture et sainteté: Colette de Corbie* (1381–1447) (Saint-Etienne, 1994), 21–67; Bynum, *Holy Feast and Holy Fast*, 137–38.

27. Pierre de Vaux, "Vita beatae Colettae," *AASS*, 1 March, 566.

28. Perrine de Baumes, "Virtutes et miracula beatae Colettae," *AASS*, 1 March, 611.

29. "Videlicet, quod aliquando torquebatur in igne, sicut B. Laurentius . . . et illud martyrium communiter per spatium unius integre noctis protendebatur. Interdum vero torquebatur velut S. Vincentius, aliquando vero crucifigebatur; aliquando autem excoriabatur ut S. Bartholomeus, aliquotiens minutatim confricabatur, nonnumquam vero bulliebatur. Nihilominus interdum sibi videbatur quod cor ejus aperiretur. . . . Aliquando sibi videbatur et sensibiliter experiebatur, quod infra ventrem haberet titionem ardentem, ipsam totaliter incendentem; altera vice quod in oculorum radicibus haberet carbonem ignitum illos inflammantem, et penitus consumentem; alias autem quod ferramentis acutissimis, per medium totius corporis et omnium membrorum de extremo in extremum transpungeretur." Pierre de Vaux, "Vita beatae Colettae," 567.

30. Ibid., 561–62. The same episode is present also in Perrine de Baumes's biography. Perrine de Baumes, "Virtutes et miracula beatae Colettae," 608.

31. Perrine de Baumes, "Virtutes et miracula beatae Colettae." See also Lopez, *Culture et sainteté*, 89–92.

32. Perrine de Baumes, "Virtutes et miracula beatae Colettae," 609.

33. For this view, see Aviad M. Kleinberg, *Prophets in Their Own Country: Living Saints and the Making of Sainthood in the Later Middle Ages* (Chicago, 1992), 121–24.

34. Margaretha Ebner, *Margaretha Ebner und Heinrich von Nördlingen: Ein Beitrag zur Geschichte der deutschen Mystik*, ed. Philipp Strauch (Amsterdam, 1966), 1; English translation in *Margaret Ebner, Major Works*, trans. Leonard P. Hindsley, Classics of Western Spirituality (New York, 1993), 85.

35. *Margaret Ebner, Major Works*, 85.

36. "Und den wetagen het ich biz in daz trit jar, daz ich min selbs uneweltig was. und wen ez mir in daz haupt gieng, so lachet ich oder wainet vier tag oder mer emslichen." Ebner, *Margaretha Ebner und Heinrich von Nördlingen*, 2.

37. Ibid., 3.

38. "Also was ich in daz trit jar, daz ich nie trit von mir selber tet und aller menclich sprach, ich wer erlamet. Do huob ich ain ander siechtag an mir, der weret driezehen wochen; daz was, daz ich von den als ez taget alle morgen lag biz daz ez naht wart, daz ich min selbes ungewaltig was, und lag als ich tod wär, daz ich niht auzze noch trank." Ibid.

39. Ibid., 5: "und haun grosser üebung mit disciplinen und mit andern grossen dingen niht gehebt wan als ez mir got von siner güet gab mit grossem siechtagen."

40. Debra L. Stoudt, "The Production and Preservation of Letters by Fourteenth-Century Dominican Nuns," *Mediaeval Studies* 53 (1991): 309–26.

41. Ebner, *Margaretha Ebner und Heinrich von Nördlingen*, 119–30.

42. Ibid., 134–35. For previous eating disorders, see ibid., 102.

43. For analyses of Ebner's religious life, see Uhlinka Rublack, "Female Spirituality and the Infant Jesus in Late Medieval Dominican Convents," *Gender and History* 6 (1994): 37–57; Rosemary Drage Hale, "Rocking the Cradle: Margaretha Ebner (Be)Holds the Divine," in *Performance and Transformation: New Approaches to Late Medieval Spirituality*, ed. Mary A. Suydam and Joanna E. Ziegler (London, 1999), 211–35.

44. Albrecht Classen, "The Literary Treatment of the Ineffable: Mechthild von Magdeburg, Margaret Ebner, Agnes Blannbekin," *Studies in Spirituality* 8 (1998): 162–87.

45. Margarete Weinhandl, ed., *Deutsches Nonnenleben: Das Leben der Schwestern zu Töss und der Nonne von Engeltal Büchlein von der gnaden Überlast* (Munich, 1921).

46. Ibid., 120–31.

47. On the subject of Suso's pastoral care of nuns, especially Stagel, see Frank Tobin, "Henry Suso and Elsbeth Stagel: Was the *Vita* a Cooperative Effort?" in *Gendered Voices: Medieval Saints and Their Interpreters*, ed. Catherine M. Mooney (Philadelphia, 1999), 118–35; Jeffrey F. Hamburger, "The Use of Images in the Pastoral Care of Nuns: The Case of Heinrich Suso and the Dominicans," *Art Bulletin* 71 (1989): 20–46; Ulrike Wiethaus, "Thieves and Carnivals: Gender in German Dominican Literature of the Fourteenth Century," in *The Vernacular Spirit: Essays on Medieval Religious Literature*, ed. Renate Blumenfeld-Kosinski, Duncan Robertson, and Nancy Bradley Warren (London, 2002), 209–38.

48. Suso, *Deutsche Schriften*, 11–12; *Exemplar*, 3–4.

49. Weinhandl, *Deutsches Nonnenleben*, 126–28.

50. Amy Hollywood, "Beatrice of Nazareth and Her Hagiographer," in *Gendered Voices: Medieval Saints and Their Interpreters*, ed. Catherine M. Mooney (Philadelphia, 1999), 78–117; Amy Hollywood, *Sensible Ecstasy: Mysticism, Sexual Difference, and the Demands of History* (Chicago, 2002), 241–73.

51. Richard Kieckhefer, "Holiness and the Culture of Devotion: Remarks on Some Late Medieval Male Saints," in *Images of Sainthood in Medieval Europe*, ed. Renate Blumenfeld-Kosinski and Timea Szell (Ithaca, NY, 1991), 295.

52. Richard Rolle, *The* Passio Domini *Theme in the Works of Richard Rolle: His Personal Contribution in Its Religious, Cultural, and Literary Context*, ed. Mary F. Madigan, Salzburg Studies in English Literature, Institut für englische Sprache und Literatur (Salzburg, 1978), 236–77.

53. E.g., Bernardino of Siena, *Prediche volgari (1425)*, ed. Ciro Cannarozzi, 5 vols. (Florence, 1958), 5:345–84; Fiona Somerset, "Excitative Speech: Theories of Emotive Response from Richard Fitzralph to Margery Kempe," in *The Vernacular Spirit: Essays on Medieval Religious Literature*, ed. Renate Blumenfeld-Kosinski, Duncan Robertson, and Nancy Bradley Warren (London, 2002), 59–79.

54. Rulman Merswin, *Vier anfangende Jahre: Des Gottesfreundes Fünfmannenbuch (Die sogenannten Autographa)*, ed. Philipp Strauch, Altdeutsche Texbibliothek 23; Schriften aus der Gottesfreund-Literatur 2 (Halle, 1927). English translation in *Mystical Writings of Rulman Merswin*, ed. Thomas S. Kepler (Philadelphia, 1960), 39–52.

55. For a small selection of the secondary literature on the subject, see R. N. Swanson, "Passion and Practice: The Social and Ecclesiastical Implications of Passion Devotion in the Late Middle Ages," in *The Broken Body: Passion Devotion in Late Medieval Culture*, ed. A. A. MacDonald, H. N. B. Ridderbos, and R. M. Schlusemann, Medievalia Groningana 21 (Groningen, 1998), 1–30; Bynum, *Wonderful Blood*; Michael Camille, "Mimetic Identification and Passion Devotion in the Later Middle Ages: A Double-Sided Panel by Meister Francke," in *Broken Body*, 183–210; Rachel Fulton, *From Judgment to Passion: Devotion to Christ and the Virgin Mary, 800–1200* (New York, 2002); Richard Kieckhe-

fer, "Major Currents in Late Medieval Devotion," in *Christian Spirituality: High Middle Ages and Reformation*, ed. Jill Raitt (New York, 1987), 75–108; Anke E. Passenier, "The Suffering Body and the Freedom of the Soul: Medieval Women's Ways of Union with God," in *Begin with the Body: Corporeality, Religion, and Gender*, ed. Jonneke Bekkenkamp and Maaike de Haardt (Leuven, 1998), 264–87.

56. Passenier, "Suffering Body"; Heather Webb, "Catherine of Siena's Heart," *Speculum* 80 (2005): 802–17; Caroline W. Bynum, *Fragmentation and Redemption: Essays on Gender and the Human Body in Medieval Religion* (New York, 1992), 53–78.

57. Karma Lochrie, *Margery Kempe and Translations of the Flesh* (Philadelphia, 1991), 167–202; Ellen Ross, "'She Wept and Cried Right Loud for Sorrow and for Pain': Suffering, the Spiritual Journey, and Women's Experience in Late Medieval Mysticism," in *Maps of Flesh and Light: The Religious Experience of Medieval Women Mystics*, ed. Ulrike Wiethaus (Syracuse, NY, 1993), 45–59; Kleinberg, *Prophets in Their Own Country*, 149–51.

58. Nagy, *Don de larmes*.

59. *Les quinze joies de mariage*, ed. Jean Rychner (Geneva, 1963), 18–26.

60. Savonarola, *Ad mulieres Ferrarienses*, 109.

61. Ibid., 111–12, 116, 121.

62. María del Carmen García Herrero, *Las mujeres en Zaragoza en el siglo XV*, 2 vols. (Zaragoza, 1990), 2:293–95: "doloreandose de los dolores del prenyado que tenia," "siempre doloreandose," "aquexandose los dolores de su parto," "con los dolores del parto y esprimiendose del cuerpo," "despues de muchos dolores grandes que laquexavan a la dita Ysabel de la Cavalleria"; previously published in Universidad de Zaragoza, *Homenaje al Profesor Emerito Antonio Ubieto Arteta* (Zaragoza, 1989), 290–92.

63. The quotations in the text are from "Public Record of the Labour of Isabel de la Cavalleria, January 10, 1490, Zaragoza," trans. Monserrat Cabre, http://www.the-orb .net/birthrecord.html (accessed 10 March 2009).

64. Rublack, "Pregnancy, Childbirth and the Female Body," 91.

65. The one exception is the behavior of people considered insane. In that case, behavior is a symptom, but for the sane it is not considered as such.

66. Handerson, *Gilbertus Anglicus*, 46. See also Gilbertus Anglicus, *Healing and Society*.

67. Jean-Claude Schmitt, *Les revenants: Les vivants et les morts dans la société médiévale*, Bibliothèque des histoires (Paris, 1994), 115–46; Caesarius of Heisterbach, *Dialogus miraculorum*, ed. Joseph Strange, 2 vols. (Cologne, 1851), 2:315–63, distinctio XI de praemio mortuorum.

68. See, in addition to the episodes cited in the references in n. 67, Margaret Jennings, "Tutivillus: The Literary Career of the Recording Demon," *Studies in Philology* 74 (1977): 1–93; Kathy Cawsey, "Tutivillus and the 'Kyrkchaterars': Strategies of Control in the Middle Ages," *Studies in Philology* 102 (2005): 434–51.

69. Baldus de Ubaldis, "Tractatus de carceribus," in *Decimum volumen tractatuum e variis iuris interpretibus collectorum* (Lyons, 1599), 614: "audires prima hora noctis inter catervas debilium, stridorem ossium, crepitum nervorum in modum restis se extendentium, sibilium energumenorum, et diversorum aegrorum prae dolore non minimum ululatum."

70. Ronald C. Finucane, *Miracles and Pilgrims: Popular Beliefs in Medieval England* (London, 1977), 83–100.

71. E.g., Giovanni Mattiotti, "Vita et acta sancta Franciscae Romanae," *AASS*, 2 March, 100: "detentus dolore maximo capitis"; William of Canterbury, *Miracula gloriosi martyris Thomae archiepiscopi Cantuariensis*, vol. 1 of *Materials for the History of Thomas Becket, Archbishop of Canterbury*, ed. James C. Robertson, Rolls Series 67 (repr., London, 1965), 507, 6:118: "Dolore capitis peracuto vexabarit"; "Liber miraculorum," in *Processus canonizationis et legendae variae sancti Ludovici OFM*, Analecta Franciscana, sive Chronica aliaque varia documenta ad historiam fratrum minorum 7 (Florence, 1951), bk. 4. chap. 13: "dolorem vehementissimum in capite paciebatur." Cf. Constantine the African, "De morborum cognitione et curatione," 7–11, bk. 1, chaps. 10–12: "de dolore capitis."

72. Geoffroy de la Tour Landry, *Le livre du chevalier de la Tour Landry pour l'enseignement de ses filles*, ed. Anatole de Montaiglon (Paris, 1854); German translation: *Der Ritter vom Thurn*, trans. Marquard vom Stein, ed. Ruth Harvey, Texte des späten Mittelalters und der frühen Neuzeit 32 (Berlin, 1988); anonymous English translation: *The booke of the enseygnementes and techynge that the Knyght of the Towre made to his doughters*, Early English Text Society (London, 1902), subsequently translated by William Caxton.

73. Francesco Barberino, *Del reggimento e costumi di donna*, ed. Carlo Baudi di Vesme, Collezione di opere inedite o rare dei primi tre secoli della lingua (Bologna, 1875); Bonvesin da Riva, "De quinquaginta curialitatibus ad mensam," in *Poeti del duecento*, ed. Gianfranco Contini (Milan, 1960); *"Book of Courtesy": A Fifteenth Century Courtesy Book*, ed. R. W. Chambers, Early English Text Society (London, 1937); Ingrid Bennewitz, "'Darumb lieben Toechter/seyt nicht zu gar fürwitzig . . .': Deutschsprachige moralisch-didaktische Literatur des 13.–15. Jahrhunderts," in *Geschichte der Mädchen- und Frauenbildung*, vol. 1, *Vom Mittelalter bis zur Aufklärung*, ed. Elke Kleinau and Claudia Opitz (Frankfurt, 1996), 23–41; Mark Addison Amos, "'For Manners Make Man': Bourdieu, de Certeau, and the Common Appropriation of Noble Manners in the *Book of Courtesy*," in *Medieval Conduct*, ed. Kathleen Ashley and Robert L. A. Clark, Medieval Cultures 29 (Minneapolis, MN, 2001), 23–48; Anna Dronzek, "Gendered Theories of Education in Fifteenth-Century Conduct Books," in *Medieval Conduct*, 135–59; Ann Marie Rasmussen, "Fathers to Think Back Through: The Middle High German Mother-Daughter and Father-Son Advice Forms Known as *Die Winsbeckin* and *Der Winsbecke*," in *Medieval Conduct*, 106–34.

74. Humbert de Romans, Gilbert de Tournai, and Stephen of Bourbon, *Prediche alle donne del secolo XIII*. Cf. Franco Mormando, *The Preacher's Demons: Bernardino of Siena and the Social Underworld of Early Renaissance Italy* (Chicago, 1999), 1–40.

75. William of Canterbury, *Miracula gloriosi martyris Thomae archiepiscopi Cantuariensis*, 272, 349, 375; Benedict of Peterborough, *Miracula sancti Thomae Cantuariensis*, vol. 2 of *Materials for the History of Thomas Becket*, ed. James C. Robertson, Rolls Series 67 (repr., London, 1965), 234.

76. "In primo igitur basilicae ingressu ad corpus beati Otmari perveniens, puer ipse, tendentibus sese compagum retinaculis, vehiculo decidens, in pavimentum provolvitur,

et vocibus horrendis tecta ecclesiae complens, nimio se dolore urgeri insolito clamoris strepitus protestatur. Senior autem noster Grimaldus his diebus in monasterio positus, cum ipsa hora pro foribus basilicae infra claustrum consisteret, audito huiuscemodi strepitu Salomonem episcopum una cum Augensis coenobii abbate, qui ipso die ibidem forte convenerant, secum assumens, ecclesiam intrat, causamque tam horrendi atque insoliti clamoris interrogat. Quid plura? Abbates cum episcopo propius accedunt, flebili ululatu puerum huc illucque in pavimento volutari cernunt, seque ipsum propriis unguibus cogente molestia lacerare et quasi discerpere perspiciunt. Post longam huiuscemodi vexationem sinistra manus in volam contracta extenditur, incurvata cervix erigitur, . . . et planta pedis dextri ab ipsis natibus quibus impressa fuerat, fracto genu cum sanguinis effusione prosiliens—episcopo autem astante hymnumque *Te Deum laudamus* canente—corrigitur." Yso, "De miraculis S. Otmari libri II," in MGH, SS, ed. G. H. Pertz (Hannover, 1829), 2:52.

77. "Stuperes insanientis horribiles mugitus, calcitrantis strepitum, dentium stridorem, oculorum vertiginem, tociusque immoderatam corporis distortionem, cum miser, intolerabiliter passus, hac illacque preceps ferebatur." *Liber miraculorum sancte Fidis,* ed. Auguste Bouillet (Paris, 1897), 64, bk. 1, chap. 24. English translation in *The Book of Sainte Foy,* trans. Pamela Sheingorn (Philadelphia, 1995), 91.

78. Benedict of Peterborough, *Miracula sancti Thomae Cantuariensis,* 46: "non a phantastica illusione, sed a vero et vehementi dentium dolore, mirabiliter ereptus est; erat enim tumor maxillae maximum, dolor immoderatus, adeo ut gestus et clamoris causam ignoranti furere potius videretur quam dolere." Benedict of Peterborough, *Miracula sancti Thomae Cantuariensis,* 63: "vertebat se in latera, volutabatur clamans; resurgebat saepius, sed gradu instabili stare non poterat: corruebat in faciem, allidebatur ad petram, malo suo venisse videbatur." "Liber miraculorum [sancti Ludovici]," 290: "Adam Iohannis . . . quadam nocte dolorem vehementissimum paciebatur in capite, et in tantum quod sensum amisit, visum et auditum, nec aliquem cognoscebat, ymo continue inania loquebatur, nec erat spes quod videret."

79. William of Canterbury, *Miracula gloriosi martyris Thomae archiepiscopi Cantuariensis,* 504–5.

80. Pierre de Vaux, "Vita beatae Colettae," 586: "per integrum annum et semis angebatur dolore capitis, passione scilicet, quae gutta malogranata vulgariter nuncupatur, quod nullo modo refici poterat corporaliter absque doloris horribilis et indicibilis afflictione. Nam saepe surgebat de mensa, ambulans per hortum, ejulans et clamans lamentabiliter, sibi loqui volentibus intendere non valens prae nimia doloris afflictione."

81. Giovanni Boccaccio, *Decameron,* ed. Vittore Branca (Florence, 1999), 54–65.

82. For a survey of plague chronicles and their descriptions, see Gabrielle Zanella, "Italia, Francia e Germania: Una storiografia a confronto," in *La peste nera: Dati di una realtà ed elementi di una interpretazione; Atti del XXX convegno storico internazionale, Todi,* 10–13 *ottobre,* 1993 (Spoleto, 1994), 49–136.

83. Procopius, *History of the Wars,* trans. H. B. Dewing, Loeb Library of the Greek and Roman Classics (London, 1914; repr., Cambridge, MA, 1961), 1:460–61, bk. 2, chaps. 23–29.

84. The idea that experiencing no pain in situations in which one ought to feel pain indicates a sick mind goes back to Hippocratean medicine.

85. See below, chap. 5.

86. Gerson, "Médecine de l'âme."

87. I know of no death manual that describes a woman dying, but I have not examined enough to make a categorical statement.

88. Nancy Caciola, *Discerning Spirits: Divine and Demonic Possession in the Middle Ages* (Ithaca, NY, 2003); Alberto Tenenti, *La vie et la mort à travers l'art du XVe siècle*, 2nd ed. (Paris, 1983).

89. See below, chap. 6.

90. *Trattato de l'arte di bien morire, attributo al Cardinale di Fermo Domenico Capranica* (Florence, 1477); *Fratri Alberti magni ordinis predicatorum quondam episcopi Ratisponensis.* These are in fact two incunabulum editions of the same text.

91. "Cum enim infirmus doloribus cruciatur corpore, tunc diabolus dolorem dolori superaddit. . . . Proinde ad confidentiam veram: quam precipue infirmus in deum habere debet in agone inducere cum debet dispositio Cristi in cruce. Tertia temptatio est inpatientia que est contra caritatem. Nam moriturus maxime dolor accidit corporis: hi precipue qui non morte naturali que rata est, sicut manifeste docet experientia, sed frequenter ex accidentibus, puta febre vel apostemate: aut alia infirmitate gravi et afflictiva atque longa dissoluuntur . . . ut plerumque ex nimio dolore et in patientia amentes et insensati videntur." *Trattato de l'arte di bien morire, attributo al Cardinale di Fermo Domenico Capranica; Fratri Alberti magni ordinis predicatorum quondam episcopi Ratisponensis.*

92. For exemplary good deaths of kings in Germany and Spain, see Peter Schmid, "Sterben-Tod-Leichenbegängnis König Maximilian I.," 185–215, and Ariel Guiance, "La mort du roi: Sacralité et pouvoir politique dans la Castille médiévale," 299–320, both in *Der Tod des Mächtigen: Kult und Kultur des Todes spätmittelalterlicher Herrscher*, ed. Lothar Kolmer (Paderborn, 1997).

93. Huizinga, *Autumn of the Middle Ages*, 54–56.

94. Gerd Althoff, "*Ira Regis*: Prolegomena to a History of Royal Anger," in *Anger's Past: The Social Uses of an Emotion in the Middle Ages*, ed. Barbara H. Rosenwein (Ithaca, NY, 1998), 59–74; Gerd Althoff, "The Variability of Rituals in the Middle Ages," in *Medieval Concepts of the Past: Ritual, Memory, Historiography*, ed. Gerd Althoff, Johannes Fried, and Patrick J. Geary (Cambridge, 2002), 71–88.

95. Christine de Pizan, *Le livre des faits et bonnes moeurs du roi Charles V le Sage*, trans. Eric Hicks and Thérèse Moreau, ed. Danielle Regnier-Bohler (Paris, 1997), 312–13, bk. 3, chap. 71.

96. Religieux de Saint-Denys, *Chroniques*, ed. M. L. Bellaguet, 3 vols. (Paris, 1842; repr., Paris, 1994), 2:86–89.

97. Raymond Van Dam, *Saints and Their Miracles in Late Antique Gaul* (Princeton, NJ, 1993), 99, citing Gregory of Tours, *Historiarum libri X*, 154, 4.21: "Wa! Quid potatis, qualis est illi rex caelestis, qui sic tam magnos regis (sic) interfecit?"

98. Einhard, *Vita Karoli magni*, ed. O. Holder-Egger, MGH, SSRG in usum scholarum (Hannover, 1911; repr., Hannover, 1927), 35.

99. Benedict VIII [dubious], "Bulla Benedicti papae VIII qua Henrico sanitatem a S. Benedicto restitutam esse testatur, monasterioque Casinensi asserit dona ab imperatore delata," PL 139:1636.

100. Adam of Bremen, *Gesta Hammaburgensis ecclesiae pontificum*, ed. Bernhard Schmeider, MGH, SSRG in usum scholarum 2 (Hannover, 1917), 215.

PART II

1. The utter helplessness and dissolution of the self, so eloquently analyzed by Scarry, are rarely mentioned in medieval discourses. See Elaine Scarry, *The Body in Pain: The Making and Unmaking of the World* (Oxford, 1985), 3–11.

2. Aydede, *Pain*, 1–4.

CHAPTER FIVE

1. I owe this insight to Omri Herzog.

2. Guy de Chauliac, *Chirurgia*, 1:306.

3. Arnau de Villanova, *Commentum*, 181–82.

4. "Hippocratis aphorismi et Galeni in eos commentarii II," in Galen, *Opera*, 17/2:560. E.g., Francesco de Piedmont, *Suplementum in secundum librum secretorum remediorum Iuannis Mesuae, quem vocant de appropriatis* (Venice, 1531), chap. 16: "Signa autem doloris sunt sensus corruptus, quia nocivae rei praesentis perceptio, quod si fortiter imprimat, et dolor non sentiatur, mens aegrotat, ut voluit Hippocrates cum ait: Quicumque dolentes aliquid corporis plerum doloris non sentiunt, his mens aegrotat."

5. Hippocrates, *Aphorismi*, ed. and trans. Carolus Gottlob Kühn, Medicorum Graecorum opera quae extant 23 (Leipzig, 1827), 13; Avicenna, *Liber canonis*, fol. 40v; Avicenna, *Canon of Medicine*, 248.

6. The hypochondrium is the upper part of the abdomen.

7. Handerson, *Gilbertus Anglicus*, 37.

8. Ibid., 39, 59.

9. Avicenna, *Liber canonis*, fols. 38v–411; Avicenna, *Canon of Medicine*, 249.

10. Rey, *History of Pain*, 17–23.

11. Modern research on pain has also devoted a great deal of attention to vocabulary and categories. See Anthony Diller, "Cross-cultural Pain Semantics," *Pain* 9 (1980): 9–26.

12. Henri de Mondeville, *Chirurgie*, 176, 193. As a surgeon, Mondeville's first thought concerned treatment and sedation.

13. Ibid., 394.

14. Ibid., 395. Cf. Bernard de Gordon, *Lilio de medicina*, 1:187; Bernard de Gordon, *Lilium medicinae*, 73.

15. Savonarola, *De gotta*.

16. Galen, *Opera*, 8:81–82; English translation from the Greek: *On the Affected Parts*, trans. Rudolph E. Siegel (Basel, 1976), 48.

17. Galen, *Opera*, 8:88–89, 121–37; *On the Affected Parts*, 43–70, 205–9.

18. By *dulcis*, Archigenes probably meant "weak," but Arnau deliberately took the term to mean "sweet" in order to criticize Archigenes.

19. "Quod si res non solum convenit nominare secundum modum usitatum a sapientibus, set eciam modo vulgi, nondum excusatur Archigenes ab errore. Nam licet aliqui

pacientes vocent aliquem dolorem rabidum vel acutum, tamen nullus conqueritur se pati dolorem acetosum aut salsum sive viscosum et consimilis. Si vero propter nominum penuriam hec nomina transumpserit ad denotandum species dolorum, adhuc erravit inconvenienter transumendo. Nam licet dolor qui est cum constriccione maiori vel minori possit per similitudinem ad saporem ponticum vel stipticum sic nominari, tamen nulla similitudine potest dolor aliquis dulcis vocari, cum omnis dolor affligat et de se non delectet. Quod si dulcem nominet dolorem, ideo quia parum affligit, tunc conveniencius debilis nominabitur." Arnau de Villanova, *Doctrina Galieni de interioribus,* 337.

20. "Hippocratis aphorismi et Galeni in eos commentarii II," in Galen, *Opera,* 17/2:459, aphorism 5.2. Galen does indeed cite there only three types of pain.

21. Gotthard Strohmaier, "Constantine's Pseudo-classical Terminology and Its Survival," in *Constantine the African and 'Ali ibn al-'Abbas al-Maǧūsī: The "Pantegni" and Related Texts,* ed. Charles Burnett and Danielle Jacquart, Studies in Ancient Medicine 10 (Leiden, 1994), 90–98.

22. Constantine the African, "De morborum cognitione et curatione," 157–58, bk. 7, chap. 14, "de labore et dolore."

23. Maurus of Salerno, "In Hippocratis aphorismos commentarium," in *Collectio Salernitana,* ed. Salvatore de Renzi (Naples, 1856), 4:539–40. On Maurus of Salerno, see Morris H. Saffron, "Maurus of Salerno: Twelfth-Century 'Optimus Physicus' with His Commentary on the Prognostics of Hippocrates," *Transactions of the American Philosophical Society,* n.s., 62 (1972): 5–104.

24. Danielle Jacquart, "'Theorica' et 'practica' dans l'enseignement de la médecine à Salerno au XIIᵉ siècle," in *La science médicale occidentale entre deux renaissances (XIIᵉ s.–XVᵉ s.),* by Danielle Jacquart (Aldershot, UK, 1997).

25. Avicenna, *Liber canonis,* fols. 43v, 173r–80v; Avicenna, *Canon of Medicine,* 249–51. For general complaints about Gerard's translations, see Roger French, *Canonical Medicine: Gentile da Foligno and Scholasticism* (Leiden, 2001), 186–93.

26. Arnau de Villanova, *Tractatus,* 219: "maiorem partem medicorum Latinorum infatuat."

27. For the loss of meanings during translation in pharmacological medieval work, see Riddle, "Theory and Practice in Medieval Medicine," 179–83.

28. "Et iterum species doloris multae sunt secundum Avicennam; sed secundum Galenum omnem possunt reduci ad 3 aut 4. . . . Galen super aphorismum 5um, 2ae partis, 'labores spontanei etc.'" Bernard de Gordon, *Lilio de medicina,* 1:186. This arbitrary citation of Galen's commentary to the Hippocratic *Aphorisms* is misleading. Galen's writings are littered with descriptions of pain, but he considers them merely adjectives, not accurate descriptors. Avicenna was not well accepted in Montpellier, where Bernard taught, and his work did not become obligatory reading until 1340; see Danielle Jacquart, "La reception du Canon d'Avicenne: Comparaison entre Montpellier et Paris aux XIIIᵉ et XIVᵉ siècles," in *Histoire de l'école médicale de Montpellier* (Paris, 1985), 69–77.

29. Cited in Siraisi, *Taddeo Alderotti,* 223.

30. Ibid.

31. Henri de Mondeville, *Chirurgie*, 396: "dolor a sanguine fixivus tolerabilis non inflammativus," "dolor ex colera est deambulativus, intercutaneus, pungitivus, pruritum faciens."

32. Siraisi, *Taddeo Alderotti*, 225–26.

33. Alain de Lille, "Compendiosa in Cantica canticorum ad laudem deiparae virginis Mariae elucidatio," PL 210:59.

34. Jacquart and Thomasset, *Sexualité et savoir médical*, 68.

35. I am not sure what the antonyms of the last two words are; all four words were used in "Consilia magistri Bartolomei Montagnane," MS Vat. Lat. 2471, fols. 56r–v (*consilium* 20), 101r (*consilium* 57), 199r (*consilium* 129); Barzizza, *Introductorium practicae medicinae*, fols. 141v ("dolor pungitivus vel mordicativus vel ulcerativus"), 156v ("dolor extensivus cum gravitate").

36. Indeed, Mondeville clearly stated that he had much more theoretical material on pain but refrained from writing it partly because he feared the wrath of the Paris faculty of medicine. Henri de Mondeville, *Chirurgie*, 397.

37. Arderne, *Treatises*, 100–101.

38. Demaitre, "Medieval Notions of Cancer," 624.

39. Chiara Crisciani, "Histories, Stories, Exempla, and Anecdotes: Michele Savonarola from Latin to Vernacular," in *Historia: Empiricism and Erudition in Early Modern Europe*, ed. Gianna Pomata and Nancy G. Siraisi (Cambridge, MA, 2005), 297–324. I am grateful to Gianna Pomata for drawing my attention to this work, and to Chiara Crisciani for allowing me to read her work before publication and for introducing me to Savonarola's vernacular treatise.

40. The motif of the Spider and the Gout, each of whom complains of his habitation, goes back to Petrarch's letters. Francesco Petrarca, *Le familiari*, ed. V. Rossi and U. Bosco, 4 vols. (Florence, 1933–42), 3:72–77.

41. Savonarola, *De gotta*, canto 1: "il dolor non sia altro che uno affannoso e alla natura molesto sentire; . . . siche il soluere di continuo o vero mala complexio como dicono philosophi et medici dello dolore sono cagion factiua."

42. Ibid.

43. In the last few decades, present-day researchers on pain have come to the same conclusion. See Ronald Melzack, "The McGill Pain Questionnaire," in *Pain Measurement and Assessment*, ed. Ronald Melzack (New York, 1983), 41–47.

44. Galen, *Opera*, 8:75–76, 113; Arnau de Villanova, *Doctrina Galieni de interioribus*, 345.

45. Galen, *Opera*, 8:21. Cf. Arnau de Villanova, *Commentum*, 307.

46. Avicenna, *Liber canonis*, fol. 38v; Avicenna, *Canon of Medicine*, 250–51.

47. Saffron, "Maurus of Salerno," 43, 46, 49, 51.

48. Bernard de Gordon, *Lilium medicinae*, 72–73: "si quis sentiat conquassationem et aggrauationem ac si cum acubus pungeretur, aut cum vrticis, et sentit motum deambulatiuum inter cutem et carnem pungitiuum, pruritiuum, perforatiuum, signum est humores cholericos, acutos aut salsos adustos dominari in corpore, qui dissoluti in vapores cum vadunt ad membra sensibilia, inducunt dolores acutos. Si autem sentiat extensionem in membro, ac si essent rigida et tensa, sicut chorda arcus, tunc sunt hi melancholici, quos natura non potest bene regere, aut ventosi. Si vero dolor sit affixus, humores sunt. Si dea-

mbulatiuus, ventus est. Si grauativus, ac si sentiret magnum pondus, ita etiam quod non audet se expandere, est signum humoris et multi et malae qualitatis. Primus autem dolor significat humores malos, secundus multos, tertius utrunque. [sic] Quarta autem species doloris potest vocari dolor inflammatus, videtur enim homini quaedam flamma caloris transire per spatulas, et in paratis ad febres putridas et potissimum de sanguine, et in tali dolore sic grauatiuo, sic confractiuo, sic inflammatiuo competit statim phlebotomia." See also *Lilio de medicina,* 1:186–87. I have chosen here to follow the Latin, rather than the Castilian, version, for it seems more consistent with Bernard's previously elaborated theories of pain taxonomy.

49. Arnau de Villanova, *Doctrina Galieni de interioribus,* 325.

50. "Consilia magistri Bartolomei Montagnane," MS Vat. Lat. 2471, fol. 59r (*consilium* 21). Baverio Maghinardo de Bonetti described an almost identical case—headache, impediments of hearing and speech, dizziness, pain in shoulders and arms—also arising from cold and humid humors in the brain. Bonetti, *Consiliorum liber,* fol. 67v (*consilium* 10).

51. Arnaldus de Villanova, "Speculum medicinale," Rome, Biblioteca apostolica Vaticana, MS Pal. Lat. 1175, fols. 259v–261r. Not surprisingly, Arnau recommended a regimen of healthy living (drawn from Pseudo-Mesue), phlebotomy, and a mild painkiller. Two folios further on, Arnau cites an almost-identical case, only this time the knight who fell off his horse was German (263r).

52. See above, n. 19.

53. See above, chap. 2.

54. Fiorelli, *Tortura giudiziaria nel diritto commune,* 1:182–91; Sbriccoli, "Tormentum id est torquere mentem"; *Dig.* 14.18.18.

55. *Dig.* 48.18.7.

56. *Dig.* 48.18.18; Accursius, *Accursii glossa in "Digestum novum,"* Corpus glossatorum iuris civilis 9 (Turin, 1487; repr., Venice, 1968), 479.

57. *Dig.* 48.18.15.

58. *Registre criminel du Châtelet de Paris du 6 septembre 1389 au 18 mai 1392,* ed. H. Duplès-Agier, 2 vols. (Paris, 1861–64), 1:502–8, 2:137–47.

59. See above, chap. 2.

60. Grillandus, *Tractatus de hereticis,* fol. 28r.

61. Hieronymus, *Dialogus contra Pelagianos,* ed. Claudio Moreschini, CCSL 80 (Turnhout, 1990), bk. 3, par. 11; Catherine Conybeare, "The Ambiguous Laughter of Saint Laurence," *Journal of Early Christian Studies* 10 (2002): 175–202. Centuries later, Ivo of Chartres cited Ambrose's heroic view of fortitude; Ivo of Chartres, *Panormia,* 20, bk. 8, chap. 34, provisional edition, ed. Bruce Brasington and Martin Brett, http://wtfaculty .wtamu.edu/~bbrasington/panormia.html (accessed 10 March 2009).

62. Augustine, "Sermo 276 in festo martyris Vincentii III," PL 38:1255–57. See also "De sancto Vincentio Martyre," *AASS,* 2 January, 393–97; Jacobus de Voragine, *Legenda aurea,* 174–79; Jacobus de Voragine, *Registrum in sermones de sanctis,* sermon 70; Leonardo de Utino [Udine], *Sermones aurei (anni 1446) de sanctis fratris Leonardi de Utine sacre theologie doctoris ordinis predicatorum* (Strasbourg, 1481), fols. 77r–79v.

63. William of Saint-Thierry, "De natura corporis et animae libri duo," PL 180:718.

64. *ST,* pt. 2a–2ae, qq. 123–24.

65. Franciscus Brunus, *Tractatus de indicijs et tortura*, fol. 226r.

66. See above, chap. 2.

67. Bonifacius de Vitalinis, "Tractatus maleficij," 452–53: "si quis ultro et sine tormentis confiteatur, secundum quosdam non potest damnari, nisi perseveret, et saepe interrogetur per diversos dies, si velit perseverare vel non. . . . Tu dic contra, secundum Azo, et haec est communis opinio, quod si quis confiteatur *sponte* [my italics], statim est carcerandum et sine alia praesumptione damnandum. . . . Sed tutius puto, si iudex faciat eum perseverare in confessione sua. . . . Sed si confiteatur in tormentis, vel formidine tormentorum, tunc non statur dicto eius, nec debet haberi pro confesso, nisi postea sponte perseveret."

68. Ibid., 453: "nisi postea sponte perseveret." Ibid., 456: "vel perseveret sponte et non coacte." Baldus de Ubaldis, *Consiliorum sive responsorum*, 3:364:6: "nisi perseveretur sponte." Henrico de Segusio [Hostiensis], *Summa aurea* (Basel, 1573), 471: "Ideo dicit versus sponte. Hoc autem ideo dictum est: quia si prae magna angustia tormentorum quis confiteatur, non obest ei, nisi in confessione perseverarit post depositionem tormentorum."

69. Joseph Ziegler, *Medicine and Religion c. 1300: The Case of Arnau de Vilanova*, Oxford Historical Monographs (Oxford, 1998), 46.

70. Peter Biller and Joseph Ziegler, eds., *Religion and Medicine in the Middle Ages*, York Studies in Medieval Theology 3 (York, UK, 2001); Peter Biller, "Words and the Medieval Notion of 'Religion,'" *Journal of Ecclesiastical History* 36 (1985): 351–69; Ziegler, *Medicine and Religion*, 46–113.

71. The marginal character of pain discourse in scholastic disciplines tends to be underplayed. Pain is not really amenable to scholastic taxonomies.

CHAPTER SIX

1. The term *theologia* for a separate discipline was probably invented by Abelard, but what is now considered theology goes back to the second century. See Clanchy, *Abelard*, 264–77.

2. Bynum, *Resurrection of the Body*.

3. Nemesius, *De natura hominis*.

4. Thomas Aquinas, *On Spiritual Creatures (De spiritualibus creaturis)*, trans. Mary C. Fitzpatrick, Mediaeval Philosophical Texts in Translation 5 (Milwaukee, WI, 1949), 52–64.

5. "Ea enim natura corporum est, ut ex consortio animae in sensum quendam animae sentientis animata, non sit haebes inanimis que materies, sed et adtacta sentiat et conpuncta doleat et algens rigeat et confota gaudeat et inaedia tabescat et pinguescat cibo. Ex quodam enim obtinentis se penetrantis que animae transcursu, secundum ea in quibus erit, aut oblectatur aut laeditur. Cum igitur conpuncta aut effossa corpora dolent, sensum doloris transfusae in ea animae sensus admittit." Hilary of Poitiers, *De trinitate*, ed. P. Smulders, CCSL 62 (Turnhout, 1980), 469, bk. 10, chap. 14; English translation in *On the Trinity*, trans. C. S. Gayford, Nicene and Post-Nicene Fathers, 2nd ser., 9 (Edinburgh, 1898; repr., Grand Rapids, MI, 1983), 9:15.

6. Esther Cohen, "The Animated Pain of the Body," *American Historical Review* 105 (2000): 36–68. For another interpretation of Augustine's stance, see Pasquale Porro, "Fisica Aristotelica e escatologia cristiana: Il dolore dell'anima nel dibatitto scolastico del XIII secolo," in *Enosis kai filia—unione e amicizia: Omaggio a Francesco Romano* (Catania, 2002), 617–42. I am grateful to Carla Casagrande for bringing this article to my attention.

7. Cf. Peter Lombard, *Sententiae in IV libris distinctae*, 2 vols., Spicilegium Bonaventurianum 5 (Quaracchi and Grottaferrata, 1971–81), bk. 3, qq. 15–16. For a biography of John of Damascus, see J. Nasrallah, *Saint Jean de Damas* (Harissa, Lebanon, 1950).

8. Unlike other scholars, who assume that *primus homo* meant humanity in general, regardless of gender, I am convinced that indeed theologians were thinking quite specifically of gendered man; see Clark, "Adam's Engendering."

9. John of Damascus, *De fide orthodoxa: Versions of Burgundio and Cerbanus*, ed. Eligius M. Buytaert (St. Bonaventure, NY, 1955), chaps. 26–35.

10. "Non igitur passio est dolor, sed passionis sensus." Ibid., 132, chap. 36.

11. Augustine defined pain in *De ciuitate Dei*, ed. Bernard Dombart and Alphonse Kalb, 2 vols., CCSL 47–48 (Turnhout, 1955), 438, bk. 14, chap. 15, as "Dolor . . . dissensio est ab his rebus, quae nobis nolentibus accidunt."

12. *ST*, pts. 1a–2ae, q. 35, art. 1: "Dolor, qui dicitur corporis, est corruptio repentina salutis ejus rei, quam male utendo anima corruptioni fecit obnoxiam." Duns Scotus, *Quaestiones*, 576: "Dolor causatur ab absoluto disconvenientiae sic, quod in tali absoluto prius est relatio disconvenientis terminata ad potentiam, cui disconvenit tale absolutum." Matthew of Acquasparta, *Quaestiones disputatae selectae*, 2 vols., BFSMA 1–2 (Quaracchi, 1914), 2:114: "Dolor, qui est sensus divisionis continui." Aegidius Romanus, *In tertium librum sententiarum eruditissima commentaria cum questionibus* (Rome, 1623), 507–12, claimed that pain was in the touch "nam si dolor est immutatio sensibilium per quem percipit lesivum et corruptivum." See also Aegidius Romanus, *Quodlibeta castigatissima* (Venice, 1504), fol. 17v.

13. Henry of Ghent claimed that (externally motivated) change was also necessary for the sensation of pain. Duns Scotus disagreed, claiming that only the soul's apprehension mattered. Henry of Ghent, *Quotlibeta*, fol. 459v, quodlibet 11, q. 8; Duns Scotus, *Quaestiones*, 568–77. See also Francesco Piro, "Sensi interni e eziologia degli affetti: A proposito di due *Quaestiones* sul dolore di Enrico di Gand," in *Corpo e anima, sensi interni e intelletto dai secoli XIII–XIV ai post-Cartesiani e Spinoziani*, ed. Graziella Federici Vescovini, Valeria Sorge, and Carlo Vinti, Textes et études du Moyen Âge 30 (Turnhout, 2005), 189–210, who situates the question of internal apprehension of pain within the history of contemporary science.

14. "Dolor est solutio continuitatis." Alexander of Hales, *Glossa*, art. 8:27. Alexander claims to quote Aristotle, but modern editors have not found such a statement in Aristotle's writings. The Latin translation of Avicenna, though, does define pain in almost identical terms: "Dicimus igitur quod dolor est sensibilitas rei contrarie. Omnes vero doloris cause in duobus comprehenduntur generibus, scilicet genere mutationis complexionis cito facte et est malitia complexionis diverse, et genere solutionis continuitatis." See above, chap. 5.

15. William of Auvergne, *The Soul*, ed. and trans. Roland J. Teske, Mediaeval Philosophical Texts in Translation 37 (Milwaukee, WI, 2000), 403–6, chap. 6, pt. 38.

16. The most comprehensive discussions of the soul, largely based upon Aristotle's *De anima*, are in Thomas Aquinas, *Questiones disputatae*, ed. Raymond Spiazzi and P. Bazzi, 2 vols. (Turin, 1964–65), 1:480–510, q. 26, "De passionibus animae"; and Thomas Aquinas, *Questiones de anima*, ed. James H. Robb (Toronto, 1968). For the sensitive appetite in the twelfth century, see Odon Lottin, *Psychologie et morale aux XIIe et XIIIe siècles*, vol. 2, *Psychologie et morale: Les mouvements premiers de l'appétit sensitif de Pierre Lombard a saint Thomas d'Aquin* (Gembloux, 1948), 493–589. For the thirteenth and fourteenth centuries, see Peter of Tarentaise [Pope Innocent V], *Innocentii Quinti pontificis maximi, ex ordine Praedicatorum assumpti, qui antea Petrus de Tarantasia dicebatur, in IV librum sententiarum commentaria*, 4 vols. (1649–52; repr., Ridgewood, NJ, 1964), 3:109; *ST*, pts. 1a–2ae, q. 35, art. 1; Thomas Aquinas, *Questiones disputatae*, 1:505; Thomas Aquinas, *In quatuor libros sententiarum*, ed. Robertus Busa, *Sancti Thomae Aquinatis opera omnia qui sont in indice Thomistico* 1 (Stuttgart, 1980), 314, ad dist. 15, q. 2, art. 1b; Alexander of Hales, *Quaestiones disputatae antequam esset frater*, BFSMA 19 (Quaracchi, 1960), 224; William of Ockham, *Quodlibeta septem*, 251, 253; English translation in William of Ockham, *Quodlibetal Questions*, trans. Alfred J. Freddoso and Francis E. Kelley, 2 vols. (New Haven, CT, 1991), 1:224; Durand de St. Pourçain, *Petri Lombardi sententias theologicas commentariorum libri IIII* (Venice, 1571), fol. 240v.

17. Matthew of Acquasparta, *Quaestiones disputatae selectae*, 2:191–94. Thomas Aquinas, *In quatuor libros sententiarum*, 316, mentions that "etiam dicunt quod inferior ratio compatiebatur et ut est natura et ut est ratio," but neither he nor Matthew of Acquasparta agrees or disagrees with the idea.

18. Bonaventura, *Commentaria in quatuor libros sententiarum magistri Petri Lombardi* (Quaracchi, 1887), 3:353–54, ad dist. 16, q. 1, art. 2.

19. E.g., Peter of Tarentaise, *In IV librum sententiarum commentaria*, 3:109: "et sic magis patitur anima secundum vires sensibiles appetitivas, in quibus aliqua delectatio obijcitur, quam secundum cognitivas in quibus sola rei similitude seu intentio recipitur."

20. *ST*, pts. 1a–2ae, q. 44, art. 1 ad 3; Thomas Aquinas, *Sententia libri ethicorum* (Rome, 1969), bk. 4, l. 17, n. 4. I thank Barbara Rosenwein for this reference.

21. Walter Chatton, *Reportatio super sententias, libri III–IV*, ed. Joseph C. Wey and Girard J. Etzkorn, Studies and Texts 149 (Toronto, 2005), 127.

22. For a full list, see Friedrich Stegmüller, *Repertorium commentariorum in sententias Petri Lombardi*, 2 vols. (Würzburg, 1947).

23. For a detailed discussion, see Joseph Ziegler, "Medicine and Immortality in Terrestrial Paradise," in *Religion and Medicine in the Middle Ages*, ed. Peter Biller and Joseph Ziegler (York, UK, 2001), 201–42.

24. Augustine, *De ciuitate Dei*, bk. 14, chap. 1. Henry of Ghent concurred, centuries later: "in statu innocentiae hominis, qua potuit non mori per diuturnam conservationem a morte." Henry of Ghent, *Quodlibet IX*, ed. R. Macken, vol. 13 of *Henrici de Gandavo opera omnia* (Leuven, 1983), 271.

25. Augustine, *De ciuitate Dei*, bk. 14, chap. 9.

26. "De tristitia uero, quam Cicero magis aegritudinem appellat, dolorem autem Vergilius, ubi ait: 'Dolent gaudentque,' (sed ideo malui tristitiam dicere, quia aegritudo uel dolor usitatius in corporibus dicitur), scrupulosior quaestio est, utrum inueniri possit in bono." Ibid., bk. 14, chap. 7.

27. Hugh of Saint Victor, "De sacramentis christiane fidei," PL 176:275, bk. 1, chap. 18.

28. "Primus homo . . . habuit se ad utrumque, non mori et non pati, et mori et pati. Passibilis et mortalis potestate, non actu; immortalis et impassibilis iterum potestate, et non actu. Unde quidam dicunt eum fuisse immortalem et impassibilem ante casum inobedientie." Anselm of Laon, "Sentences du liber Pancrisis," no. 38, in *Psychologie et morale aux XIIe et XIIIe siècles*, vol. 5, *L'école d'Anselme de Laon et de Guillaume de Champeaux*, by Odon Lottin (Gembloux, 1959), 36.

29. Jacquart, "Hildegard et la physiologie de son temps"; Hildegard of Bingen, *Causae et curae*, 33, 36, cited in Ziegler, "Medicine and Immortality," 209n23.

30. Bonaventura, *Commentaria*, 351, ad dist. 16, q. 3, art. 1.

31. Matthew of Acquasparta, *Quaestiones disputatae*, 99, q. 6.

32. Alexander of Hales, *Quaestiones disputatae*, 224–70, q. 16: "De passibilitate animae Christi et Adae"; Alexander of Hales, *Summa theologica*, 5 vols. (Quaracchi, 1928), 2:631–40, bk. 2:1, tract. 3, chaps. 1–3: "De coniuncto humano."

33. Matthew of Acquasparta, *Quaestiones disputatae selectae*, 2:271–72.

34. Augustine, *In Iohannis euangelium tractatus*, ed. Radbod Willems, CCSL 36 (Turnhout, 1954), 96–97, tract. 9, chap. 10: "Eua de latere dormientis, ecclesia de latere patientis." See also Augustine, *Enarrationes in Psalmos*, ed. Eligius Dekkers and Johannes Fraipont, CCSL 40 (Turnhout, 1956), 190–91.

35. De Moulin, *De heelkunde in de vroege Middeleeuwen*, 124.

36. John of Damascus and Peter Lombard did discuss Eve within the context of creation, but not of the Fall. I am grateful to Rita Copeland for pointing this out.

37. Honorius Augustodunensis, "Elucidarium," in *L'elucidarium et les lucidaires*, ed. Yves Lefèbvre, Bibliothèque des Écoles françaises d'Athènes et de Rome 180 (Paris, 1954), 374: "Quali modo pareret? sine dolore et absque sorde." Only one manuscript has "mulier" as the subject of the sentence.

38. "Sine sorde et sine dolore." Ibid., 384.

39. Anselm of Canterbury, *Cur Deus homo: Prima forma inedita*, ed. Eugenius Druwé (Rome, 1933).

40. Bonaventura, *Commentaria*, 353: "ex contrariis agentibus et patientibus constiti sumus, ita quod continua in corpore nostro sit resolutio. . . . Patimur enim, nolimus velimus."

41. Bonaventure's editors attributed this quotation to *De ciuitate Dei*, bk. 14, chap. 15, par. 2: "Dolor est dissensus ab iis quae accidunt [nobis] nolentibus." This is not quite what Augustine wrote; like many scholars, Bonaventure was probably quoting Augustine from memory.

42. Augustine, *De libero arbitrio*, 316, 3:23: "Quid est enim aliud dolor nisi sensus diuisiones uel corruptionis in patiens?" Alexander of Hales, *Glossa*, 151, ad dist. 15, art. 4: "Dolor est sensus propriae corruptionis."

43. Hildegard of Bingen, *Causae et curae*, 36, 43–44.

44. Ziegler, "Medicine and Immortality," 210.

45. E.g., "certe omni animae laborare molestum est." Augustine, "Sermones de sanctis," no. 280, PL 38:1282; Georges Duby, "Réflexions sur la douleur physique au Moyen Âge," in *Mâle Moyen Âge* (Paris, 1988), 203–9.

46. Henry of Ghent, *Quotlibeta*, fol. 337v, quodlibet 8, q. 32. The disputation took place at Christmas 1284, and the very phrasing of the question raises the possibility that the perception of the earth as a round body was common at the time. Henry's answer, though, intimates that he held the Ptolemaic view concerning the shape of the earth: "Infimum autem universi corporis medium terrae est, quot etiam cor terrae nominatur."

47. "Stabilitio loci, qui vocatur infernus." "Infimum autem universi corporis medium terrae est, quod etiam cor terrae nominatur." William of Auvergne, "De universo," in *Opera omnia*, 1:635.

48. The subject of unbaptized babies and their fate was of great concern to scholars. See Donald C. Mowbray, "A Community of Sufferers and the Authority of Masters: The Development of the Idea of *Limbo* by Masters of Theology at the University of Paris (c. 1230–c. 1300)," in *Authority and Community in the Middle Ages*, ed. Donald C. Mowbray, Rhiannon Purdie, and Ian P. Wei (Stroud, UK, 1999), 43–68.

49. Gregory the Great, *Dialogi*, ed. Adalbert de Vogüé, 3 vols., Sources chrétiennes 265 (Paris, 1980), 3:158–60.

50. Thomas Aquinas, *Questiones disputatae*, 1:483. The *questiones disputatae* were composed between 1266 and 1269. In a quodlibetal question defended in 1270, Thomas assumed the opposite position, accepting that hellfire was contrary to fire's natural virtue but was acting as an instrument of divine justice. Thomas Aquinas, *Questiones de quolibet*, 2 vols. (Rome, 1996), 2:281, quodlibet 3, q. 10.

51. Henry of Ghent, *Quotlibeta*, fols. 338v–339r, quodlibet 8 (1284), q. 34.

52. Bernstein, "Esoteric Theology."

53. Aegidius Romanus, *Quodlibeta castigatissima*, fol. 17r–v, bk. 2, q. 9: "utrum demones possint pati ab igne inferni."

54. William of Auvergne, "De universo," in *Opera omnia*, 1:835.

55. Alain Boureau, *Satan the Heretic: The Birth of Demonology in the Medieval West*, trans. Teresa L. Fagan (Chicago, 2006), 93–116; Thomas B. De Mayo, *The Demonology of William of Auvergne: By Fire and Sword* (Lewiston, NY, 2007), 162–90.

56. "Si autem consideremus diligentius, dolor, qui dicitur corporis, magis ad animam pertinet. Animae est enim dolere, non corporis, etiam quando ei dolendi causa existit a corpore, cum in eo loco dolet, ubi laeditur corpus. Sicut ergo dicimus corpora sentientia et corpora uiuentia, cum ab anima sit corpori sensus et uita: ita corpora dicimus et dolentia, cum dolor corpori nisi ab anima esse non possit. Dolet itaque anima cum corpore in eo loco eius, ubi aliquid contingit ut doleat; dolet et sola, quamuis sit in corpore, cum aliqua causa etiam inuisibili tristis est ipsa corpore incolumi; dolet etiam non in corpore constituta." Augustine, *De ciuitate Dei*, 2:760, bk. 21, chap. 3; English translation from 2:453.

57. Gregory the Great, *Dialogi*, 3:99–100, bk. 4, chap. 30; Aelred of Rievaulx, "Dialogus de anima," in *Opera omnia*, ed. A. Hoste and C. H. Talbot, CCCM 1 (Turnhout, 1971), 1:737–38; Peter Abelard, "Commentaria in Epistulam Pauli ad Romanos," in *Petri*

Abaelardi opera theologica, ed. Eligius M. Buytaert, CCCM 11 (Turnhout, 1969), 81–82, bk. 1, chap. 2; Peter Lombard, *Sententiae,* 1:92–98; *ST,* pts. 1a–2ae, q. 35, art. 1.

58. For a summary concerning the views on hellfire, see Jérôme Baschet, *Les justices de l'au-delà: Les représentations de l'enfer en France et en Italie (XIIᵉ–XVᵉ siècle)* (Rome, 1993), 50–52.

59. Le Goff, *Naissance du purgatoire.*

60. Claude Carozzi, "Structure et fonction de la vision de Tnugdal," in *Faire croire: Modalités de la diffusion et de la réception des messages religieux du XIIᵉ au XVᵉ siècle,* Collection de l'École française de Rome 51 (Rome, 1981), 223–34; Thomas Aquinas, *Questiones de anima,* 271–73.

61. See above, chap. 1.

62. "Ardet igitur anima humana se ipsa teste, cum nihil caloris in se habeat. . . . Quid ergo mirum, si sola imaginatione ignis ardere sibi videatur, et ardere se iudicet, cum ipsa imaginatio substantiae animae vicinior sit quam sensus, et solummodo spirituale sit . . . ? sed hoc ei videtur propter fortissimam coniunctionem et unionem qua corpori unita est et inde est, quod sibi videtur et se iudicat pati quod ipsum corpus patitur, quia non solum in corpore est, sed corpus, ut multi ex philosophis dixerunt, potius in ea . . . non vere dolet ipsa anima huiusmodi passionibus, tanquam suis propriis; sed magis condolet, tanquam alienis." William of Auvergne, "De universo," in *Opera omnia,* 1:643.

63. William stressed the total connection of body and soul also in his treatise on the soul. William of Auvergne, *Soul,* 403–6, chap. 6, pt. 38.

64. Thomas Aquinas, *Questiones disputatae,* 1:480–510, 2:359–62; Thomas Aquinas, *Questiones de quolibet,* 2:231–33.

65. Thomas Aquinas, *Questiones de quolibet,* 2:232.

66. Thomas Aquinas, *Questiones disputatae,* 1:482: "Tertio vero modo quo nomen passionis transumptive sumitur, anima potest pati eo modo quo eius operatio potest impediri." Thomas Aquinas, *Questiones de anima,* 269: "Oportet ergo dicere quod secundum rei veritatem ille ignis corporeus animae sit nocivus." Thomas Aquinas, *Questiones de quolibet,* 2:232: "Alio modo dicitur pati proprie loquendo, secundum contarietatem agentis ad paciens, protus scilicet pati dicimur cum aliquid nobis adveniat quod est contrarium vel nature vel voluntati nostra; et secundum hoc infirmitas et tristicia passiones dicuntur."

67. Thomas Aquinas, *Questiones de anima,* 269–73.

68. Henry of Ghent, *Quodlibet XII: Quaestiones 1–30,* ed. J. Decorte, vol. 16 of *Henrici de Gandavo opera omnia* (Leuven, 1987), 47–50.

69. Matthew of Acquasparta, *Quaestiones disputatae,* 93–134, qq. 6–7.

70. Ibid., p. 103: "utpote vel ligati vel in carcere inclusi." In this, Matthew was following Augustine's own definition of pain as something contrary to our will. See Augustine's definition, as attributed by Bonaventure, above, n. 41.

71. Matthew of Acquasparta, *Quaestiones disputatae,* 101, 103, 105–6.

72. Ibid., 108–9: "anima enim sive spiritus separatus habet suum sensum, non corporeum, sed spiritualem, quo non tantum speculative, sed experimentaliter sentit."

73. See Alain Boureau, "Miracle, volonté et imagination: La mutation scolastique (1270–1320)," in *Miracles, prodiges et merveilles au Moyen Âge* (Paris, 1995), 159–72.

74. Matthew of Acquasparta, *Quaestiones disputatae*, 95, 114.

75. The rebuttals also contain other statements that flatly contradict the solution, such as ad 13th, which claims that incorporeal souls accepted passions in all three meanings of the word (ibid., 116).

76. Ibid., 120–34.

77. Baschet, *Justices de l'au-delà*, 52–59.

78. Jacobus de Voragine, *Sermones quadragesimales*, 296.

79. Glucklich, *Sacred Pain*.

80. Weinhandl, *Deutsches Nonnenleben*, 126–27; Suso, *Deutche Schriften*, 18–19; Ebner, *Margaretha Ebner und Heinrich von Nördlingen*; Passenier, "Suffering Body"; Stoudt, "Production and Preservation of Letters"; Wiethaus, "Thieves and Carnivals."

81. See above, chap. 1.

82. John 7:23. Jacobus de Voragine, *Sermones quadragesimales*, 293–97.

83. Rudolph Arbesmann, "The Concept of Christus Medicus in St. Augustine," *Traditio* 10 (1954): 1–28.

84. See above, chap. 4.

85. Herolt, *Sermones discipuli*, sermon 128, "De infirmitatibus."

86. For the original text of Francesca's visions, see Giovanni Mattiotti, *Il dialetto romanesco del quattrocento: Il manoscritto quattrocentesco di G. Mattiotti*, ed. Giorgio Carpaneto (Rome, 1995); for the Latin text, see Giovanni Mattiotti, *Santa Francesca Romana: Edizione critica dei trattati latini di Giovanni Mattiotti*, ed. Alessandra Bartolomei Romagnoli, Storia e attualità 14 (Vatican City, 1994). See also O. Moroni, "Le visioni di S. Francesca Romana tra medioevo e umanesimo," *Studi romani* 21 (1973): 160–78. For Francesca's education and life, see D. Mazzuconi, "Pauca quedam de vita et miraculis beate Francisce de Pontianis: Tre biografie quattrocentenesche di santa Francesca Romana," in *Una santa tutta romana: Saggi e ricerche nel VI centenario della nascità di Francesca Bussa dei Ponziani (1384–1984)*, ed. Giorgio Picasso (Siena, 1984), 95–199; Vittorio Bartoccetti, "Le fonti della visione di S. Francesca Romana," *Rivista storica benedettina* 13 (1922): 13–40; Lugano, *Pocessi inediti per Francesca Bussa*; Arnold Esch, "Tre sante ed il loro ambiente sociale a Roma: S. Francesca Romana, S. Brigida di Svezia e S. Caterina da Siena," in *Atti del simposio internazionale Cateriniano-Bernardiniano(Siena, 17–20 aprile 1980)*, ed. Domenico Maffei and Paolo Nardi (Siena, 1982), 89–120.

87. Manuele Gragnolati, *Experiencing the Afterlife: Soul and Body in Dante and Medieval Culture* (Notre Dame, IN, 2005), does convincingly embed Dante's work in the context of contemporary Italian writing. I still find that the *Divine Comedy* is intrinsically different from the usual visionary model.

88. There is a widespread literature on visions of hell. See, among others, Peter Dinzelbacher, *Vision und Visionsliteratur im Mittelalter* (Stuttgart, 1981); Le Goff, *Naissance du purgatoire*; Alan E. Bernstein, *The Formation of Hell: Death and Retribution in the Ancient and Early Christian Worlds* (Ithaca, NY, 1993); Carol Zaleski, *Otherworld Journeys: Accounts of Near-Death Experience in Medieval and Modern Times* (Oxford, 1987). For English translations of visions, see Eileen Gardiner, ed., *Visions of Heaven and Hell before Dante* (New York, 1989).

89. Most narratives of otherworld experiences insist upon the suddenness and involuntary character of the traveler's death; the *Purgatory of Saint Patrick* is unusual in the sense that the knight Owain knew what to expect and had chosen to visit purgatory. Late medieval visionaries sometimes asked to experience hell in life, and their prayers were answered. See Barbara Newman, *From Virile Woman to WomanChrist: Studies in Medieval Religion and Literature* (Philadelphia, 1995), 108–36; McNamara, "The Need to Give."

90. E.g., *Visio Tnugdali*, ed. Albrecht Wagner (Erlangen, 1882), 6–9, 55; Van der Zanden, *Étude sur le "Purgatoire de saint Patrice,"* 23.

91. "La vie de saint Jehan Paulus," in *The German Legends of the Hairy Anchorite*, ed. Charles A. Williams and Louis Allen, University of Illinois Studies in Language and Literature 6 (Urbana, 1935), 83–140; L. Karl, "La vie de St. Jehan Paulus," *Revue des langues romaines* 56 (1913): 425–45.

92. Baschet, *Justices de l'au-delà*, 66–83.

93. Peter Dinzelbacher, "The Way to the Other World in Medieval Literature and Art," *Folklore* 97 (1986): 70–87.

94. See above, n. 86; Dante Alighieri, *The Divine Comedy*, trans. and ed. Robert M. Durling (New York, 1996), 1:xvi, Inferno; *Visio Tnugdali*, 33–39; Van der Zanden, *Étude sur le "Purgatoire de saint Patrice,"* 4–24.

95. *Visio Tnugdali*, 10–12, 19–23; Zaleski, *Otherworld Journeys*, 52–69.

96. Mattiotti, *Dialetto*, 270–71.

97. Roger of Wendover, *Liber qui dicitur flores historiarum ab anno domini MCLIV annoque Henrici Anglorum regis*, ed. Henry Hewlett, 2 vols., Rolls Series 84 (London, 1887), 2:261; Mattiotti, *Dialetto*, 269, 272.

98. Martha Himmelfarb, *Tours of Hell: An Apocalyptic Form in Jewish and Christian Literature* (Philadelphia, 1983); Bernstein, *Formation of Hell*, 267–335.

99. "Et in his tamen, nihil nisi corporale, vel corporalibus simile recitasse: flumina, flammas, pontes, naves, domos, nemora, prata, flores, homines nigros et candidos, et caetera qualia in hoc mundo solent, vel ad gaudium amari, vel ad tormentum timeri; se quoque solutas corporibus, manibus trahi, pedibus duci, collo suspendi, flagellari, praecipitari, et multa hujusmodi, quae naturae minime repugnant, narrat." "Tractatus de purgatorio sancti Patricii," PL 180:975–76.

100. See Jan S. Emerson, "Harmony, Hierarchy, and the Senses in the Vision of Tundal," in *Imagining Heaven in the Middle Ages: A Book of Essays*, ed. Jan S. Emerson and Hugo Feiss (New York, 2000), 3–46.

101. *Visio Tnugdali*, 28.

102. E.g., Roger of Wendover, *Flores historiarum*, 260.

103. "Avevano anche l'altre pene generale sopradicte." "Avevano anche tucte l'altre generale pene." Mattiotti, *Dialetto*, 273–75.

104. Baschet, *Justices de l'au-delà*, 293–96.

105. It is sometimes assumed that those descriptions of hell were based upon contemporary punitive methods. This is patently untrue, for judicial torture was conducted in private, and most judicial executions were public hangings. The only cases I know of drawing and quartering belong to the very rare and spectacular English punishments for treason in the fourteenth century.

106. Gobi, *Scala coeli*, nos. 619, 339-45; Herolt, *Sermones discipuli*, sermon 125, "De penis inferni."

107. Ronald E. Pepin, "*Nouem Species Poenae:* The Doctrine of Nine Torments in Honorius Augustodunensis, Alain de Lille, Pastoralia, and Bernard de Morlas (al. Morval)," *Latomus: Revue d'études latines* 47 (1988): 668-74; Honorius Augustodunensis, "Elucidarium," 447-48, bk. 3, chap. 4; Bernard of Clairvaux, "Sermo 42 de diversis," in *Sancti Bernardi opera*, vol. 6/1, *Sermones III*, ed. Jean Leclercq and H. M. Rochais (Rome, 1970), 259; Baschet, *Justices de l'au-delà*, 61-66.

108. Thomas of Chobham, *Summa*, 33. Thomas also tried to correlate pains with sins: darkness for infidelity; chains of fire for all kinds of sin; whips for perennial complainants who lacked patience to accept God's chastisement; cold for the malicious and avaricious; fire for lust (*concupiscentia*); fear for those who took pleasure in the suffering of others; worms for the jealous; confusion for the stubborn who refused to confess and repent; and stench for *luxuria*. Ibid., 38-42. Herolt counted fire, cold, stench, hunger, and thirst (for gluttons and drunks), the horrible sight of demons (for those who watched women dancing), chains and darkness (for the lustful and those who liked dancing), noise, perpetual despair, and the privation of heavenly vision. Herolt, *Sermones discipuli*, sermon 125. Guillaume Péraud listed fire, the worm, stench, cold, hunger, the devils, horror of devils and the place, darkness, and chains. Guilielmus Peraldus, *Sermones moralissimi super epistolas dominicales totius anni multas materias predicabiles complectentes . . .* (Avignon, 1519), 1:fols. 79v-80r; Guilielmus Peraldus, *Summa aurea* (Brescia, 1494), fol. 172v.

109. Caesarius of Heisterbach, *Dialogus miraculorum*, 2:315: "Pix, nix, nox, vermis, flagra, vincula, pus, pudor, horror." Stephen of Bourbon, *Tractatus*, 1:69, 83, 90, 101, 115. See also Bromyard, *Summa praedicantium*, s.v. "pena," art. 1: "Illius insuper penarum multitudo versibus ostenditur frequentibus: Iudice [sic] scriptura caligo iuncta flagella frigus flamma timor vermis confusio fetor."

110. Thomas of Chobham, *Summa*, 33: "Omnes pene simul sunt."

111. Bromyard, *Summa praedicantium*, s.v. "pena," art. 7.18.

112. "Alphabetum narrationum," MS Harley 268, fol. 13or; Arnold of Liège, *Alphabet of Tales*, 265. Also in Bromyard, *Summa praedicantium*, s.v. "pena," art. 9:25; and in Stephen of Bourbon, *Tractatus*, 1:22-23. See also Jacques Le Goff, "Le vocabulaire des exempla d'après l'Alphabetum narrationum (début XIVe siècle)," in *La lexicographie du Latin médiéval: Colloque du CNRS* (Paris, 1981), 321-32.

113. E.g., "De poena Lodewici Landgravii," "De poena Wilhelmi comitis Juliacensis"; Caesarius of Heisterbach, *Dialogus miraculorum*, 2:316-22.

114. Herolt, *Sermones discipuli*, sermon 125. For a similar story, see also Gobi, *Scala coeli*, no. 249; Stephen of Bourbon, *Tractatus*, 1:79.

115. Gobi, *Scala coeli*, no. 784.

116. "Alphabetum narrationum," MS Harley 268, fol. 13or-v; Arnold of Liège, *Alphabet of Tales*, 265.

117. Pseudo-Augustine, "De uera et falsa penitentia," PL 40:1127. Pseudo-Augustine does not say what Stephen quotes. Presumably, Stephen took it from the attribution to Augustine in Gratian, *Decretum*, 94, I, D. 25, c. 5, *palea*. Stephen of Bourbon, *Tractatus*, 1:87.

118. Herolt, *Sermones discipuli*, sermon 125; despite Herolt's assertion, I could not find the comparison in any of Bernard of Clairvaux's works nor in any pseudo-Bernardian work.

119. "Quantus sit ille dolor aliquantulum experte lotrices pannorum sciunt, que in tempore hyemis de riparia congelata veniunt ad ignem." Stephen of Bourbon, *Tractatus*, 1:73.

120. This is the only case I have found in which a preacher indicates a lifetime's hardening as an ameliorating circumstance in hell. The hardening against torture and pain, said to be typical of "criminals," was a common motif among jurists. See below, chap. 8.

121. Stephen of Bourbon, *Tractatus*, 1:67; Bromyard, *Summa praedicantium*, s.v. "pena," art. 4.

122. Thomas of Chobham, *Summa*, 47–48.

123. "Secundus locus est infernus ubi erit fames perpetua. tanta sc. quod pre nimia fame eorum caro erit consumpta. . . . Tanta quod fames intra costas eorum erit inclue; et imo erit perpetua. Quod de costis eorum nunquam exire poterit. . . . Tanta quod linguas proprias manducabunt. . . . Tanta quod sua et aliorum brachia devorabunt. . . . Tanta quod pre nimia fame diabolum et deum blasphemabunt." Jacobus de Voragine, *Registrum in sermones de tempore*, "Dominica xxv post festum trinitatis sermo iii."

124. Herolt, *Sermones discipuli*, sermon 125.

125. Pelbart of Themeswar, *Pomerium sermonum de sanctis per anni circulum tam hyemalium quam estivalium* (Hagenau, 1520), pars aestivalis, sermon 88, "In commemoratione defunctorum sermo iii, sc. de purgatorij iudicij loco ac acerba pena": "in hoc mundo propter occupationem sui corporis est sicut quod occupatur in bello et in periculo ubi non precipit laborem vel lesionem suam; sed in purgatorio est apprehensionis fortioris ubi libere sentit cruciatum suum; unde idem Algazel dicit quod in purgatorio est cruciatus ineffabilis, sed omnis pena huius vite est effabilis." For Pelbart's history and sermons, see Zoltan J. Kosztolnyik, "Pelbartus of Temesvár: A Franciscan Preacher and Writer of the Late Middle Ages in Hungary," *Vivarium: A Journal for Mediaeval Philosophy and the Intellectual Life of the Middle Ages* 5, no. 2 (1967): 100–110.

126. Pelbart of Themeswar, *Pomerium sermonum de sanctis*, sermon 88: "Superat ei omnem penam quam unque passus est aliquis in hac vita vel pati potest. Numquam inquit in carne tanta inventa est pena. licet mirabilia martyres passi sunt tormenta et multi nequiter quanta sustinuerunt supplicia." "gravius esse in purgatorio ad ictum occuli quam fuerit pena sancti Laurentii in cracitula et quicquid pene in hac vita potest excogitari." Petrus de la Palude [attr.], *Sermones thesauri novi de sanctis* (Nürenberg, 1496), fol. 149: "Ignis purgatorij est durior quam quicquid excogitari posset, licet enim martyres innumerabilia passi sunt tormenta, ut Laurentius, Petrus, Katherina, Ursula etc. numque in eis talis pena inventa est."

127. Jacobus de Voragine, *Registrum in sermones de tempore*, "Dominica xxii post festum trinitatis sermo primus": "in inferno est una pena substantialis per modum damni; scilicet carentia visionis dei. et alia per modum sensus, scilicet ignis et vermis." Herolt, *Sermones discipuli*, sermon 125: "sexta pena sunt vincula et tenebre. Unde in verbis pessimis. Ligatis manibus et pedibus etc. Sciendum quod illi principaliter ligantur manibus et pedibus que hec in mundo per illicitos tactus et gressus deum offenderunt,

sc. amplexando et osculando et alios et se ipsos illicite tangendo. Similiter chorisando et saltando et superbe cum pedibus incedendo. Et tales maledicunt tunc sibi et membris suis . . . maledicte manus mee . . . pedes mei maledicti . . . maledicti oculi quod nunquam pro peccatis meis unam lacrimam fundistis . . . maledictum cor meum. . . . Octava pena est mors eterna et perpetua tristitia sine omni consolatione. . . . Et si presens et temporalis mors quod sermone Aristotele nihil aliud est quod recessus anime a corpore; ita homines cruciat quod nec stare nec sedere nec quicque facere potent pro dolore; o quod tunc facit perpetua mors in damnatis. . . . Utinam damnati mori possent; sed heu nesciunt mori . . . si enim damnatus haberet omnia regna mundi libenter daret ut semel mori posset; Nona pena est separatio a deo et beata virgine Maria et ab omnibus sanctis et angelis. . . . Excludi a bonis eternis et alienum effici ab his qui preparata sunt sanctis tantum cruciatum et tantum dolorem infert ut si nulla extrinsecus pena torqueret hec sola sufficeret."

128. Gregory the Great, *Moralia in Iob*, ed. Marcus Adriaen, CCSL 143 (Turnhout, 1979), 527, bk. 9, chap. 66: "In huius vitae tormentis timor dolorem habet, dolor timorem non habet, quia nequaquam mentem metus cruciat cum pati iam coeperit quod metuebat. Infernum vero et umbra mortis obscurat, et sempiternus horror inhabitat quia eius ignibus traditi, et in suppliciis dolorem sentiunt, et in doloris angustia pulsante se semper pavore feriuntur; ut et quod timent tolerent, et rursus quod tolerant sine cessatione pertimescant. . . . Hic metus amittitur cum tolerari iam coeperit quod timebatur; illic et dolor dilaniat et pavor angustat. Horrendo igitur modo erit tunc reprobis dolor cum formidine, flamma cum obscuritate . . . dolor cruciat, sed nullatenus pavorem fugat." Centuries later, Thomas of Chobham (*Summa*, 37–42) substituted fear for the ligatures in the sixth pain of hell.

129. Herolt, *Sermones discipuli*, sermon 125; Jacobus de Voragine, *Registrum in sermones de sanctis*, "Dominica xxii post festum trinitatis sermo primus."

CHAPTER SEVEN

1. On the structure of quodlibetal questions, see Palémon Glorieux, *La littérature quodlibétique de 1260 à 1320*, 2 vols., Bibliothèque Thomiste (Paris, 1925–35), 1:1–55. On the social and intellectual context, see Ian P. Wei, "The Self-Image of the Masters of Theology at the University of Paris in the Late Thirteenth and Early Fourteenth Centuries," *Journal of Ecclesiastical History* 46 (1994): 398–431.

2. G. P. Sijen, "La passibilité du Christ chez Philippe de Harveng," *Analecta Praemonstratensia* 14 (1938): 193–94.

3. Ibid., 194–95.

4. Gillian Evans, "*Mens Devota*: The Literary Community of the Devotional Works of John of Fécamp and St. Anselm," *Medium Aevum* 43 (1974): 105–15.

5. Fulton, *From Judgment to Passion*, 177–88.

6. Anselm of Canterbury, *Cur Deus homo*; Southern, *Saint Anselm and His Biographer*.

7. Hugh of Saint Victor, "De quatuor voluntatibus in Christo libellus," PL 176:841–46.

8. William of Auvergne, *Soul*, 403–6, chap. 6, pt. 38.

9. The fact that the two English archbishops who condemned scholastic positions as heretical—Robert Kilwardby and John Pecham—were both noted scholars who had joined

the church hierarchy after long and fruitful academic careers, only emphasizes the tensions that shook the academic world. Thomas Aquinas was posthumously condemned in 1277, Giles of Rome was denied his master's degree in the same year, and Richard Knapwell of Oxford mobilized the entire academic world on both sides of the Channel in his appeal to the pope, above Archbishop Pecham's head, in 1286. See Alain Boureau, *Théologie, science et censure au XIIIᵉ siècle: Le cas de Jean Peckham* (Paris, 1999), 10, 12–17.

10. The most important analysis of the debate is ibid., 118–27. For specific scholars, see Godfrey of Fontaines, *Les quatre premiers quodlibets de Godefroid de Fontaines*, ed. Maurice de Wulf and A. Pelzer, Les philosophes du Moyen Âge, 1st ser., 2 (Louvain, 1904), q. 6; Aegidius Romanus, *Quodlibeta castigatissima*, fol. 13r–v: "ut sic facile sit ostendere quod Christus mortuus sit vere et naturaliter sicut alii homines"; Henry of Ghent, *Quodlibet XII*, 21–22, q. 3; Henry of Ghent, *Quotlibeta*, fols. 403v–413r, quod. 10: "Unum ad questionem simpliciter dicendum est quod Christi corpus vivus et Petri corpus vivus sunt idem corpus specie, sicut et corpus Petri vivus et corpus Pauli vivus. Aliter enim Christus non haberet univoce humanam naturam nobiscum, nec esset univoce homo nobiscum" (fol. 404r).

11. Peter Lombard, *Sententiae*, 2:92–93.

12. "Non corpus sentit, sed anima per corpus, quo velut nuntio utitur ad confirmandum in seipsa quod extrinsecus nuntiatur. Sicut ergo anima quod foris est per corpus tanquam per instrumentum videt vel audit, ita etiam per corpus quaedam sentit mala quae sine corpore non sentiret, ut famem, et sitim et hujusmodi." This text, or one close to it, is what Migne presumably used for his edition of the *Sententiae*. See Peter Lombard, "Sententiarum libri quatuor," PL 192:790; Peter Lombard, *Sententiae*, 2:93n3.

13. Peter Lombard, "Sententiarum libri quatuor," PL 192:785.

14. Peter Lombard, *Sententiae*, 2:96–98.

15. Peter Abelard, *Sic et non: A Critical Edition*, ed. Blanche B. Boyer and Richard McKeon (Chicago, 1977), 283–96, q. 80.

16. Peter Lombard, *Sententiae*, 2:103–5.

17. Thomas Aquinas, *Quaestiones de anima*, 264–73; Thomas Aquinas, *Questiones disputatae*, 2:359–62.

18. Alexander of Hales attributed four roughly equivalent meanings to *passio:* the ability to receive sensory information, the ability to receive emotional information, the extent of the change caused by the information, and the necessity of the change. Alexander of Hales, *Summa theologica*, 2:631–40.

19. Thomas Aquinas, *Scriptum super sententiis magistri Petri Lombardi*, ed. R. P. Mandonnet and Marie Fabien Moos (Paris, 1947), 3:492–502, ad dist. 15, q. 2, art. 3.

20. Thomas Aquinas, *Quaestiones de anima*, 264–73; Thomas Aquinas, *Questiones disputatae*, 1:480–86, 2:359–62.

21. Godfrey of Fontaines, *Les quatre premiers quodlibets*, 212–13. Godfrey himself, though answering the quodlibetal question posed to him, condemned it as stemming more from curiosity than from devotion.

22. Aegidius Romanus, *Quodlibeta castigatissima*, fol. 13r-v.

23. Henry of Ghent, *Quotlibeta*, fols. 403v–413r, q. 10.

24. Aegidius Romanus, *Quodlibeta castigatissima*, fol. 13r-v; Bonaventura, *Commentaria*, 350–51, dist. 16, q. 3, art. 1; Henry of Ghent, *Quodlibet XII*, 9–22, quod. I;

Roger Marston, *Quodlibeta quaestiones,* ed. G. I. Etzkorn and Ignatius C. Brady, BFSMA 26 (Quaracchi, 1968), 390–92; John Pecham, *Quodlibeta quatuor,* ed. G. I. Etzkorn and Fernandus Delorme, BFSMA 25 (Quaracchi, 1989), 139–40, quod. 3, q. 4; Boureau, *Théologie, science et censure,* 243–44.

25. The same distinction is current in thirteenth-century medical literature. See Gil-Sotres, "Derivation and Revulsion."

26. *ST,* pt. 3a, q. 46, art. 5.

27. Ibid., pt. 3a, q. 46, arts. 6–7; Thomas Aquinas, *Questiones disputatae,* 1:504–7, q. 26, art. 9.

28. Thomas Aquinas, *Scriptum super sententiis magistri Petri Lombardi,* bk. 3, dist. 15, q. 2, art. 1, qc3co.

29. Joan Gibson, "Could Christ Have Been Born a Woman? A Medieval Debate," *Journal of Feminist Studies in Religion* 8 (1992): 65–82. See also Alastair J. Minnis, "*De Impedimento Sexus:* Women's Bodies and Medieval Impediments to Female Ordination," in *Medieval Theology and the Natural Body,* ed. Peter Biller and Alastair J. Minnis, York Studies in Medieval Theology 1 (York, UK, 1997), 109–39.

30. Bonaventura, *Commentaria,* 3:348–51; Durand de St. Pourçain, *Sent8entias theologicas commentariorum libri IIII,* fol. 240v; Duns Scotus, *Quaestiones,* 591; Gabriel Biel, *Collectorium circa quattuor libros sententiarum,* ed. Wilfrid Werbeck and Udo Hofman, 6 vols. (Tübingen, 1979), 4:266.

31. Durand de St. Pourçain, *Sentenias theologicas commentariorum libri IIII,* fol. 239v, q. 2.

32. Anselm of Laon had already noted the similarity between Adam and Christ in the twelfth century. Anselm of Laon, "Sentences du liber Pancrisis," 19–20: "De Adam et Christo: Adam est forma Christi. . . . Et hoc est: similes sunt Christus et Adam. Sed non sicut delictum ita et donum." See also Alexander of Hales, *Quaestiones disputatae,* 224–74, "De passibilitate animae Christi et Adae."

33. Durand de St. Pourçain, *Sentenias theologicas commentariorum libri IIII,* fol. 239v, q. 2.

34. Bonaventura, *Commentaria,* dist. 16, q. 3, art. 1.

35. Thomas Aquinas, *Scriptum super sententiis magistri Petri Lombardi,* bk. 3, dist. 15, qq. 1–2.

36. Thomas Aquinas, *Scriptum super sententiis magistri Petri Lombardi,* bk. 3, dist. 15, q. 2, art. 2, 1–2. See also Riccardo Quinto, "Per la storia del trattato tomistico *De passionibus animae:* Il *timor* nella letteratura teologica tra il 1200 e il 1230s," in *Thomistica,* ed. E. Manning, Recherches de théologie ancienne et médiévale, Supplementa (Leuven, 1995), 35–87, who places the notion of fear within the psychological theology of the thirteenth century; Thomas Prügl, "Tristitia: Zur Theologie der *Passiones Animae* bei Thomas von Aquin," in *Die Einheit der Person: Beiträge zur Anthropologie des Mittelalters; Richard Heinzmann zum 65. Geburtstag,* ed. Martin Thurner (Stuttgart, 1998), 143–44; Stephen Loughlin, "The Complexity and Importance of *Timor* in Aquinas' *Summa theologiae,*" in *Fear and Its Representations in the Middle Ages and Renaissance,* ed. Anne Scott and Synthia Kosso (Turnhout, 2002), 1–16.

37. Alexander of Hales, *Glossa,* 150–70; Alexander of Hales, *Quaestiones disputatae,* 247; Robert Kilwardby, *Quaestiones in librum tertium sententiarum,* ed. Elisabeth

Gössman (Munich, 1982), 194–216; Matthew of Acquasparta, *Quaestiones disputatae selectae*, 2:191–94.

38. The belief in Christ's voluntary assumption of human defects goes back to John of Damascus, *De fide orthodoxa*, 132. All scholastic authorities stress this point. Peter Lombard, *Sententiae*, 2:95–96, bk. 3, dist. 15, q. 1, art. 8; Bonaventura, *Commentaria*, 3:334–35; Alexander of Hales, *Glossa*, 168–69; Durand de St. Pourçain, *Sententias theologicas commentariorum libri IIII*, fol. 239r; Aegidius Romanus, *In tertium librum sententiarum*, 508–10; William of Ockham, *Quaestiones variae*, ed. G. I. Etzkorn, Francis E. Kelley, and Joseph C. Wey, Opera philosophica et theologica 8 (Saint Bonaventure, NY, 1984), q. 6, art. 9.

39. Hilary of Poitiers, *De trinitate*, 35, bk. 10, chap. 23.

40. Chatton, *Reportatio super sententias*, 125–34.

41. Bonaventura, *Commentaria*, 348–55; Durand de St. Pourçain, *Sententias theologicas commentariorum libri IIII*, fol. 240r–v; Duns Scotus, *Quaestiones*, 563–623; Kilwardby, *Quaestiones in librum tertium sententiarum*, 217–26; Matthew of Acquasparta, *Quaestiones disputatae*, 191–94; Peter of Tarentaise, *In IV librum sententiarum commentaria*, 3:110–15; Thomas Aquinas, *Questiones disputatae*, 1:501–10, q. 26, arts. 8–10; Thomas Aquinas, *Scriptum super sententiis magistri Petri Lombardi*, bk. 3, dist. 15, qq. 1–2; *ST*, pt. 3a, q. 46, arts. 5–7.

42. Chatton, *Reportatio super sententias*, 125–34.

43. Biel, *Collectorium*, 4:273–76.

44. Ibid., 276–80.

45. See, among many other excellent works, Sarah Beckwith, *Christ's Body: Identity, Culture and Society in Late Medieval Writings* (London, 1993); Bynum, *Fragmentation and Redemption*, 79–117; Kieckhefer, "Major Currents in Late Medieval Devotion"; James Marrow, *Passion Iconography in Northern European Art of the Late Middle Ages and the Early Renaissance* (Kortrijk, Belgium, 1979); Ellen M. Ross, *The Grief of God: Images of the Suffering Jesus in Late Medieval England* (Oxford, 1997); Miri Rubin, *Corpus Christi: The Eucharist in Late Medieval Culture* (Cambridge, 1991), 302–12; Swanson, "Passion and Practice."

46. Pseudo-Beda, "De meditatione passionis Christi per septem diei horas libellus," PL 94:563; Pseudo-Anselm, "Dialogus beatae Mariae et Anselmi de passione Domini," PL 159:277, 281; John of Caulibus, *Meditaciones vite Christi, olim S. Bonaventuro attributae*, ed. M. Stallings-Taney, CCCM 153 (Turnhout, 1997), 261–63; English translation in John of Caulibus, *Meditations on the Life of Christ*, trans. F. X. Taney, A. Miller, and C. M. Stallings-Taney (Asheville, NC, 1999), 243–45; Ludolph of Saxony, *Vita Jesu Christiex evangelio et aprobatis ab ecclesia Catholica doctoribus sedule collecta, editio novissima*, ed. L. M. Rigollot, 4 vols. (Paris, 1878), 4:96; Marrow, *Passion Iconography*, 68–94.

47. Ludolph of Saxony, *Vita Jesu Christi*, 4:138–39; Caroline W. Bynum, "The Blood of Christ in the Later Middle Ages," *Church History* 71 (2002): 685–714; Bynum, *Wonderful Blood*.

48. See Fulton, *From Judgment to Passion*, 53–59, 62.

49. F. J. E. Raby, ed., *The Oxford Book of Medieval Latin Verse* (Oxford, 1966), 6, 109. For a short survey of early medieval attitudes toward the Passion, see Thomas H. Bestul,

Texts of the Passion: Latin Devotional Literature and Medieval Society, Middle Ages Series (Philadelphia, 1996), 34–36.

50. Celia Chazelle, *The Crucified God in the Carolingian Era: Theology and Art of Christ's Passion* (Cambridge, 2001), 161.

51. Fulton, *From Judgment to Passion,* passim.

52. E.g., Jean Gerson, "Requeste pour les condamnes a mort," in *Oeuvres complètes,* ed. Palémon Glorieux (Paris, Tournai, and Rome, 1968), 7/1:341–43; Michael T. Clanchy, "Images of Ladies with Prayer Books: What Do They Signify?" *Studies in Church History* 38 (2004): 106–22; David L. D'Avray, "Sermons to the Upper Bourgeoisie by a Thirteenth-Century Franciscan," *Studies in Church History* 16 (1979): 187–99; Darleen Pryds, "Court as *Studium:* Royal Venues for Academic Preaching," in *Medieval Sermons and Society: Cloister, City, University,* ed. Jacqueline Hamesse et al., Textes et études du Moyen Âge 9 (Louvain-la-Neuve, 1998), 343–56.

53. Erich Auerbach, "*Passio* as Passio," *Criticism* 43 (2001): 288–308.

54. Jacobus de Voragine, *Legenda aurea,* 336–38. Though the *Legenda aurea* is not, properly speaking, a preachers' manual, it was used as such.

55. *ST,* pt. 3a, q. 15, art. 5.

56. John Bromyard, *Summa praedicantium,* s.v. "Passio Christi," intro.

57. Ibid., art. 2:5–8.

58. *ST,* pt. 3a, q. 15, art. 5. Cf. Pelbart of Themeswar, *Pomerium sermonum de sanctis,* sermon 67, "In die parasceve sermo II de passione Christi."

59. Jacobus de Voragine, *Sermones quadragesimales.*

60. Jacobus de Voragine, *Legenda aurea,* 336–53.

61. Jean Gerson, "Sermon sur la passion," in *Oeuvres complètes,* ed. Palémon Glorieux (Paris, Tournai, and Rome, 1968), 7/2:450. The sermon was preached on Holy Friday, 13 April 1403, in the presence of a great audience and thereafter became a best-seller. See Daniel Hobbins, "The Schoolman as Public Intellectual: Jean Gerson and the Late Medieval Tract," *American Historical Review* 108 (2003): 1328–29: "We know, for instance, that six copies of Gerson's famous Passion sermon of 1403 (*Ad Deum vadit*) belonged to ecclesiastical owners, while eleven belonged to lay owners. These lay owners spanned a wide social range: the dukes of Burgundy and Bourbon and the queen of France, lower-ranking nobles and courtiers, a medical master, and two widows, including Jeanne de Velle, a middle-class widow from Tournai who died in 1434. This general pattern of distribution also holds for Gerson's other popular French works." For the text of the sermon, see Gerson, "Sermon sur la passion," 449–93. Later, Gerson used this sermon as the basis for his biography of Christ: Jean Gerson, *La vie de Nostre Benoit Sauveur Ihesuscrist & la saincte vie de Nostre Dame, translatee a la requeste de tres hault et puissant prince Iehan, duc de Berry,* ed. Millard Meiss and Elizabeth H. Beatson (New York, 1977). For a general analysis of Gerson's French sermons and this one in particular, see Dorothy C. Brown, *Pastor and Laity in the Theology of Jean Gerson* (Cambridge, 1987), 24–25.

62. Gerson, "Sermon sur la passion," 459.

63. Ibid., 477.

64. Ibid., 454.

65. Bernardino of Siena, *Prediche volgari,* 5:347–48.

66. Gerson, "Sermon sur la passion," 492–93; Pelbart of Themeswar, *Pomerium sermonum quadragesimalium tripartitus*, sermon 68, "In parasceve sermo iii de passionis Christi generalitate et vulnerum multitudine"; Bernardino of Siena, *Prediche volgari*, 5:345–84, "Quaresimale del 1425, della passione di Gesù Cristo"; Richard C. Trexler, "Gendering Jesus Crucified," in *Iconography at the Crossroads*, ed. Brendan Cassidy, Index of Christian Art Occasional Papers 2 (Princeton, NJ, 1993), 107–20.

67. Pelbart of Themeswar, *Pomerium sermonum quadragesimalium tripartus*, sermon 68, "In parasceve sermo iii de passionis Christi generalitate et vulnerum multitudine."

68. Bernardino of Siena, *Prediche volgari*, 5:347–54.

69. There are other counts of wounds as well. Ludolph of Saxony counted 5,490 wounds.

70. Gerson, "Sermon sur la passion," 489.

71. Pseudo-Beda, "De meditatione passionis Christi"; Pseudo-Anselm, "Dialogus"; Pseudo-Bernard, "Meditatio in passionem et resurrectionem Domini," PL 184:741–68.

72. Ubertino da Casale, *Arbor vitae crucifixae Jesu*, ed. Charles T. Davis, Monumenta politica et philosophica rariora, ser. 1, no. 4 (Venice, 1485; repr., Turin, 1962). The book was written in 1305.

73. "Quanto quid tenerius, tanto patitur gravius; nunquam autem fuit corpus ita tenerum ad sustinendum passiones, sicut corpus Salvatoris. Corpus enim mulieris tenerius est quam corpus viri: caro autem Christi tota virginea fuit, quia de Spiritu sancto concepta et de Virgine nata: igitur passio Christi fuit omnium passionum acerbior, quia omnium virginum tenerior." Bonaventura, "Opusculum VI de perfectione vitae ad sorores," 121; English translation from Bonaventura, *The Works of Bonaventure*, vol. 1, *Mystical Opuscula*, trans. José de Vinck (Paterson, NJ, 1960), 242. See also Humbert de Romans, Gilbert of Tournai, and Stephen of Bourbon, *Prediche*, 43–45; Edward T. Brett, *Humbert de Romans: His Life and Views of 13th-Century Society*, Pontifical Institute Studies and Texts 67 (Toronto, 1984); Simon Tugwell, "Humbert de Romans's Material for Preachers," in *De Ore Domini: Preachers and the Word in the Middle Ages*, ed. Thomas L. Amos, Eugene B. Green, and Beverly M. Kienzle (Kalamazoo, MI, 1989), 105–17. The same theme recurs in sermons and meditations as well.

74. Caroline W. Bynum, "Jesus as Mother and Abbot as Mother: Some Themes in Twelfth-Century Cistercian Writing," in *Jesus as Mother: Studies in the Spirituality of the High Middle Ages* (Berkeley, CA, 1984), 110–69.

75. See M. Stallings-Taney's introduction to the critical edition of John of Caulibus, *Meditaciones vite Christi*, xi.

76. Bestul, *Texts of the Passion*, 44–45. For authorship of the *Meditaciones vite Christi*, see Sarah McNamer, "The Origins of the *Meditationes vitae Christi*," *Speculum* 84 (2009): 905–56.

77. For the medieval English version, see Nicholas Love, *The Mirror of the Blessed Life of Jesus Christ*, ed. Michael G. Sargent, Exeter Medieval Texts and Studies (Exeter, 2004). The Italian version was translated into modern English in *Meditations on the Life of Christ*, trans. Isa Ragusa and Rosalie B. Green (Princeton, NJ, 1961).

78. Ludolph of Saxony, *Vita Jesu Christi*. See also Charles Abbot Conway, *The Vita Christi of Ludolph of Saxony and Late Medieval Devotion Centred on the Incarnation: A Descriptive Analysis*, Analecta Cartusiana 34 (Salzburg, 1976).

79. "Plange igitur et dole, et satage, anima mea, et deducant oculi tui lacrymas, et non taceat pupilla oculi tui super fratrem tuum. . . . Dolebis enim, si consideras lacrymas mulierum . . . lacrymas patientis, et lacrymas genitricis." Ludolph of Saxony, *Vita Jesu Christi*, 4:158.

80. Fulton, *From Judgment to Passion*, 142–92.

81. Ibid., 187, 197.

82. Pseudo-Beda, "De meditatione passionis Christi," 563.

83. Pseudo-Anselm, "Dialogus," 282.

84. Pseudo-Beda, "De meditatione passionis Christi," 566; Pseudo-Anselm, "Dialogus," 282.

85. Pseudo-Anselm, "Dialogus," 272–73.

86. The same theme was echoed later by Cavalca, *Lo specchio della croce*, 166.

87. Pseudo-Anselm, "Dialogus," 283; Pseudo-Beda, "De meditatione passionis Christi," 568.

88. "In matutinis castigatus, in mane accusatus, in tertia acclamatus, in sexta condemnatus, in nona cum clamore et lacrymas expirasti." Ludolph of Saxony, *Vita Jesu Christi*, 4:158; John of Caulibus, *Meditaciones vite Christi*, 255–89. See also Rolle, *The Passio Domini Theme*; alternatively, one could begin at compline and end at vespers. See Pseudo-Beda, "De meditatione passionis Christi," 561–68.

89. Goscelin of Saint Bertin, "The *Liber confortatorius* of Goscelin of Saint Bertin," ed. C. H. Talbot, *Studia Anselmiana*, 3rd ser., 37 (1955): 83; English translation from *Writing the Wilton Women: Goscelin's Legend of Edith and "Liber confortatorius,"* trans. W. R. Barnes and Rebecca Hayward, ed. Stephanie Hollis et al. (Turnhout, 2004), 166.

90. Suso, *Deutsche Schriften*, 195–96.

91. Cavalca, *Lo specchio della croce*.

92. Margery Kempe, *The Book of Margery Kempe*, ed. Barry Windeatt (Harlow, Essex, 2000), 202–4.

93. Janel M. Mueller, "Autobiography of a New 'Creatur': Female Spirituality, Self-hood, and Authorship in *The Book of Margery Kempe*," in *Women in the Middle Ages and the Renaissance: Literary and Historical Perspectives*, ed. Mary Beth Rose (Syracuse, NY, 1986), 151.

94. Rolle, *The Passio Domini Theme*, 236–77.

95. Julian of Norwich, *A Book of Showings to the Anchoress Julian of Norwich*, ed. Edmund Colledge and James Walsh, 2 vols. (Toronto, 1978), 1:207–9.

96. Ibid., 210.

97. See Mills, *Suspended Animation*, 177–99.

98. Angela of Foligno, *Il libro della beata Angela da Foligno*, 294–97.

99. "O santa Maria . . . dime di quela pena del tuo Fiolo, de la quale non oldo memoria; inperzioché tu vedesti de quela passione più che nessuno santo; poi ch'io vezo che tu la vedesti con li ochi del capo e con la inmaginazione. . . . È nessuno santo che me sapia dire niente de questa pasione [*sic*] de la qualle non ascolto né parlare né dire parolla, la quale vide l'anima mia et è tanta ch'io non la posso dire? Tanta pasione vide l'anima mia!" Ibid., 293.

100. Ebner, *Margaretha Ebner und Heinrich von Nördlingen*, 1–2; English translation in *Margaret Ebner, Major Works*, 85–86, 118–19, 149–50.

101. Ebner, *Margaretha Ebner und Heinrich von Nördlingen*, 52.

102. Ibid., 51–52: "zwe wochen vor ostern, da ward ich gar krank von der gebunden swige und auch von der rede, die ich emsseklichen het biz an den antlatztag ze metin. do ich die metin an fienk, do kom mir in daz hertz der aller gröst smercz und daz bitterst laid, as ob ich gegenwertiklichen bi minem geminten hertzeklichen liebsten lieb gewesen wer und smerzelichez liden mit minen augen sehe und ze der zit allez vor mir geschehen wer, und wart auch rehtes laides alle min tag nie me innan biz an die zit. ez was auch min smertz und daz bitter laid as gross, daz mich duht, daz kainem menschen uf ertrich ie laider gescheh, ich maht snat Maren Magdalen nit usse genemen." English translation in *Margaret Ebner, Major Works*, 113.

103. Julian of Norwich, *Showings*, 1:234.

104. See above, chap. 4.

105. Kempe, *Book of Margery Kempe*, 162–63.

106. Constable, "Ideal of the Imitation of Christ," 205. The translation of the first part of the quotation is his; PL 184:1167.

107. Bonaventura, "Opusculum VI de perfectione vitae ad sorores," 122; Bonaventura, "Vitis mystica, seu tractatus de passione Domini," in *Doctoris seraphici S. Bonaventurae opera omnia*, edited by Aloysius Lauer (Quaracchi, 1898), 8:169. English translation in Bonaventura, *Mystical Opuscula*, 145–206. For the entire *Vitis mystica*, see Bestul, *Texts of the Passion*, 45–50.

108. Cavalca, *Lo specchio della croce*, 131–37.

109. Angela of Foligno, *Il libro della beata Angela da Foligno*, 421: "Ne la croxe comenzò, ne la croxe almezò, e ne la croxe fenì." Ibid., 481: "ma lo re di re, avegnaché tuta la vita sua fosse crose invizibile per lo dolore inefabile e continuo lo qual portò." Antonio Blasucci, "La theologia del dolore nelle beata Angela da Foligno," *Miscellanea Francescana* 59 (1959): 497.

110. *Margaret Ebner, Major Works*, 133; Ebner, *Margaretha Ebner und Heinrich von Nördlingen*, 87: "siner aller süezzesten besnidunge, daz ich dar uz niezzen sölt sin aller creftigostes minnenwallendez hailigez bluot."

111. Ebner, *Margaretha Ebner und Heinrich von Nördlingen*, 99–101: "min aller liebstez kint, wie maht si die grossen genade ie gehaben order dertragen in menschlichem libe? . . . ez set mir auch, daz ez des nahtez grossen frost lide. . . . kint mins, sie sprechent, du weret as arm, ist ez war? Ez sprach: 'ez ist war.' . . . kint mins, ist daz auch war, daz dich Joseph want in sin hosen? . . . ez sprach: 'er want mich in waz er gehaben moht, er het nit daz mir zem.' ich had auch lang lust und begirde gehebt zuo siner hailigen besnidunge . . . ez sprach: 'Josep [*sic*] huob mich, wan ez min muoter nit getuon maht vor sere, des siu enphant. siu wainet auch bitterlichen, und ich wainet auch und enphieng grossen smerzen und vergosse auch vil bluotes. dar nach nam mich min muoter zuo ir mit grosser minne und geswaiget min kinthet."

112. "Tempestive enim cepit pro nobis pati . . . compatere tu ei et plora cum illo, quia fortiter hodie plorauit. Nam in solemnitatibus istis multum gaudere debemus propter nostram salutem, sed multum compati et dolere propter suas angustias et dolores.

Audistis in nativitate quantam affliccionem et penuriam habuerit. Et inter alia hoc eciam fuit, quod quando mater posuit eum in presepio ad caput eius posuit quendam lapidem interposito forte feno. . . . Audis et hodie quia sanguinem suum fudit. Fuit enim caro ipsius cum cultello lapideo a matre incisa. Nonne ergo compati debet ei? . . . Plorauit ergo puer Iesus hodie propter dolorem quem sensit in carne sua: nam veram carnem et passibilem habuit sicut ceteri homines . . . quod forte sepe puerorum more faciebat ad ostendendam miseriam nature humane quam vere assumperat, et ad occultandum se, ne a demonio cognosceretur." John of Caulibus, *Meditaciones vite Christi*, 30.

113. Ibid., 37–38.

114. "Merito sane dum circumciditur Puer qui natus est nobis, Salvator vocatur; quod videlicet ex hoc jam coeperit operari salutem nostram, immaculatum, illum pro nobis sanguinem fundens." Bernard of Clairvaux, "In circumcisione Domini sermo 1," in *Sancti Bernardi opera*, vol. 4, *Sermones I*, ed. J. Leclerq and H. Rochais (Rome, 1966), 275.

115. Ludolph, *Vita Jesu Christi*, 3:317: "sciendum est, quod si nos omnia quae Christus in mundo passus est, vellemus enarrare, innumerabilia utique essent, praesertim, cum tota vita Christi in terris quaedam passio fuerit. . . . Exordiendo enim a primordio Nativitatis suae, inspice quam pauper natus fuit, qui nec domicilium neque vestes habuit, sed in vili diversorio natus, in praesepi super foeno exiguo ante bruta animalia reclinatus, pannis vilibus involutus fuit; octavo die circumcisus fuit, et jam sanguinem suum pro nobis fundere coepit; deinde persecutionem Herodis fugiens in Aegyptum deportatus, et inde rediens per totam pueritiam et adolescentiam suam parentibus subjectus, et non dubium in magna paupertate educatus fuit. Dehinc, adveniente tempore ostensionis suae, inspice quomodo tempore magni frigoris baptizatus in aquis frigidis mergi voluit, et quomodo, tempore jejunii quadraginta dierum continuato, maceratus fuit, et quantas tunc a diabolo tentationes sustinuit, quantas etiam injurias et contumelias a Judaeis frequenter passus fuit. . . . Inspice etiam cum quanto labore vixerit, quia quotidie erat praedicans in templo, et in synagoga, et de civitate in civitatem, de terra in terram perambulavit, in oratione saepe pernoctavit, infirmos multos curavit, obsessos a daemone liberavit, mortuos suscitavit, multitudinem esurientem pavit; et nihilominus in his omnibus naturae legibus subjectus, fami, siti, et ceteris infirmitatibus hominis, absque tamen peccato, expositus fuit."

116. "Want hi began vroech te doghene doen hi gheboren was: dat was armoede ende coude. Hi wert besneden ende storte sijn bloet: hi wert ghevlocht in vremden landen: hi diende heren Josephe ende sire moeder; hi leet hongher ende dorst, scande ende versmaetheit, onwerdighe woorde ende werke der joden; his vaste, hi waecte ende hi wert becort vanden viant. Hi was onderworpen allen mesnchen. Hi ghinc van lande te lande ende van stede te stede, met groten arbeyte ende met groten ernste, prediken dat evangelium." Jan van Ruusbroec, *Die geestelijke brulocht*, trans. H. Rolfson, ed. J. Alaerts, CCCM 103, Opera omnia 1 (Turnhout, 1988), 182–85. I have used Rolfson's English translation.

117. "Et commenca des son enfance en povrete, en doleur, en pleur, en faim, en soif, en froit, en pelerinage estrange en Egypte, en veilles, en tentations, en reproches des mauvais, en persecutions mortelles." Gerson, "Sermon sur la passion," 449.

118. Heiko Oberman, *The Harvest of Medieval Theology: Gabriel Biel and Late Medieval Nominalism* (Cambridge, 1963), 266–67, cites Biel's *Sermones de festivitatibus Christi* (Hagenau, 1510), no. 24, *in fine*, noting that Biel transposed the entire section to

his commentary on *Sententiae*, bk. 3, dist. 15, q. 1, art. 2. See Biel, *Collectorium*, 4:276–80. Oberman's argument, that Biel's view was part of Biel's argument for concentration on Christ as healer and precursor of Protestantism, rather than as a dying figure, does not hold in view of the tradition Biel was simply copying.

119. The theme of tracing Christ's suffering back to the womb also appears in several Dutch fifteenth-century anonymous Passion tracts; see Marrow, *Passion Iconography*, 210–11.

120. For Crucifixion iconography, see Merback, *The Thief, the Cross, and the Wheel*. For a different interpretation of Crucifixion iconography, see Sara Lipton, "'The Swet Lean of His Head': Writing about Looking at the Crucifix in the High Middle Ages," *Speculum* 80 (2005): 1172–1208.

121. For summaries of such visions, see Kieckhefer, *Unquiet Souls*, 94–95; for the wounds and blood, see Constable, "Ideal of the Imitation of Christ," 209–11.

122. For live reenactments of the Crucifixion, see Jody Enders, *The Medieval Theater of Cruelty: Rhetoric, Memory, Violence* (Ithaca, NY, 1999), 202–12.

CHAPTER EIGHT

1. Evagrius Ponticus, *Traité pratique, ou, Le moine*, ed. Antoine Guillaumont and Claire Guillaumont, 2 vols., Sources chrétiennes 170–71 (Paris, 1971), 1:98–108.

2. Ibid., 2:537–81.

3. David Brakke, "The Lady Appears: Materializations of 'Woman' in Early Monastic Literature," *Journal of Medieval and Early Modern Studies* 33 (2003): 397.

4. Hieronymus, *Epistolae*, 246.

5. Barbara H. Rosenwein, *Emotional Communities in the Early Middle Ages* (Ithaca, NY, 2006), 95–99; Nagy, *Don de larmes*, 135–52.

6. Eusebius, *Historia ecclesiastica*, ed. Eduard Schwartz and Theodor Mommsen, Die griechischen christlichen Schriftsteller der ersten drei Jahrundert 9 (Leipzig, 1908), 2:340–51; English translation from *A New Eusebius: Documents Illustrating the History of the Church to AD 337*, ed. J. Stevenson and W. H. C. Frend (London, 1987), 23.

7. Eusebius, *New Eusebius*, 27.

8. Eusebius, "Acta martyrum Palaestinae," in *Historia ecclesiastica*, trans. Gustave Bardy, Sources chrétiennes 55 (Paris, 1956), 3:162, bk. 11, chap. 17.

9. Eusebius, *Historia ecclesiastica*, 2:996, bk. 10, par. 37.

10. Peter Brown, *Authority and the Sacred: Aspects of the Christianization of the Roman World* (Cambridge, 1995); Peter Brown, *The Cult of the Saints: Its Rise and Function in Latin Christianity* (Chicago, 1981); Salisbury, *Blood of Martyrs*, 9–30.

11. Cavalca, *Lo specchio della croce*, 164–65.

12. Bromyard, *Summa praedicantium*, s.v. "Passio Christi," art. 1.

13. For the different types of martyrs, see Hippolyte Delehaye, *Les passions des martyrs et les genres littéraires*, Subsidia hagiographica 13B (Brussels, 1921), 140–50.

14. For Prudentius, see Anne-Marie Palmer, *Prudentius on the Martyrs* (Oxford, 1989); Michael Roberts, *Poetry and the Cult of the Martyrs: The "Liber Peristephanon" of Prudentius* (Ann Arbor, MI, 1993). Jacobus was not the most extreme in depicting human pain. Jean de Mailly went much farther in making his martyrs passible, but his work had

fewer echoes. See Jean de Mailly, *Abregé des gestes et miracles des saints*, trans. Antoine Dondaine (Paris, 1947), passim; Sherry L. Reames, *The "Legenda aurea": A Reexamination of Its Paradoxical History* (Madison, WI, 1985), 204–5.

15. This is the model that Shaw identified as *andreia*. Brent D. Shaw, "Body/Power/Identity: Passions of the Martyrs," *Journal of Early Christianity* 4 (1996): 269–312. Shaw saw this as the pre-Christian model, while Christianity provided a different model of courage. However, I consider the standards of late antique martyrs as a continuation of *andreia*.

16. "Nam ubi erat illa femina, quando ad asperrimam uaccam se pugnare non sensit, et quando futurum esset quod iam fuerat, inquisiuit? ubi erat? quid uidens, ista non uiderat? quo fruens, ista non senserat? quo amore alienata, quo spectaculo auocata, quo poculo inebriata?" Augustine, "Sermones de sanctis," no. 280, PL 38:1282. See also Brent D. Shaw, "The Passion of Perpetua," *Past and Present* 139 (1993): 3–45.

17. Paul Fouracre, "Merovingian History and Merovingian Hagiography," *Past and Present* 127 (1990): 3–38.

18. *Vita vel passio Haimhrammi episcopi et martyris Ratisbonensis*, 481–501.

19. The seventh tribulation was yet to come. See Alan Friedlander, *The Hammer of the Inquisitors: Brother Bernard Délicieux and the Struggle against the Inquisition in Fourteenth-Century France* (Leiden, 2000), 288–91. Bernard Délicieux himself was subjected to torture once during his trial for conspiracy to poison the pope, but the torture was hedged about with warnings not to cause the suspect any irremediable damage and certainly not to kill him. The notary at the trial, though, says that "et vocem et clamorem eiusdem fratris Bernardi audientibus, ipsum, ut apparebat ex vocibus et clamoribus supradictis, quaestionibus supposuit." Bernard did not confess under torture but later, under questioning, he did. See Alan Friedlander, ed., "Processus Bernardi Delitiosi: The Trial of Fr. Bernard Délicieux, 3 September–8 December 1319," *Transactions of the American Philosophical Society*, n.s., 86, no. 1 (1996): 142–43.

20. Angelo Clareno, *Liber chronicarum*, 606.

21. Ibid., 608: "locum sequestratum et maleficiis aptum." "Et ipse cum suis apparitoribus domum illam ingressus."

22. See above, chap. 2.

23. Angelo Clareno, *Liber chronicarum*, 618.

24. "Ad tantam enim, cum esset vir sapiens et de nobili genera natus, devenerat insaniam, ut agitatus propriis manibus minaretur inferre tormenta." Ibid., 610.

25. Marjorie Reeves, *The Influence of Prophecy in the Later Middle Ages: A Study in Joachimism* (Oxford, 1969; repr., Oxford, 2000), 181–83; Kevin H. Hughes, "Eschatological Union: The Mystical Dimension of History in Joachim of Fiore, Bonaventure, and Peter Olivi," *Collectanea Franciscana* 72 (2002): 105–43.

26. The basic sources for the late antique and early medieval narratives are the following. For St. Agatha, see "Acta S. Agathae," *AASS*, 1 February, 615–18; Ambrosius, "De S. Agathe," PL 17:1210–11; Beda Venerabilis, "Martyrologium," PL 94:834–35; Jacques Dubois and Geneviève Renaud, eds., *Le martyrologe d'Adon: Ses deux familles, ses trois recensions* (Paris, 1984), 27, 80. See also Carla Morini, "La *passio S. Agathae:* La tradizione latina tardo antica e alto-medievale," *Cultura et scuola* 137 (1996): 94–105; Carla Morini, "La *passio S. Agathae:* La tradizione medievale inglese," *Rivista di cultura*

classica e medioevale 42 (2000): 49–60. For St. Agnes, see "Gesta sancte Agnetis," *AASS*, 2 January, 351–54; Ambrosius, "De virginibus ad Marcellinam sororem suam libri tres," PL 16:189–91. The hymn and sermon attributed to [Pseudo-]Ambrose are later (PL 17: 701–5); Prudentius, *Peristefanon*, 294–313; Alexander J. Denomy, *The Old French Lives of Saint Agnes and Other Vernacular Versions of the Middle Ages* (Cambridge, 1938). For St. Lawrence, see "Acta alia ex martyrologio Adonis ad diem X Augusti," *AASS*, 2 August, 518–19. For the *Passio Polychronii*, see Hippolyte Delehaye, ed., "Recherches sur le légendier romain," *Analecta Bollandiana* 51 (1933): 34–98. An earlier version was published by Giovanni Nino Verrando, "Passio SS. Xysti Laurenti et Yppoliti: La trasmissione manoscritta delle varie recensioni della considdetta *Passio vetus*," *Recherches augustiniennes* 25 (1991): 181–221. For patristic literature, see Ambrosius, *De officiis*, ed. Maurice Testard, CCSL 15 (Turnhout, 2000), 23–184; Augustine, "Sermo 303 in natali Laurentii II," PL 38:1394; Prudentius, *Peristefanon*, 257–77; Pseudo–Maximus of Turin, "Homiliae in natali sancti Laurentii Levitae et martyris," PL 57:407–12; Dubois and Renaud, *Martyrologe d'Adon*, 258–64; Nigel of Canterbury, *The Passion of St. Lawrence, Epigrams and Marginal Poems*, ed. and trans. Jan Ziolkowski (Leiden, 1994). For St. Vincent, see "Acta S. Vincentii martyris archidiaconi Caesaragustani . . . passio brevior," *Analecta Bollandiana* 1 (1882): 259–62; Augustine, "Sermo 276 in festo martyris Vincentii III," PL 38:1255–57; Prudentius, *Peristefanon*, 33–40; Salisbury, *Blood of Martyrs*, 173–87.

27. Guy Philippart, *Les légendiers latins et autres manuscrits hagiographiques*, TSMA 24–25 (Turnhout, 1977); Donna C. Trembinski, "Narratives of (Non) Suffering in Dominican Legendaries: Explorations and Explanations" (Ph.D. diss., University of Toronto, 2004), 3–22.

28. Jacobus de Voragine, *Legenda aurea*, xx. Donna C. Trembinski, "[Pro] passio Doloris: Early Dominican Conceptions of Christ's Physical Pain," *Journal of Ecclesiastical History* 59 (2008): 630–56, and "Insensate Saints: Contextualizing Non-Suffering in Early Dominican Legendaries," *Florilegium* 23 (2007): 123–42.

29. Barbara Fleith, "Le classement des quelque 1000 manuscrits de la *Legenda aurea* latine . . . ," in *Legenda aurea: Sept siècles de diffusion*, ed. Brenda Dunn-Lardeau (Montreal, 1986), 19–24; Laura Gaffuri, "Du texte au texte: Réflexions sur la première diffusion de la *Legenda aurea*," in *De la sainteté à l'hagiographie: Genèse et usage de la "Légende dorée*," ed. Barbara Fleith and Franco Morenzoni, Publications romanes et françaises 229 (Geneva, 2001), 139–46. As a source for saints' lives, the *Legenda aurea* has come under a great deal of criticism. See Reames, *The "Legenda aurea*," 197–212. Even Reames admits that the *Legenda* was the most popular legendary of the later Middle Ages.

30. Jacobus de Voragine, *Golden Legend* (London, 1487).

31. Alain Boureau, *La légende dorée: Le système narratif de Jacques de Voragine (d. 1298)* (Paris, 1984).

32. "Si consideremus perturbationem torquentis et tranquillitatem tormenta patientis, videre facillimum est quis erat sub poenis, and quis supra poenas." "Tanta in Vincentio penarum asperitas seviebat in membris et tanta securitas resonabat in verbis ut putaremus alium loqui et alium torqueri. Et vere sic erat. Caro enim patiebatur et spiritus loquebatur." Augustine, "Sermo 276 in festo martyris Vincentii III," 1255–56.

33. The need for interpretation is not a purely late medieval phenomenon. It belongs far more to the genre of sermons throughout the ages. Thus, Augustine of Hippo and

Maximus of Turin both tried to understand the martyrs they were discussing in their sermons.

34. Miri Rubin, "Choosing Death? Experiences of Martyrdom in Late Medieval Europe," in *Martyrs and Martyrologies*, Studies in Church History 30 (Oxford, 1993), 153–83; Esther Cohen, "Who Desecrated the Host?" in *De Sion exibit lex et verbum domini de Hierusalem: Essays on Medieval Law, Liturgy, and Literature in Honor of Amnon Linder*, ed. Yitzhak Hen (Turnhout, 2001), 197–210.

35. Boureau, *La légende dorée*, 38.

36. Augustine, letter 38, in *Sancti Aurelii Augustini epistulae*, 156–57.

37. Augustine, "Soliloquiorum libri duo," PL 32:880–81; Augustine, *Confessionum*, 140, bk. 9, chap. 4(12).

38. "Interim autem, ut refert in libro soliloquiorum, tam uehementissimo dolore dentium torqueri cepit ut fere, sicut ipse ait, ad credendam opinionem Cornelii philosophi duceretur, qui summum bonum sapientiam, summum uero malum dolorem corporis posuerat. Tam uehemens autem ille dolor fuit quod etiam loquelam amisit. Quocirca, ut in libro confessionum refert, in tabulis cereis scripsit ut omnes pro eo orarent ut dolorem illum dominus mitigaret.Ipse igitur genua cum aliis flexit et subito sanum se sensit." Jacobus de Voragine, *Legenda aurea*, 846–47, 857. For Augustine's story of the miraculously aborted hemorrhoid operation (not his own), see Augustine, *De ciuitate Dei*, 2: 816–18.

39. Leonardo de Utino, *Sermones aurei*, fol. 269v.

40. "Notandum est quod passio sancti Laurentii inter ceteras sanctorum martyrum passiones excellentima uidetur esse." "Neque enim beatus Laurentius ignium tormenta uisceribus sentire poterat, qui sensibus paradisi refrigerium possidebat." Jacobus de Voragine, *Legenda aurea*, 765, 771.

41. Karen A. Winstead, ed. and trans., *Chaste Passions: Medieval English Virgin Martyr Legends* (Ithaca, NY, 2000), 27–31, translates the fairly tame Middle English epithet *bouke* as "asshole." See also Beth Crachiolo, "Seeing the Gendering of Violence: Female and Male Martyrs in the *South English Legendary*," in *"A Great Effusion of Blood"? Interpreting Medieval Violence*, ed. Mark D. Meyerson, Daniel Thiery, and Oren Falk (Toronto, 2004), 147–63. For the original, see *The South English Legendary*, ed. Charlotte D'Evelyn and Anna J. Mill, 3 vols., Early English Text Society (London, 1956–59), 1:54, 58.

42. Anne B. Thompson, "The Legend of St. Agnes: Improvisation and the Practice of Hagiography," *Exemplaria* 13 (2001): 355–97. For vernacular versions of Agnes's life, see Denomy, *Old French Lives of Saint Agnes*, 3–11; Robert Taylor, "Sermon anonyme sur sainte Agnès, texte du XIIIe siècle," *Travaux de linguistique et de littérature* 7 (1969): 241–53.

43. "Acta S. Agathae," 615–16.

44. "O felicem me, quo mihi irasci te gravius putas, modo melius incipis misereri. Insurge ergo, miser, et toto malignitatis spiritu debacchare: Videbis me dei virtute plus posse, dum torquor, quam possis ipse, qui torques. Ad hoc praeses coepit clamare et carnifices virgis et fustibus verberare. Et ait Vincentius: 'Quid dicis, Dacianuse! Ecce, tu ipse me vindicas de apparitoribus meis.'" Jacobus de Voragine, *Legenda aurea*, 175.

45. "Ego in hiis penis ita delector sicut qui bonum nuntium audit aut qui videt quem diu desiderauit aut qui multos thesauros invenit. Non enim potest triticum in horreum

poni nisi theca eius fuerit fortiter conculcata et in paleas redacta. Sic anima mea non potest intrare in paradisum cum palma martyrii nisi diligenter feceris corpus meum a carnificibus attrectari." Ibid., 258.

46. Cohen, *Crossroads of Justice.*

47. Jean de Mailly, *Abregé des gestes et miracles des saints,* 119.

48. "Istud certamen superavit per refrigerantes dei gratiam que sibi refrigerium prestitit." Leonardo de Utino, *Sermones aurei,* fol. 76v. None of the earlier vernacular versions cited by Denomy or Taylor (see above, n. 42) mention more than one fire.

49. Jacobus de Voragine, *Legenda aurea,* 754, 770-72; Jacobus de Voragine, *Registrum in sermones de sanctis,* sermon 205; Pseudo-Maximus, "Homiliae in natali sancti Laurentii"; Maximus of Turin, *Maximi episcopi Taurinensis sermones,* ed. Almut Mutzenbecher, CCSL 23 (Turnhout, 1962), 13–15; Prudentius, *Peristefanon,* 257–77. For later medieval versions, see Pelbart of Themeswar, *Pomerium sermonum de sanctis,* pars aestivalis, sermon 46.

50. "Soror nostra parva et ubera non habet." Song of Songs 8:8.

51. Ambrosius, "De virginibus ad Marcellinam sororem suam libri tres," 190.

52. For a summary of feminist analysis of the different tortures of men and women in martyrologies, see Gail Ashton, *The Generation of Identity in Late Medieval Hagiography: Speaking the Saint* (London, 2000), 145–57. Ashton interprets the cutting of breasts as an alternative penetration.

53. Pelbart of Themeswar, *Pomerium sermonum de sanctis,* pars aestivalis, sermons 67–68.

54. Taylor, "Sermon anonyme sur sainte Agnès," 246–53. See also Leonardo de Utino, *Sermones aurei,* fol. 76v.

55. The erotic imagery of the wound in Christ's breast surfaces in women's mystical writings of the time. See esp. Elizabeth Alvilda Petroff, *Body and Soul: Essays on Medieval Women and Mysticism* (New York, 1994), 51–65; Mary A. Suydam, "Writing Beguines: Ecstatic Performances," *Magistra* 2 (1996): 137–69.

56. Joan Mueller, "Clare of Assisi and the Agnes Legend: A Franciscan Citing of St. Agnes of Rome as *Mulier Sancta,*" *Studies in Spirituality* 8 (1998): 145.

57. Ambrosius, *De officiis,* 85–86: "Hic Laurentium sanctum ad hoc nullus urgebat, nisi amor devotionis; tamen et ipse post triduum, cum illuso tyranno, impositus super craticulam exureretur *Assum est,* inquit, *versa et manduca.* Ita animi virtute vincebat ignis naturam." Augustine, "Sermo 303 in natali Laurentii II," 1394: "*Jam,* inquit, *coctum est; quod superest, versate me, et manducate.*" Prudentius, *Peristefanon,* 271, ll. 406-8: "coctum est, deuora et experimentum cape, sit crudum an assum suauius!"

58. "Gaudeo plane quia ostia Christi effici merui." Verrando, "Passio SS. Xysti Laurentii et Yppoliti," 208, 216.

59. "Ego me obtuli sacrificium deo in odorem suavitatis, quia sacrificium deo est spiritus contribulatus." Delehaye, "Recherches sur le légendier romain," 92; Dubois and Renaud, *Martyrologe d'Adon,* 263.

60. "Moyses, Leviti[cus], vi: ix, dicit hec est lex holocausti, cremabitur in altari nocte usque mane ignis ex eodem altari erit. Decius cesar dixit beato Laurentio, aut sacrifica dijs aut nox ista in te cum suppliciis expendetur. Et beatus Laurentius ait, gaudeo plane quod hostia Christi effici merui, ego me obtuli sacrificium deo in odorem suavitatis. Et

ibidem dicitur, Omnem sacrificium quod coquitur in clibano et quiquid in craticula vel in sartagine preparatur, eius erit sacerdotis, a quo offertur [7:9]. Et de beato Laurentio dicitur, meruit esse hostia Christi levita Laurentius, qui dum in craticula positus assertur non negavit dominum, et ideo inventus est sacrificium laudabilis." Leonardo de Utino, *Sermones aurei*, fol. 278r. See also Olivier Maillard, *Summarium quoddam sermonum de sanctis per totum anni circulum, simul et de communi sanctorum et pro defunctis* (Paris, 1507): "Felices illi sunt qui de proprio corpore deo possunt offerre olocausta atque sacrificia."

61. "Infelix, has epulas ego semper optaui." It is Decius's answer that makes it clear that Lawrence is the food: "Si epule iste sunt, tibi similes pande profanos ut tecum pariter epulentur." Jacobus de Voragine, *Registrum in sermones de tempore*, sermon 204; Jacobus de Voragine, *Legenda aurea*, 759; Pelbart of Themeswar, *Pomerium sermonum de sanctis*, pars aestivalis, sermon 46.

62. Jacobus de Voragine, *Legenda aurea*, 769; Jacobus de Voragine, *Registrum in sermones de sanctis*, sermon 206: "in qua longa morte quod *bene manducaverat* et *bene biberat* tamquam illa esca *saginatus* et illo calice *ebrius* tormenta non sensit" (my italics). Jacobus is quoting Augustine, *In Iohannis euangelium tractatus*, 270, tract. 27.

63. See Pio Franchi de' Cavalieri, "Assum est, versa et manduca," *Note agiografiche (Studi e testi 27)* 5 (1915): 66–70. In several versions, Lawrence was also quoted as saying, "Being roasted, I thank [God]." Jacobus de Voragine, *Legenda aurea*, 760; Norman Cohn, *Warrant for Genocide: The Myth of the Jewish World-Conspiracy and the "Protocols of the Elders of Zion"* (London, 1967).

64. Jacobus de Voragine, *Registrum in sermones de sanctis*, sermon 204.

65. Jacobus de Voragine, *Legenda aurea*, 764–65; Johannes Herolt, *Sermones discipuli*, sermon 31.

66. Jacobus de Voragine, *Registrum in sermones de sanctis*, sermon 69.

67. Ibid., sermon 70. See also Leonardo de Utino, *Sermones aurei*, fol. 79r.

68. Delehaye, "Recherches sur le légendier romain," 91–92; Jacobus de Voragine, *Legenda aurea*, 759.

69. "Et notandum quod beatus Laurentius post beatum Stephanum inter ceteros martyres primatum tenere dicitur." Jacobus de Voragine, *Legenda aurea*, 766; Verrando, "Passio SS. Xysti Laurentii et Yppoliti," 209.

70. Jacobus de Voragine, *Registrum in sermones de sanctis*, sermons 65–68.

71. "Primum certamen fuit in Eculeo in quo fecit eum dacianus toto corpore distendi distentum diversis vulneribus cruciari, cruciatum ferreis pectinibus laniari et carnifices ad seviendum crudelius verberibus fecit urgeri. Secundum certamen habuit in craticulae incendio ubi totum corpus ungulis ferreis aperitur ardentes lamine infiguntur, sale ignis aspergitur, telis viscera extraiaciuntur. Tercium certamen habuit in carceris ergastulo. Nam tirannus fecit ipsum in obscuro carcere includi. Ibi testas acutissimas congeri. In ligno pedes affigi et sine omni humano solatio derelinqui. Quartus certamen habuit in molli lectulo. Postquam enim tirannus vidit se eum per asperitates tormentorum vincere non posse, in lecto mollissimo eum reclinare fecit, putans per delicias ipsam allicere posse. Vicit autem ista certamina maxima mentis constantia." Leonardo de Utino, *Sermones aurei*, fol. 79r.

72. "Quodsi illi fidei calore et beati martyrii gloria timere nesciunt quae timentur, Christus etiamsi uitiorum nostrorum origine esset conceptus, tamen per crucem mansurus Deus et mundum iudicaturus et rex aeternorum saeculorum futurus, tristis metu crucis esset?" Hilary of Poitiers, *De trinitate*, 499.

73. Augustine, *In Iohannis euangelium tractatus*, 537, tract. 84: "martyr Christi longe impar est Christo."

74. Henry of Ghent, *Quodlibet IX*, 270–79, q. 16.

75. See above, chap. 6.

76. William of Auxerre, *Summa aurea*, ed. Jean Ribailler, 5 vols., Spicilegium Bonaventurianum 16–20 (Paris, 1986), 3:560–72; *ST*, pts. 2a–2ae, q. 124.

77. Bernard of Clairvaux, letter 98, in *Sancti Bernardi opera*, vol. 7, *Epistolae I*, ed. J. Leclercq and C. H. Talbot (Rome, 1974), 249–53.

78. William of Auxerre, *Summa aurea*, 3:570.

79. Ibid., 560–64. Ibid., 564: "in instanti, in quo patitur, patitur voluntarie; sed ante fuit invita, et ita voluntate paciendi meretur, et non passione."

80. Ibid., 564: "dicimus igitur cum Prepositino quod paciencia duos habet usu, scilicet sufferre sufferenda et respuere respuenda."

81. *ST*, pts. 2a–2ae, q. 124, art. 4.

82. "Sic ergo dicendum est quod hoc opus quod est offerre se martirio vel etiam martirium sufferre, potest facere non solum caritas perfecta, set etiam imperfecta, et, quod plus est, etiam ille qui caret caritate. . . . Set caritas perfecta hoc facit prompte et delectabiliter, sicut patet de Laurentio et Vincentio, qui in tormentis hylaritatem ostenderunt." Thomas Aquinas, *Questiones de quolibet*, 2:340–41.

83. See, e.g., Nigel of Canterbury, *Passion of St. Lawrence*, 74, ll. 17–18.

84. Thomas Aquinas, *Scriptum super sententiis magistri Petri Lombardi*, bk. 1, dist. 48, q. 1 pr.

85. *ST*, bk. 4, dist. 44, q. 2, art. 1 qc2co.

86. "Quidam dixerunt quod in innocentibus acceleratus est miraculose usus liberi aritrii, ita quod etiam voluntarie martyrium passi sunt. Sed quia hoc per auctoritatem Scripturae non comprobatur, ideo melius dicendum est quod martyrii gloriam, quam in aliis propria voluntas meretur, illi parvuli occisi per Dei gratiam sunt assecuti." *ST*, pts. 2a–2ae, q. 124, art. 1 ad 1.

87. *ST*, pt. 3a, q. 21, art. 4 ad 1.

88. Significantly, Jacobus included Peter Martyr in the *Legenda aurea* (421–42).

89. Duns Scotus, *Quaestiones*, 591.

90. Edward was mentioned as a saint already by 1001. See D. W. Rollason, "The Cult of Murdered Royal Saints in Anglo-Saxon England," *Anglo-Saxon England* 11 (1983):1–22.

91. Concerning the duty of a master to answer questions that might put him in jeopardy, see Wei, "Self-Image of the Masters of Theology," 421–30. The disputation in which this question arose took place in 1285/86, probably at Cambridge, where Marston had moved in 1284. Glorieux, *Littérature quodlibétique*, 2:264, 375.

92. Marston, *Quodlibeta quaestiones*, 439–40.

93. Durand de St. Pourçain, *Sententias theologicas commentariorum*, fol. 240v: "Utrum dolor matris in Christi passione superaverit omnes dolores martyrum." Marston, *Quodlibeta quaestiones*, 396–98; Matthew of Acquasparta, *Quaestiones disputatae*, 268.

94. *Registre criminel du Châtelet*, 1:502–8.

95. Ibid., 2:137–47.

96. See above, chap. 2, n. 96.

97. See above, chap. 2, n. 112.

98. Dyan Elliott, "Seeing Double: John Gerson, the Discernment of Spirits, and Joan of Arc," *American Historical Review* 107 (2002): 26–54; Françoise Bonney, "Autour de Jean Gerson: Opinions de théologiens sur les superstitions et la sorcellerie au début du XVᵉ siècle," *Le Moyen Âge* 71 (1971): 85–93.

99. Jean Gerson, "De distinctione verarum visionum a falsis," in *Oeuvres complètes*, ed. Palémon Glorieux (Paris, Tournai, and Rome, 1968), 3:36, 38; Jean Gerson, "On Distinguishing True from False Revelations," in *Jean Gerson: Early Works*, trans. Brian Patrick McGuire (New York, 1998), 335, 337.

100. Fiorelli, *Tortura giudiziaria nel diritto comune*, 1:295–96.

101. Ibid., 215–16; Brunus, *Tractatus de indicijs et tortura*, fol. 231v.

102. Fiorelli, *Tortura giudiziaria nel diritto comune*, 1:216.

103. Jodocus Damhouder, *Praxis rerum criminalium* (Antwerp, 1562), 38:19; Grillandus, "De questionibus & tortura tractatus," 672–74.

104. Fiorelli, *Tortura giudiziaria nel diritto comune*, 1:218–23; Grillandus, "De questionibus & tortura tractatus," 672–74.

105. Grillandus, *Tractatus de hereticis*.

106. Grillandus, "De questionibus & tortura tractatus," 672.

107. Ibid.

108. Ibid., 673.

109. Kramer, *Malleus maleficarum*, 1:623–24.

110. Fiorelli, *Tortura giudiziaria nel diritto comune*, 1:216.

BIBLIOGRAPHY

MANUSCRIPTS

London, British Library
    MS Harley 268. Arnold of Liège. "Alphabetum narrationum."
    MS Arundel 107. Humbert de Romans or Stephen of Bourbon. "De dono timoris/
        Tractatus de habundantia exemplorum."
London, Wellcome Library
    MS 617. Petrus Hispanus. "Libro della flebotomia."
Paris, Bibliothèque de l'Arsenal
    MS 1024. "Traités de medecine."
    MS 3174. Jehan Sauvage de Picquigny. "La nouvelle physique attraite de plusieurs
        autheurs par . . . secrets de medecine pour traiter maladies du corps humain."
Paris, Bibliothèque nationale de France
    Nouvelles acquisitions latines 152. "Recettes de medecine (XVᵉ siècle)."
    Nouvelles acquisitions latines 733. "Anonymi practica medicinae."
Rome, Biblioteca apostolica Vaticana
    MS Vat. Lat. 2471. "Consilia magistri Bartolomei Montagnane."
    MS Pal. Lat. 1175. Arnaldus de Villanova. "Speculum medicinale."

PRINTED SOURCES

Accursius. *Accursii glossa in "Digestum novum."* Corpus glossatorum iuris civilis 9.
    Turin, 1487. Reprint, Venice, 1968.
"Acta alia ex martyrologio Adonis ad diem X Augusti." *AASS,* 2 August, 518–19.
"Acta S. Agathae." *AASS,* 1 February, 615–18.
"Acta S. Margaritae." *AASS,* 5 July, 33–39.
"Acta S. Vincentii martyris archidiaconi Caesaragustani . . . passio brevior." *Analecta
    Bollandiana* 1 (1882): 259–62.
Adam of Bremen. *Gesta Hammaburgensis ecclesiae pontificum.* Edited by Bernhard
    Schmeider. MGH, SSRG in usum scholarum 2. Hannover, 1917.

Aegidius Romanus. *In tertium librum sententiarum eruditissima commentaria cum questionibus.* Rome, 1623.

———. *Quodlibeta castigatissima.* Venice, 1504.

Aelred of Rievaulx. "Dialogus de anima." In *Opera omnia,* edited by A. Hoste and C. H. Talbot, 1:684–754. CCCM 1. Turnhout, 1971.

Alain de Lille. "Compendiosa in Cantica canticorum ad laudem deiparae virginis Mariae elucidatio." PL 210:53–64.

Albertus Gandinus. *Tractatus de maleficiis.* Vol. 2 of *Albertus Gandinus und das Strafrecht der Scholastik.* Edited by Hermann Kantorowicz. Berlin and Leipzig, 1926.

Alcuin. "Epistolae." PL 100:139–512.

Alexander of Hales. *Glossa in quatuor libri sententiarum Petri Lombardi.* BFSMA 14. Quaracchi, 1954.

———. *Quaestiones disputatae antequam esset frater.* BFSMA 19. Quaracchi, 1960.

———. *Summa theologica.* 5 vols. Quaracchi, 1928.

Alonso de Chirino. *El menor daño de la medicina.* Edited by María Teresa Herrera. Salamanca, 1973.

Ambrosius [Ambrose]. *De officiis.* Edited by Maurice Testard. CCSL 15. Turnhout, 2000.

———. "De officiis ministrorum." PL 16:23–184.

———. "De S. Agathe." PL 17:1210–11.

———. "De virginibus ad Marcellinam sororem suam libri tres." PL 16:189–91.

———. "Expositio in psalmum David CXVIII." PL 15:1197–1526.

Angela of Foligno. *Il libro della beata Angela da Foligno.* Edited by Ludger Thier and Abele Calufetti. Grottaferrata, 1985.

Angelo Clareno. "De historia septem tribulationum ordinis minorum." *Archiv für Literatur- und Kirchengeschichte des Mittelalters* 2 (1886): 106–64, 249–336.

———. *Liber chronicarum, sive tribulationum ordinis minorum.* Translated by Marino Bigaroni. Edited by Giovanni Boccali. Pubblicazioni della Biblioteca francescana, chiesa nuova 8. Assisi, 1998.

Anselm of Canterbury. *Cur Deus homo: Prima forma inedita.* Edited by Eugenius Druwé. Rome, 1933.

———. *The Letters of Saint Anselm of Canterbury.* Edited and translated by Walter Frölich. 3 vols. Kalamazoo, MI, 1990, 1993–94.

Anselm of Laon. "Sentences du liber Pancrisis." In *Psychologie et morale aux XIIe et XIIIe siècles,* vol. 5, *L'école d'Anselme de Laon et de Guillaume de Champeaux,* by Odon Lottin. Gembloux, 1959.

Arderne, John. *De arte phisicali et de cirurgia (1412).* Translated by D'Arcy Power. Research Studies in Medical History of the Wellcome Historical Medical Museum 1. London, 1922.

———. *Treatises of Fistula in Ano, Haemorrhoids and Clysters, from an Early Fifteenth-Century Manuscript Translation.* Translated by D'Arcy Power. Early English Text Society. London, 1910.

Aristotle. *De anima.* Translated by J. A. Smith. Works of Aristotle. Oxford, 1931.

———. *De sensu et sensibili.* Translated by J. I. Beare. Works of Aristotle. Oxford, 1931.

Arnau de Villanova. *Arnaldi Villanovani philosophi et medici summi opera omnia.* Basel, 1585.

———. *Commentum super tractatum Galieni de malicia complexionis diverse*. Edited by Luis García-Ballester and Eustaquio Sánchez Salor. Arnaldi de Villanova opera medica omnia 15. Barcelona, 1985.

———. *Doctrina Galieni de interioribus secundum stilum Latinorum*. Edited by Richard J. Durling. Arnaldi de Villanova opera medica omnia 15. Barcelona, 1985.

———. *Regimen sanitatis ad regem Aragonum*. Edited by Luis García-Ballester, Michael R. McVaugh, and Pedro Gil-Sotres. Arnaldi de Villanova opera medica omnia 10/1. Barcelona, 1996.

———. *Tractatus de consideracionibus operis medicine sive de flebotomia*. Edited by Luke Demaitre and Pedro Gil-Sotres. Arnaldi de Villanova opera medica omnia 4. Barcelona, 1988.

Arnold of Liège. *An Alphabet of Tales: An English 15th-Century Translation of the "Alphabetum narrationum."* Edited by Mary M. Banks. Early English Text Society. London, 1904–5.

Augustine. *Confessionum libri tredecim*. Edited by Lucas Verheijen. CCSL 27. Turnhout, 1981.

———. "Contra Iulianum." PL 45:1049–1600.

———. *De ciuitate Dei*. Edited by Bernard Dombart and Alphonse Kalb. 2 vols. CCSL 47–48. Turnhout, 1955.

———. *De genesi ad litteram libri duodecim*. Edited by Joseph Zycha. CSEL 28/1. Vienna, 1894.

———. *De libero arbitrio*. Edited by W. M. Green. CCSL 29. Turnhout, 1970.

———. "De natura boni contra Manichaeos." PL 42:551–71.

———. *Enarrationes in Psalmos*. Edited by Eligius Dekkers and Johannes Fraipont. CCSL 40. Turnhout, 1956.

———. *Epistulae*. Edited by A. Goldbacher. CSEL 44. Vienna, 1904.

———. *In Iohannis euangelium tractatus*. Edited by Radbod Willems. CCSL 36. Turnhout, 1954.

———. *Sancti Aurelii Augustini epistulae*. Edited by K. D. Daur. CCSL 31. Turnhout, 2004.

———. "Sermones de sanctis." PL 38:1247–1484.

———. "Soliloquiorum libri duo." PL 32:869–904.

Avicenna. *Liber canonis Avicenne revisus et ab omni errore mendaque purgatus summaque cum diligentia impressus*. Venice, 1507. Reprint, Hildesheim, 1964. English translation: *The Canon of Medicine (al-Qanun fi'l-tibb)*. Translated by O. Cameron Gruner et al. Edited by Seyyed Hossein Nasr. Great Books of the Islamic World. Chicago, 1999.

Bacon, Roger. "De erroribus medicorum." In *Essays on the History of Medicine Presented to Karl Sudhoff*, translated by E. T. Wittington, edited by Charles Singer and Henry E. Sigerist, 139–57. Oxford, 1924.

Baldus de Periglis. *De questionibus et tormentis*. Paris, 1486.

Baldus de Ubaldis. *Consiliorum sive responsorum. . . .* Venice, 1580.

———. "Tractatus de carceribus." In *Decimum volumen tractatuum e variis iuris interpretibus collectorum*. Lyons, 1599.

Barberino, Francesco. *Del reggimento e costumi di donna*. Edited by Carlo Baudi di Vesme. Collezione di opere inedite o rare dei primi tre secoli della lingua. Bologna, 1875.

Bartolomaeus Caepolla. *Consilia criminalia.* Brescia, 1490.

Bartolomeo Montagnana. *Consilia magistri Bartolomei Montagnane.* Venice, 1525.

Bartolus of Sassoferrato. *Repetitio super materia quaestionum sive torturarum.* Vol. 10 of *Omnia quae extant opera.* . . . Venice, 1615.

Barzizza, Cristoforo. *Introductorium practicae medicinae.* Pavia, 1494.

Beaune, Colette, ed. *Journal d'un bourgeois de Paris.* Paris, 1990.

Beda Venerabilis. "Martyrologium." PL 94:834–35.

Benedict VIII [dubious]. "Bulla Benedicti papae VIII qua Henrico sanitatem a S. Benedicto restitutam esse testatur, monasterioque Casinensi asserit dona ab imperatore delata." PL 139:1636–38.

Benedict of Peterborough. *Miracula sancti Thomae Cantuariensis.* Vol. 2 of *Materials for the History of Thomas Becket, Archbishop of Canterbury,* edited by James C. Robertson. Rolls Series 67. Reprint, London, 1965.

Benzi, Ugo. *Consilia medica.* Venice, 1523.

Bernard de Gordon. *Lilio de medicina.* Edited by Brian Dutton and María Nieves Sánchez. 2 vols. Madrid, 1993. Latin version: *Lilium medicinae: Tractatus nimirum septem foliis sive particulis, accuratissimum omnium morborum, tam uniuersalium, quam particularium, curationem complectens.* Edited by Peter Uffenbach. Frankfurt, 1617.

Bernard of Clairvaux. "In circumcisione Domini sermo 1." In *Sancti Bernardi opera,* vol. 4, *Sermones I,* edited by J. Leclerq and H. Rochais, 273–76. Rome, 1966.

———. Letter 98. In *Sancti Bernardi opera,* vol. 7, *Epistolae I,* edited by J. Leclercq and C. H. Talbot, 249–53. Rome, 1974.

———. "Sermo 42 de diversis." In *Sancti Bernardi opera,* vol. 6/1, *Sermones III,* edited by Jean Leclercq and H. M. Rochais, 253–61. Rome, 1970.

———. "Sermon 10." In *Sancti Bernardi opera,* vol. 1, *Sermones super Cantica canticorum, 1–35,* edited by Jean Leclercq, C. H. Talbot, and H. M. Rochais, 50. Rome, 1957.

Bernardino of Siena. *Prediche volgari (1425).* Edited by Ciro Cannarozzi. 5 vols. Florence, 1958.

Biblia Latina cum glossa ordinaria. Strassburg, 1480/81. Reprint, Turnhout, 1992.

Biel, Gabriel. *Collectorium circa quattuor libros sententiarum.* Edited by Wilfrid Werbeck and Udo Hofman. 6 vols. Tübingen, 1979.

———. *Sermones de festivitatibus Christi.* Hagenau, 1510.

Boccaccio, Giovanni. *Decameron.* Edited by Vittore Branca. Florence, 1999.

Boec van medicinen in Dietsche: Een Middelnederlandse compilatie van medisch-farmaceutische literatuur. Edited by W. F. Daems. Janus, suppléments 7. Leiden, 1967.

Bonaventura. *Commentaria in quatuor libros sententiarum magistri Petri Lombardi.* Quaracchi, 1887.

———. "Opusculum VI de perfectione vitae ad sorores." In *Doctoris seraphici S. Bonaventurae opera omnia,* edited by Aloysius Lauer, 8:107–27. Quaracchi, 1898. English translation in *The Works of Bonaventure,* vol. 1, *Mystical Opuscula,* translated by José de Vinck, 209–47. Paterson, NJ, 1960.

———. "Vitis mystica, seu tractatus de passione Domini." In *Doctoris seraphici S. Bonaventurae opera omnia,* edited by Aloysius Lauer, 159–229. Quaracchi, 1898. English translation in *The Works of Bonaventure*, vol. 1, *Mystical Opuscula*, translated by José de Vinck, 145–206. Paterson, NJ, 1960.

Bonetti, Baverio Maghinardo de. *Praestantissimi medici et philosophi clarissimi D. Ioannis Bauerij de Imola consiliorum de re medica sive morborum curationibus liber*. Strasbourg, 1542.

Bonifacius de Vitalinis. "Tractatus maleficij cum additionibus & apostillis D. Hieronymi Chuchalon Hispani." In *Tractatus diversi super maleficiis, nempe Do. Alberti de Gandino, Do. Bonifacii de Vitalini, Do. Pauli Grillandi, Do. Baldi de Periglis, Do. Jacobi de Arena*, 306–608. Lyons, 1555.

Bonvesin da Riva. "De quinquaginta curialitatibus ad mensam." In *Poeti del duecento*, edited by Gianfranco Contini, 1:703–12. Milan, 1960.

"Book of Courtesy": A Fifteenth Century Courtesy Book. Edited by R. W. Chambers. Early English Text Society. London, 1937.

A Book of Showings to the Anchoress Julian of Norwich. Edited by Edmund Colledge and James Walsh. Toronto, 1978.

Bromyard, John. *Summa praedicantium*. Basel, 1480.

Brunus, Franciscus. *Tractatus de indicijs et tortura*. Siena, n.d., 1480s.

Caesarius of Heisterbach. *Dialogus miraculorum*. Edited by Joseph Strange. 2 vols. Cologne, 1851.

Caracciolo, Roberto. *Prediche de frate Roberto vulgare*. Milan, 1515.

Cavalca, Domenico. *Lo specchio della croce: Testo originale e versione in italiano corrente*. Edited by Tito Sante Centi. Bologna, 1992.

Chatton, Walter. *Reportatio super sententias, libri III–IV*. Edited by Joseph C. Wey and Girard J. Etzkorn. Studies and Texts 149. Toronto, 2005.

Christine de Pizan. *Le livre des faits et bonnes moeurs du roi Charles V le Sage*. Translated by Eric Hicks and Thérèse Moreau. Edited by Danielle Regnier-Bohler. Paris, 1997.

Chroniques du religieux de Saint-Denys. Edited by M. L. Bellaguet. 3 vols. Paris, 1842. Reprint, Paris, 1994.

Cockayne, Oswald. *Leechdoms, Wortcunning, and Starcraft of Early England, Being a Collection of Documents . . . Illustrating the History of Science in This Country before the Norman Conquest*. 3 vols. Rolls Series 35. London, 1864. Reprint, Nendeln, 1965.

Constantine the African. "De morborum cognitione et curatione." In *Opera*, 1–167. Basel, 1539.

Corpus iuris civilis. Edited by Paul Krueger, Theodore Mommsen, and Rudolph Scholl. Translated by Alan Watson. 3 vols. Berlin, 1884–95. Reprint, Philadelphia, 1985.

Corpus juris canonici emendatum et notis illustratum. Gregorii XIII. pont. max. iussu editum. 4 vols. Rome, 1582.

Corradini Bozzi, Maria Sofia, ed. *Ricettari medico-farmaceutici medievali nella Francia meridionale*. Studi della Accademia toscana di scienze e lettere 159. Florence, 1997.

Damhouder, Jodocus. *Praxis rerum criminalium*. Antwerp, 1562.

Dante Alighieri. *The Divine Comedy*. Translated and edited by Robert M. Durling. New York, 1996.

Decretales dni. Papae Gregorii IX suae integritati una cum glossis restitutae. In *Corpus juris canonici emendatum et notis illustratum.* Gregorii XIII. pont. max. iussu editum, pt. 3. Rome, 1582.

"De sancto Vincentio Martyre." *AASS,* 2 January, 393–97.

Despars, Jacques. "Summula Jacobi de Partibus per ordinem alphabeti singulorum remediorum singulis morbis conferentium." In *Supplementum in secundum librum compendii secretorum medicinae Ioannis Mesues medici celeberrimi,* by Francesco de Piedmont. Venice, 1531.

Dionysius Carthusianus. *In quatuor libros sententiarum.* Vol. 23 of *Doctoris ecstatici d. Dionysii Cartusiani opera omnia.* Tournai, 1904.

Duns Scotus, John. *Quaestiones in tertium librum sententiarum.* Vol. 14 of *Opera omnia.* Paris, 1894.

Durand de St. Pourçain. *Petri Lombardi sententias theologicas commentariorum libri IIII.* Venice, 1571.

Ebner, Margaretha. *Margaretha Ebner und Heinrich von Nördlingen: Ein Beitrag zur Geschichte der deutschen Mystik.* Edited by Philipp Strauch. Amsterdam, 1966. English translation: *Margaret Ebner, Major Works.* Translated by Leonard P. Hindsley. Classics of Western Spirituality. New York, 1993.

Einhard. "Epistolae." PL 104:509–38.

———. *Vita Karoli magni.* Edited by O. Holder-Egger. MGH, SSRG in usum scholarum. Hannover, 1911. Reprint, Hannover, 1927.

Eusebius. "Acta martyrum Palaestinae." In *Historia ecclesiastica,* translated by Gustave Bardy, 3:121–74. Sources chrétiennes 55. Paris, 1956.

———. *Historia ecclesiastica.* Vol. 2. Edited by Eduard Schwartz and Theodor Mommsen. Die griechischen christlichen Schriftsteller der ersten drei Jahrundert 9. Leipzig, 1908.

———. *A New Eusebius: Documents Illustrating the History of the Church to AD 337.* Edited by J. Stevenson and W. H. C. Frend. London, 1987.

Evagrius Ponticus. *Traité pratique, ou, Le moine.* Edited by Antoine Guillaumont and Claire Guillaumont. 2 vols. Sources chrétiennes 170–71. Paris, 1971.

Francesco de Piedmont. *Suplementum in secundum librum secretorum remediorum Iuannis Mesuae, quem vocant de appropriatis.* Venice, 1531.

Fratri Alberti magni ordinis predicatorum quondam episcopi Ratisponensis. In nomine sancte et individue trinitatis Amen. Incipit prohemium de arte bene moriendi. . . . Naples, 1476.

Friedlander, Alan, ed. "Processus Bernardi Delitiosi: The Trial of Fr. Bernard Délicieux, 3 September–8 December 1319." *Transactions of the American Philosophical Society,* n.s., 86, no. 1 (1996): 1–393.

Galen. *On the Affected Parts.* Translated by Rudolph E. Siegel. Basel, 1976.

———. *Opera omnia.* Edited by Carolus Gottlob Kühn. 20 vols. Leipzig, 1821–33.

Gardiner, Eileen, ed. *Visions of Heaven and Hell before Dante.* New York, 1989.

Gatinarius, Marcus. *De curis egritudinum particularium novi Almansoris practica uberrima.* Venice, 1521.

Gerald of Wales. *Descriptio Kambriae.* Edited by James F. Dimock. Rolls Series 21/6. Reprint, London, 1964.

Gerbert of Aurillac. "Epistolae alia Gerberti." PL 139:243–64.

Gerson, Jean. "De distinctione verarum visionum a falsis." In *Oeuvres complètes*, edited by Palémon Glorieux, 3:36–56. Paris, Tournai, and Rome, 1968. English translation: "On Distinguishing True from False Revelations." In *Jean Gerson: Early Works*, translated by Brian Patrick McGuire, 334–64. New York, 1998.

———. "La médecine de l'âme." In *Oeuvres complètes*, edited by Palémon Glorieux, 7/2:404–7. Paris, Tournai, and Rome, 1968.

———. "Requeste pour les condamnes a mort." In *Oeuvres complètes*, edited by Palémon Glorieux, 7/1:341–43. Paris, Tournai, and Rome, 1968.

———. "Sermon sur la passion." In *Oeuvres complètes*, edited by Palémon Glorieux, 7/2:449–93. Paris, Tournai, and Rome, 1968.

———. *La vie de Nostre Benoit Sauveur Ihesuscrist & la saincte vie de Nostre Dame, translatee a la requeste de tres hault et puissant prince Iehan, duc de Berry*. Edited by Millard Meiss and Elizabeth H. Beatson. New York, 1977.

"Gesta sancte Agnetis." *AASS*, 2 January, 351–54.

Gilbertus Anglicus. *Healing and Society in Medieval England: A Middle English Translation of the Pharmaceutical Writings of Gilbertus Anglicus*. Edited and introduced by Faye M. Getz. Madison, WI, 1991.

Gobi, John. *Scala coeli*. Edited by Marie-Anne Polo de Beaulieu. Paris, 1991.

Godfrey of Fontaines. *Les quatre premiers quodlibets de Godefroid de Fontaines*. Edited by Maurice de Wulf and A. Pelzer. Les philosophes du Moyen Âge, 1st ser., 2. Louvain, 1904.

Goscelin of Saint Bertin. "The *Liber confortatorius* of Goscelin of Saint Bertin." Edited by C. H. Talbot. *Studia Anselmiana*, 3rd ser., 37 (1955): 1–117. English translation in *Writing the Wilton Women: Goscelin's Legend of Edith and "Liber confortatorius,"* translated by W. R. Barnes and Rebecca Hayward, edited by Stephanie Hollis et al., 97–216. Turnhout, 2004.

Gratian. *Decretum*. Vol. 1 of *Corpus iuris canonici*, edited by Emil Friedberg. Leipzig, 1881.

Gregory of Tours. *Historiarum libri X*. Edited by Bruno Krusch and Wilhelm Levison. MGH, SSRM 1/1. Hannover, 1961. Reprint, Hannover, 1993.

———. *Liber in gloria martyrum*. Edited by Bruno Krusch. MGH, SSRM 1. Hannover, 1885. English translation: *Glory of the Martyrs*. Translated by Raymond Van Dam. Liverpool, 1988.

Gregory the Great. *Dialogi*. Edited by Adalbert de Vogüé. 3 vols. Sources chrétiennes 265. Paris, 1980.

———. *Moralia in Iob*. Edited by Marcus Adriaen. CCSL 143. Turnhout, 1979.

———. *Registrum epistolarum*. Edited by Dag Norberg. CCSL 140. Turnhout, 1982.

Grillandus, Paulus. "De questionibus & tortura tractatus." In *Tractatus diversi super maleficiis, nempe Do. Alberti de Gandino, Do. Bonifacii de Vitalini, Do. Pauli Grillandi, Do. Baldi de Periglis, Do. Jacobi de Arena*, 658–85. Lyons, 1555.

———. *Tractatus de hereticis: Et sortilegijs omnifariam coitu eorumque penis item de questionibus et torturae ac de relaxatione carceratorum Domini Pauli Grillandi Castilionei ultima hac impressione summa cura castigatus: Additis ubilibet Summariijs: prepositosque perutili: Repertorio speciales sententias aptissime continente*. Lyons, 1545.

Guido de Suzaria [attr.]. "Tractatus de tormentis sive de indicijs et tortura." In *Decimum volumen tractatuum e variis iuris interpretibus collectorum*, fols. 85r–95r. Lyons, 1599.

Guilielmus Peraldus. *Sermones moralissimi super epistolas dominicales totius anni multas materias predicabiles complectentes. . . .* Avignon, 1519.

———. *Summa aurea*. Brescia, 1494.

Guy de Chauliac. *Guigonis de Caulhiaco inventarium sive chirurgia magna*. Edited by Michael R. McVaugh. 2 vols. Studies in Ancient Medicine 14. Leiden, 1997.

Henri de Mondeville. *Die Chirurgie des Heinrich von Mondeville*. Edited by Julius Leopold Pagel. Berlin, 1892.

Henricus de Segusio [Hostiensis]. *Summa aurea*. Basel, 1573.

Henry of Ghent. *Quodlibet IX*. Edited by R. Macken. Vol. 13 of *Henrici de Gandavo opera omnia*. Leuven, 1983.

———. *Quodlibet XII: Quaestiones 1–30*. Edited by J. Decorte. Vol. 16 of *Henrici de Gandavo opera omnia*. Leuven, 1987.

———. *Quotlibeta magistri Henrici Goethals a Gandavo*. Paris, 1518.

Herman of Tournai. "De miraculis sancta Maria Laudunensis et de gestis venerabilis Bartholomaei episcopi et S. Nortberti libri tres." PL 156:961–1017.

Herolt, Johannes. *Sermones discipuli de tempore et de sanctis una cum promptuario exemplorum*. N.p., [1503?].

Hieatt, Constance B., and Robin F. Jones, eds. *La novele cirurgerie*. London, 1990.

Hieronymus. *Dialogus contra Pelagianos*. Edited by Claudio Moreschini. CCSL 80. Turnhout, 1990.

———. *Epistolae*. Edited by Isidore Hilfberg. CSEL 56/1. Vienna, 1996.

———. *St. Jerome: Letters and Select Works*. Translated by W. H. Fremantle. Nicene and Post-Nicene Fathers 6. Edinburgh, 1893.

Hilary of Poitiers. *De trinitate*. Edited by P. Smulders. CCSL 62. Turnhout, 1980. English translation: *On the Trinity*. Translated by C. S. Gayford. Nicene and Post-Nicene Fathers, 2nd ser., 9. Edinburgh, 1898. Reprint, Grand Rapids, MI, 1983.

Hildebert of Lavardin. "Epistolae." PL 171:141–312.

Hildegard of Bingen. *Causae et curae*. Edited by P. Kaiser. Leipzig, 1903.

———. *Epistolarium*. Edited by L. Van Acker. 3 vols. CCCM 91. Turnhout, 1991–2001.

———. *The Letters of Hildegard of Bingen*. Translated by Joseph L. Baird and Radd K. Ehrman. 3 vols. New York, 1994–2004.

Hippocrates. *Aphorismi*. Edited and translated by Carolus Gottlob Kühn. Medicorum Graecorum opera quae extant 23. Leipzig, 1827.

Honorius Augustodunensis. "Elucidarium." In *L'elucidarium et les lucidaires*, edited by Yves Lefèbvre, 341–478. Bibliothèque des Écoles françaises d'Athènes et de Rome 180. Paris, 1954.

———. "Gemma animae." PL 172:541–738.

Hugh of Saint Victor. "De quatuor voluntatibus in Christo libellus." PL 176:841–46.

———. "De sacramentis Christiane fidei." PL 176:173–616. English translation: *On the Sacraments of the Christian Faith*. Translated by Roy Deferrari. Cambridge, MA, 1951.

Humbert de Romans, Gilbert of Tournai, and Stephen of Bourbon. *Prediche alle donne del secolo XIII.* Translated by Carla Casagrande. Edited by Maria Corti. Nuova corona 9. Milan, 1978.

Isidore of Seville. *Etymologiarum sive originum libri XX.* Edited by W. M. Lindsay. 2 vols. Oxford, 1911.

Ivo of Chartres. "Decretum." PL 161:48–1022.

———. *Panormia.* Edited by Bruce Brasington and Martin Brett. http://wtfaculty.wtamu .edu/~bbrasington/panormia.html.

Jacobus de Voragine. *Legenda aurea.* Edited by Giovanni Paolo Maggioni. Millennio medievale 6, testi 3. Florence, 1998. Original English translation: *Golden Legend.* London, 1487. Modern English translation (of the Graesse edition): *The Golden Legend.* Translated by William Granger Ryan. 2 vols. Princeton, NJ, 1993.

———. *Registrum in sermones de sanctis.* Lyons, 1520.

———. *Registrum in sermones de tempore.* Lyons, 1520.

———. *Sermones quadragesimales.* Edited by Giovanni Paolo Maggioni. Florence, 2005.

Jean Beleth. *Summa de ecclesiasticis officiis.* Edited by Herbert Douteil. 2 vols. CCCM 41. Turnhout, 1976.

Jean de Mailly. *Abregé des gestes et miracles des saints.* Translated by Antoine Dondaine. Paris, 1947.

Jean de Saint-Amand. *Die Concordanciae des Johannes de sancto Amando: Nach einer Berliner und zwei Erfurter Handschriften.* Edited by Julius Pagel. Berlin, 1894.

Jocelyn of Furness. "The Life of Saint Kentigern." Edited and translated by Cynthia Whiddon Green. M.A. thesis, University of Houston, 1998. http://www.gypsyfire .com/Translation.htm.

Johann of Werden [attr.]. *Sermones dormi secure vel dormi sine cura.* Strasbourg, 1485.

Johannes Diaconus. "Imagines beati Gregorii magni ejusque parentum." PL 75:461–78.

John of Caulibus. *Meditaciones vite Christi, olim S. Bonaventuro attributae.* Edited by C. M. Stallings-Taney. CCCM 153. Turnhout, 1997. English translation: *Meditations on the Life of Christ.* Translated by F. X. Taney, A. Miller, and C. M. Stallings-Taney. Asheville, NC, 1999. English translation from the Italian version: *Meditations on the Life of Christ.* Translated by Isa Ragusa and Rosalie B. Green. Princeton, NJ, 1961.

John of Damascus. *De fide orthodoxa: Versions of Burgundio and Cerbanus.* Edited by Eligius M. Buytaert. St. Bonaventure, NY, 1955. English translation in *Writings,* translated by Frederic H. Chase. Fathers of the Church. Washington, DC, 1958.

John of Mirfield. *Surgery [Breviarium Bartholomaei, Part IX].* Translated by J. B. Colton. New York, 1969.

John Pecham. *Quodlibeta quatuor.* Edited by G. I. Etzkorn and Fernandus Delorme. BFSMA 25. Quaracchi, 1989.

John of Salisbury. *Policraticus.* Edited by K. S. B. Keats-Rohan. CCCM 118. Turnhout, 1993.

Joubert, Laurent. *The Second Part of the Popular Errors.* Translated by Gregory David de Rocher. Tuscaloosa, AL, 1995.

Julian of Norwich. *A Book of Showings to the Anchoress Julian of Norwich.* Edited by Edmund Colledge and James Walsh. 2 vols. Toronto, 1978.

Kempe, Margery. *The Book of Margery Kempe*. Edited by Barry Windeatt. Harlow, Essex, 2000.

Kramer [Institoris], Heinrich. *Malleus maleficarum*. Edited and translated by Christopher S. Mackay. 2 vols. Cambridge, 2006.

La Tour Landry, Geoffroy de. *Le livre du chevalier de la Tour Landry pour l'enseignement de ses filles*. Edited by Anatole de Montaiglon. Paris, 1854. German translation: *Der Ritter vom Thurn*. Translated by Marquard vom Stein. Edited by Ruth Harvey. Texte des späten Mittelalters und der frühen Neuzeit 32. Berlin, 1988. English translation: *The booke of the enseygnementes and techynge that the Knyght of the Towre made to his doughters*. Early English Text Society. London, 1902.

Leonardo de Utino [Udine]. *Sermones aurei (anni 1446) de sanctis fratris Leonardi de Utine sacre theologie doctoris ordinis predicatorum*. Strasbourg, 1481.

"Liber miraculorum." In *Processus canonizationis et legendae variae sancti Ludovici OFM*, 275–331. Analecta Franciscana, sive Chronica aliaque varia documenta ad historiam fratrum minorum 7. Florence, 1951.

Liber miraculorum sancte Fidis. Edited by Auguste Bouillet. Paris, 1897. English translation: *The Book of Sainte Foy*. Translated by Pamela Sheingorn. Philadelphia, 1995.

Liber sextus Decretalium d. Bonifacii papae VIII. In *Corpus juris canonici emendatum et notis illustratum*. Gregorii XIII. pont. max. iussu editum, part 3. Rome, 1582.

Love, Nicholas. *The Mirror of the Blessed Life of Jesus Christ*. Edited by Michael G. Sargent. Exeter Medieval Texts and Studies. Exeter, 2004.

Ludolph of Saxony. *Vita Jesu Christi ex evangelio et aprobatis ab ecclesia Catholica doctoribus sedule collecta, editio novissima*. Edited by L. M. Rigollot. 4 vols. Paris, 1878.

Lugano, Placido T., ed. *I pocessi inediti per Francesca Bussa dei Ponziani (santa Francesca Romana), 1440–1453*. Studi e testi 120. Vatican City, 1945.

Maillard, Olivier. *Summarium quoddam sermonum de sanctis per totum anni circulum, simul et de communi sanctorum et pro defunctis*. Paris, 1507.

Marston, Roger. *Quodlibeta quaestiones*. Edited by G. I. Etzkorn and Ignatius C. Brady. BFSMA 26. Quaracchi, 1968.

Matthew of Acquasparta. *Quaestiones disputatae*. BFSMA 18. Quaracchi, 1959.

———. *Quaestiones disputatae selectae*. 2 vols. BFSMA 1–2. Quaracchi, 1914.

Mattiotti, Giovanni. *Il dialetto romanesco del quattrocento: Il manoscritto quattrocentesco di G. Mattiotti*. Edited by Giorgio Carpaneto. Rome, 1995.

———. *Santa Francesca Romana: Edizione critica dei trattati latini di Giovanni Mattiotti*. Edited by Alessandra Bartolomei Romagnoli. Storia e attualità 14. Vatican City, 1994.

———. "Visioni di santa Francesca Romana: Testo romanesco del secolo XV." Edited by A. Pelaez. *Archivio della Società romana di storia patria* 14 (1891): 365–409; 15 (1892): 251–73.

———. "Vita et acta sancta Franciscae Romanae." *AASS*, 2 March, 88–216.

Maurus of Salerno. "In Hippocratis aphorismos commentarium." In *Collectio Salernitana*, edited by Salvatore de Renzi, 4:513–57. Naples, 1856.

Maximus of Turin. Homilia 74. PL 51:407–10.

————. *Maximi episcopi Taurinensis sermones.* Edited by Almut Mutzenbecher. CCSL 23. Turnhout, 1962.

Mechthild von Magdeburg. *Das fliessende Licht der Gottheit: Nach der Einsiedler Handschrift in kritischem Vergleich mit der gesamten Überlieferung.* Edited by Hans Neumann and Gisela Vollmann-Profe. 2 vols. Münchener Texte und Untersuchungen zur deutschen Literatur des Mittelalters 100–101. Munich, 1990–93.

Merswin, Rulman. *Neun-Felsen-Buch (Das sogenannte Autograph).* Edited by Philipp Strauch. Altdeutsche Textbibliothek 27; Schriften aus der Gottesfreund-Literatur 3. Halle, 1929. English translation in *Mystical Writings of Rulman Merswin.* Edited by Thomas S. Kepler. Philadelphia, 1960.

————. *Vier anfangende Jahre: Des Gottesfreundes Fünfmannenbuch (Die sogenannten Autographa).* Edited by Philipp Strauch. Altdeutsche Texbibliothek 23; Schriften aus der Gottesfreund-Literatur 2. Halle, 1927. English translation in *Mystical Writings of Rulman Merswin.* Edited by Thomas S. Kepler. Philadelphia, 1960.

Mondino de Liuzzi. *Practica de accidentibus.* Edited by Giuseppe Caturegli. Scientia veterum: Collana di studi di storia della medicina 107. Pisa, 1967.

Montaigne, Michel de. *Essais.* Edited by Maurice Rat. 2 vols. Paris, 1962.

Musurillo, Herbert, ed. *The Acts of the Christian Martyrs.* Oxford, 1972.

The Myroure of Oure Ladye, Containing A Divotional Treatise on Divine Service. . . . Edited by J. H. Blunt. Early English Text Society. London, 1873.

Nemesius of Emesa. *De natura hominis: Traduction de Burgundio de Pise.* Edited by G. Verbeke and J. R. Moncho. Corpus Latinum commentariorum in Aristotelem Graecorum, suppl. 1. Leiden, 1975.

Nicolas de Tudeschis [Panormitanus]. *Consilia, quaestiones et tractatus Panormitani.* Lyons, 1534.

Nigel of Canterbury. *The Passion of St. Lawrence: Epigrams and Marginal Poems.* Edited and translated by Jan Ziolkowski. Leiden, 1994.

Pape, Gui. *Consilia domini Guidonis Pape cum repertorio. . . .* Lyons, 1533.

Paré, Ambroise. *Oeuvres complètes.* 3 vols. Paris, 1628. Reprint, Geneva, 1970.

Pelbart of Themeswar. *Pomerium sermonum de sanctis per anni circulum tam hyemalium quam estivalium.* Hagenau, 1520.

————. *Pomerium sermonum quadragesimalium tripartitus.* Hagenau, 1509.

Perrine de Baumes. "Virtutes et miracula beatae Colettae." *AASS,* 1 March, 601–19.

Peter Abelard. "Abelard's Letter of Consolation to a Friend." Edited by J. T. Muckle. *Mediaeval Studies* 12 (1950): 195–202.

————. "Commentaria in Epistulam Pauli ad Romanos." In *Petri Abaelardi opera theologica,* edited by Eligius M. Buytaert, 1–340. CCCM 11. Turnhout, 1969.

————. *Sententie magistri Petri Abaelardi.* Edited by David Luscombe. In *Petri Abaelardi opera theologica,* edited by Eligius M. Buytaert. CCCM 14. Turnhout, 2006.

————. *Sic et non: A Critical Edition.* Edited by Blanche B. Boyer and Richard McKeon. Chicago, 1977.

Peter de la Palude [attr.]. *Sermones thesauri novi de sanctis.* Nürenberg, 1496.

Peter Lombard. *Sententiae in IV libris distinctae.* 2 vols. Spicilegium Bonaventurianum 5. Quaracchi and Grottaferrata, 1971–81.

————. "Sententiarum libri quatuor." PL 192:785–964.

Peter of Tarentaise [Pope Innocent V]. *Innocentii Quinti pontificis maximi, ex ordine praedicatorum assumpti, qui antea Petrus de Tarantasia dicebatur, in IV librum sententiarum commentaria.* 4 vols. 1649–52. Reprint, Ridgewood, NJ, 1964.

Petrarca, Francesco. *A Dialogue between Reason and Adversity: A Late Middle English Version of Petrarch's "De remediis."* Edited by F. N. M. Diekstra. Assen, 1968.

————. *Le familiari.* Edited by V. Rossi and U. Bosco. 4 vols. Florence, 1933–42.

Petrus de la Palude [attr.]. *Sermones thesauri novi de sanctis.* Nürenberg, 1496.

Petrus Hispanus. "Thesaurus pauperum." In *Obras médicas de Pedro Hispano,* edited by Maria Helena Da Rocha Pereira, 77–301. Coimbra, 1973.

Pierre de Vaux. "Vita beatae Colettae." *AASS,* 1 March, 539–87.

Philippe de Harveng. "De institutione clericorum tractatus sex." PL 203:665–853.

Philippine de Porcellet. *La vie de sainte Douceline, fondatrice des Béguines de Marseille, composée au treizième siècle en langue provençale.* Edited by J.-H. Albanès. Marseille, 1879. English translation: *The Life of Saint Douceline, a Beguine of Provence.* Translated by Kathleen Garay and Madeleine Jeay. Library of Medieval Women. Cambridge, 2001.

Procopius. *History of the Wars.* Translated by H. B. Dewing. Loeb Library of the Greek and Roman Classics. London, 1914. Reprint, Cambridge, MA, 1961.

Prudentius. *Peristefanon.* In *Carmina,* edited by Maurice Patrick Cunningham, 251–389. CCSL 126. Turnhout, 1966.

————. *The Poems.* Translated by M. Clement Eagan. 2 vols. Washington, DC, 1962–65.

Pseudo-Anselm. "Dialogus beatae Mariae et Anselmi de passione Domini." PL 159: 271–88.

Pseudo–Arnau de Villanova. *Breviarium practicae medicinae.* Venice, 1494.

Pseudo-Augustine. "De uera et falsa penitentia." PL 40:1113–30.

Pseudo-Beda. "De meditatione passionis Christi per septem diei horas libellus." PL 94:561–88.

Pseudo-Bernard. "Meditatio in passionem et resurrectionem Domini." PL 184:741–68.

Pseudo–Maximus of Turin. "Homiliae in natali sancti Laurentii Levitae et martyris." PL 57:407–12.

Pseudo–Yūh'annā Ibn Māsawaih. "Grabadin, id est compendii secretorum medicamentorum liber secundum, qua propria remedia ad singularum partium corporis morbos docentur." In *Johannes Mesuae medici clarissimi opera.* Venice, 1531.

"Public Record of the Labour of Isabel de la Cavalleria, January 10, 1490, Zaragoza." Translated by Montserrat Cabre. http://www.the-orb.net/birthrecord.html.

Le purgatoire de saint Patrice. Edited by J. Vising. Gothenburg, 1916.

Les quinze joies de mariage. Edited by Jean Rychner. Geneva, 1963.

Radice, Betty, ed. *The Letters of Abelard and Heloise.* Penguin Classics. Harmondsworth, UK, 1974.

Raymond of Capua. "Vita sanctae Catharinae Senensis." *AASS,* 3 April, 861–967.

Registre criminel du Châtelet de Paris du 6 septembre 1389 au 18 mai 1392. Edited by H. Duplès-Agier. 2 vols. Paris, 1861–64.

Religieux de Saint-Denys. *Chroniques.* Edited by M. L. Bellaguet. 3 vols. Paris, 1842; repr., Paris, 1994.

Richard of Saint Victor. "Benjamin minor." PL 196:1–64.

Roger of Wendover. *Liber qui dicitur flores historiarum ab anno domini MCLIV annoque Henrici Anglorum regis.* Edited by Henry Hewlett. 2 vols. Rolls Series 84. London, 1887.

Rolle, Richard. *The Passio Domini Theme in the Works of Richard Rolle: His Personal Contribution in Its Religious, Cultural, and Literary Context.* Edited by Mary F. Madigan. Salzburg Studies in English Literature. Institut für englische Sprache und Literatur. Salzburg, 1978.

Rupert of Deutz. "Commentariorum in genesim liber quartus." PL 167:346.

Ruusbroec, Jan van. *Die geestelijke brulocht.* Translated by H. Rolfson. Edited by J. Alaerts. CCCM 103, Opera omnia 1. Turnhout, 1988.

Savonarola, Michele. *Ad mulieres ferrarienses de regimine pregnantium et noviter natorum usque ad septennium.* Published as *Il trattato ginecologico-pediatrico in volgare di Michele Savonarola.* Edited by Luigi Belloni. Milan, 1952.

———. *De gotta la preseruatione e cura per lo preclaro medico m. Michele Sauonarola ordinata: E intitulata allo illustre marchese di Ferrara S. Nicolo da Este.* Edited by Georgius Vegius. Pavia, 1505.

The South English Legendary. Edited by Charlotte D'Evelyn and Anna J. Mill. 3 vols. Early English Text Society. London, 1956–59.

Stephen of Bourbon. *Anecdotes historiques, légendes et apologues, tirés du recueil inédit d'Etienne de Bourbon, dominicain du XIII siècle.* Edited by Antoine Lecoy de la Marche. Paris, 1877.

———. *Tractatus de diversis materiis predicabilibus.* Edited by Jacques Berlioz and Jean-Luc Eichenlaub. 2 vols. CCCM 124. Turnhout, 2002–6.

Suso, Heinrich. "Büchlein der ewigen Weisheit." In *Der Mystikers Heinrish Seuse O. Pr. deutsche Schriften,* edited by Nikolaus Keller, 185–285. Regensburg, 1926.

———. *Horologium sapientiae.* Edited by Pius Künzle. Spicilegium Friburgense 23. Freiburg, 1977.

———. *Der Mystikers Heinrish Seuse O. Pr. deutsche Schriften.* Edited by Nikolaus Keller. Regensburg, 1926. English translation: *The Exemplar: Life and Writings of Blessed Henry Suso, O.P.* Translated by M. Ann Edward. 2 vols. Dubuque, IA, 1962.

———. "Una nuova versione latina delle cento meditazioni sulla passione del beato Enrico Susone, O.P." Edited by Livarius Oliger. *Archivio italiano per la storia della pietà* 2 (1959): 207–30.

Symmachus. "Epistolae." PL 18:145–406.

Tertullianus, Quintus Septimius Florens. "Apologeticum." In *Opera,* edited by Elygius Dekkers, 1:76–171. CCSL 1. Turnhout, 1954.

Theodoricus Borgognoni. *Surgery.* Translated by E. Campbell and J. B. Colton. 2 vols. New York, 1955.

The Theodosian Code and Novels and the Sirmondian Constitutions. Edited by Theodore Mommsen. Translated by Pharr Clyde. Princeton, NJ, 1952.

Thomas Aquinas. *In quatuor libros sententiarum.* Edited by Robertus Busa. Sancti Thomae Aquinatis opera omnia qui sunt in indice Thomistico 1. Stuttgart, 1980.

———. *On Spiritual Creatures (De spiritualibus creaturis).* Translated by Mary C. Fitzpatrick. Mediaeval Philosophical Texts in Translation 5. Milwaukee, WI, 1949.

————. *Questiones de anima*. Edited by James H. Robb. Toronto, 1968.

————. *Questiones de quolibet*. 2 vols. Rome, 1996.

————. *Questiones disputatae*. Edited by Raymond Spiazzi. 2 vols. Turin, 1964–65.

————. *Scriptum super sententiis magistri Petri Lombardi*. Edited by R. P. Mandonnet and Marie Fabien Moos. Paris, 1947.

————. *Sententia libri ethicorum*. Rome, 1969.

————. *Summa theologiae*. Edited by Robertus Busa. 7 vols. Sancti Thomae Aquinatis opera omnia 2. Stuttgart, 1980.

Thomas of Cantimpré. *Miraculorum et exemplorum sui temporis libri duo* [*De apibus*]. Douai, 1605.

————. "Vita Christinae Mirabilis." *AASS*, 5 July, 650–56. English translation: *The Life of Christina Mirabilis*. Translated and edited by Margot H. King. Toronto, 1986. Reprint, Toronto, 1989.

Thomas of Chobham. *Summa de arte praedicandi*. Edited by Franco Morenzoni. CCCM 82. Turnhout, 1988.

"Tractatus de purgatorio sancti Patricii." PL 180:973–1004.

Trattato de l'arte di bien morire, attributo al Cardinale di Fermo Domenico Capranica. Florence, 1477.

The Trotula: A Medieval Compendium of Women's Medicine. Edited by Monica H. Green. Philadelphia, 2001.

Ubertino da Casale. *Arbor vitae crucifixae Jesu*. Edited by Charles T. Davis. Monumenta politica et philosophica rariora, ser. 1, no. 4. Venice, 1485. Reprint, Turin, 1962.

Van der Zanden, C. M., ed. *Étude sur le purgatoire de saint Patrice*. Paris, 1927.

"La vie de saint Jehan Paulus." In *The German Legends of the Hairy Anchorite*, edited by Charles A. Williams and Louis Allen, 83–140. University of Illinois Studies in Language and Literature. Urbana, 1935.

Vincent of Beauvais. *Speculum historiale*. Douai, 1624. Reprint, Graz, 1965.

Visio Tnugdali. Edited by Albrecht Wagner. Erlangen, 1882.

"*Vita Adae et Evae*." Edited by Wilhelm Meyer. *Abhandlungen der philosophisch-philologischen Classe der Königlich bayerischen Akademie der Wissenschaften* 14 (1878): 185–250. English and Latin text: "Life of Adam and Eve." Edited by Wilfried Lechner-Schmidt. Translated by B. Custis with the assistance of G. Anderson and R. Layton. http://www.iath.virginia.edu/anderson/vita/english/vita.lat.html#per2.

Vita vel passio Haimhrammi episcopi et martyris Ratisbonensis. In *Passiones vitaeque sanctorum aevi Merovingici*, edited by Bruno Krusch, 2:452–524. MGH, SSRM 4. Hannover, 1902.

Voigts, Linda E., and Michael R. McVaugh, eds. "A Latin Technical Phlebotomy and Its Middle English Translation." *Transactions of the American Philosophical Society* 72, no. 2 (1984): 1–69.

Welter, Jean-Th., ed. *La tabula exemplorum secundum ordinem alphabeti, recueil d'exempla compilé en France à la fin du XIIIᵉ siècle*. Paris, 1926.

William de Saliceto. *Chirurgia*. Translated by P. Pifteau. Toulouse, 1898.

William of Auvergne. *Opera omnia*. 2 vols. Paris, 1674.

————. *The Soul*. Edited and translated by Roland J. Teske. Mediaeval Philosophical Texts in Translation 37. Milwaukee, WI, 2000.

William of Auxerre. *Summa aurea.* Edited by Jean Ribailler. 5 vols. Spicilegium Bonaventurianum 16–20. Paris, 1986.

William of Canterbury. *Miracula gloriosi martyris Thomae archiepiscopi Cantuariensis.* Vol. 1 of *Materials for the History of Thomas Becket, Archbishop of Canterbury,* edited by James C. Robertson. Rolls Series 67. Reprint, London, 1965.

William of Ockham. *Quaestiones variae.* Edited by G. I. Etzkorn, Francis E. Kelley, and Joseph C. Wey. Opera philosophica et theologica 8. Saint Bonaventure, NY, 1984.

———. *Quodlibeta septem.* Edited by Joseph C. Wey. Opera philosophica et theologica 9. St. Bonaventure, NY, 1980. English translation: *Quodlibetal Questions.* Translated by Alfred J. Freddoso and Francis E. Kelley. 2 vols. New Haven, CT, 1991.

William of Saint-Thierry. "De natura corporis et animae libri duo." PL 180:695–726.

Winstead, Karen A., ed. and trans. *Chaste Passions: Medieval English Virgin Martyr Legends.* Ithaca, NY, 2000.

Yso. "De miraculis S. Otmari libri II." In MGH, SS, edited by G. H. Pertz, 2:47–54. Hannover, 1829.

SECONDARY SOURCES

Abou-el-Haj, Barbara. *The Medieval Cult of Saints: Formations and Transformations.* Cambridge, 1994.

Agrimi, Jole, and Chiara Crisciani. *Les consilia médicaux.* Translated by Caroline Viola. TSMA 69. Turnhout, 1994.

Allers, R. "Microcosmus: From Anaximandros to Paracelsus." *Traditio* 2 (1944): 319–407.

Althoff, Gerd. "*Ira Regis:* Prolegomena to a History of Royal Anger." In *Anger's Past: The Social Uses of an Emotion in the Middle Ages,* edited by Barbara H. Rosenwein, 59–74. Ithaca, NY, 1998.

———. "The Variability of Rituals in the Middle Ages." In *Medieval Concepts of the Past: Ritual, Memory, Historiography,* edited by Gerd Althoff, Johannes Fried, and Patrick J. Geary, 71–88. Cambridge, 2002.

Améry, Jean. *At the Mind's Limits: Contemplations by a Survivor on Auschwitz and Its Realities.* Translated by Sidney Rosenfeld and Stella P. Rosenfeld. Bloomington, IN, 1980.

Amos, Mark Addison. "'For Manners Make Man': Bourdieu, de Certeau, and the Common Appropriation of Noble Manners in the *Book of Courtesy.*" In *Medieval Conduct,* edited by Kathleen Ashley and Robert L. A. Clark, 23–48. Medieval Cultures 29. Minneapolis, MN, 2001.

Anciaux, Paul. *La théologie du sacrement de pénitence au XIIe siècle.* Universitas Catholica Lovaniensis dissertationes, ser. 2, 41. Louvain and Gembloux, 1949.

Anderson, Gary A., and Michael E. Stone. "An Electronic Edition of the 'Life of Adam and Eve.'" http://jefferson.village.virginia.edu/anderson/iath.report.html.

Arbesmann, Rudolph. "The Concept of Christus Medicus in St. Augustine." *Traditio* 10 (1954): 1–28.

Arnold, John H. *Inquisition and Power: Catharism and the Confessing Subject in Medieval Languedoc.* Philadelphia, 2001.

Ashton, Gail. *The Generation of Identity in Late Medieval Hagiography: Speaking the Saint*. London, 2000.

Atran, Scott. *Cognitive Foundations of Natural History: Towards an Anthropology of Science*. Cambridge, 1990.

Auerbach, Erich. "*Passio* as Passio." *Criticism* 43 (2001): 288–308.

Aydede, Murat, ed. *Pain: New Essays on Its Nature and the Methodology of Its Study*. Cambridge, MA, 2005.

Baraz, Daniel. *Medieval Cruelty: Changing Perceptions, Late Antiquity to the Early Modern Period*. Ithaca, NY, 2003.

Bartlett, Robert. *Trial by Fire and Water: The Medieval Judicial Ordeal*. Oxford, 1986.

Bartoccetti, Vittorio. "Le fonti della visione di S. Francesca Romana." *Rivista storica benedettina* 13 (1922): 13–40.

Barton, Carlin A. "The Emotional Economy of Sacrifice and Execution in Ancient Rome." *Historical Reflections/Réflexions historiques* 29 (2003): 341–60.

———. *The Sorrows of the Ancient Romans: The Gladiator and the Monster*. Princeton, NJ, 1993.

Baschet, Jérôme. *Les Justices de l'au-delà: Les représentations de l'enfer en France et en Italie (XIIᵉ–XVᵉ siècle)*. Rome, 1993.

Baumgarten, Elisheva. *Mothers and Children: Jewish Family Life in Medieval Europe*. Princeton, NJ, 2004.

Baur, Marguerite L. "Recherches sur l'histoire de l'anesthésie avant 1846." *Janus* 31 (1927): 24–39, 63–90, 124–37, 170–82.

Bazàn, Bernardo, et al., eds. *Les questions disputées et les questions quodlibétiques dans les facultés de théologie, de droit et de médecine*. 2 vols. TSMA 44–45. Turnhout, 1985.

Beck, Patrice. "Le nom protecteur." *Cahiers de recherches médiévales* 8 (2001): 165–74.

Beckwith, Sarah. *Christ's Body: Identity, Culture and Society in Late Medieval Writings*. London, 1993.

Benjamins, H. S. "Keeping Marriage out of Paradise: The Creation of Man and Woman in Patristic Literature." In *The Creation of Man and Woman*, edited by Gerard P. Luttikhuizen, 93–106. Themes in Biblical Narrative: Jewish and Christian Traditions 3. Leiden, 2000.

Bennewitz, Ingrid. "'Darumb lieben Toechter/seyt nicht zu gar fürwitzig . . .': Deutschsprachige moralisch-didaktische Literatur des 13.–15. Jahrhunderts." In *Geschichte der Mädchen- und Frauenbildung*, vol. 1, *Vom Mittelalter bis zur Aufklärung*, edited by Elke Kleinau and Claudia Opitz, 23–41. Frankfurt, 1996.

Bériou, Nicole. *L'avènement des maîtres de la parole: La prédication à Paris au XIIIᵉ siècle*. 2 vols. Collection des études augustiniennes, Moyen Âge et temps modernes 31. Paris, 1998.

———. "La confession dans les écrits théologiques et pastoraux du XIIIᵉ siècle: Médication de l'âme ou démarche judiciaire?" In *L'aveu: Antiquité et Moyen Âge; Actes de la table ronde organisée par l'École française de Rome, Rome, 28–30 mars 1984*, 261–82. Rome, 1986.

Berlioz, Jacques. "Les ordalies dans les exempla de la confession (XIIIᵉ–XIVᵉ siècles)." In

L'aveu: Antiquité et Moyen Âge; Actes de la table ronde organisée par l'École française de Rome, Rome, 28–30 mars 1984, 315–40. Rome, 1986.

Bernstein, Alan E. "Esoteric Theology: William of Auvergne on the Fires of Hell and Purgatory." *Speculum* 57 (1982): 509–31.

———. *The Formation of Hell: Death and Retribution in the Ancient and Early Christian Worlds.* Ithaca, NY, 1993.

———. "Theology between Heresy and Folklore: William of Auvergne on Punishment after Death." *Studies in Medieval and Renaissance History* 5 (1982): 5–44.

Bestul, Thomas H. *Texts of the Passion: Latin Devotional Literature and Medieval Society.* Middle Ages Series. Philadelphia, 1996.

Biller, Peter. "Words and the Medieval Notion of 'Religion.'" *Journal of Ecclesiastical History* 36 (1985): 351–69.

Biller, Peter, and Joseph Ziegler, eds. *Religion and Medicine in the Middle Ages.* York Studies in Medieval Theology 3. York, UK, 2001.

Blasucci, Antonio. "La theologia del dolore nelle beata Angela da Foligno." *Miscellanea Francescana* 59 (1959): 494–507.

Bongert, Yvonne. *Recherches sur les cours laïques du Xe au XIIIe siècle.* Paris, 1948.

Bonney, Françoise. "Autour de Jean Gerson: Opinions de théologiens sur les superstitions et la sorcellerie au début du XVe siècle." *Le Moyen Âge* 71 (1971): 85–93.

Bornstein, Daniel E. *The Bianchi of 1399: Popular Devotion in Late Medieval Italy.* Ithaca, NY, 1993.

———. "Violenza al corpo di una santa: Fra agiografia e pornografia; A proposito di Douceline di Digne." *Quaderni medievali* 39 (1995): 31–46.

Boureau, Alain. *La légende dorée: Le système narratif de Jacques de Voragine (d. 1298).* Paris, 1984.

———. "The Letter-Writing Norm, a Mediaeval Invention." In *Correspondence: Models of Letter-Writing from the Middle Ages to the Nineteenth Century,* edited by Roger Chartier, Alain Boureau, and Cécile Dauphin, 24–58. London, 1997.

———. "Miracle, volonté et imagination: La mutation scolastique (1270–1320)." In *Miracles, prodiges et merveilles au Moyen Âge,* 159–72. Paris, 1995.

———. *Satan the Heretic: The Birth of Demonology in the Medieval West.* Translated by Teresa L. Fagan. Chicago, 2006.

———. *Théologie, science et censure au XIIIe siècle: Le cas de Jean Peckham.* Paris, 1999.

Brakke, David. "The Lady Appears: Materializations of 'Woman' in Early Monastic Literature." *Journal of Medieval and Early Modern Studies* 33 (2003): 387–402.

Bremond, Claude, Jacques Le Goff, and Jean-Claude Schmitt, eds. *L'exemplum.* TSMA 40. Turnhout, 1982.

Brett, Edward T. *Humbert de Romans: His Life and Views of Thirteenth-Century Society.* Pontifical Institute Studies and Texts 67. Toronto, 1984.

Brévart, Francis B. "Between Medicine, Magic, and Religion: Wonder Drugs in German Medico-Pharmaceutical Treatises of the Thirteenth to Sixteenth Centuries." *Speculum* 83 (2008): 1–57

Briscoe, Marianne G. *Artes praedicandi.* TSMA 61. Turnhout, 1992.

Browe, Petrus. *De ordaliies.* 2 vols. Rome, 1933.

Brown, Dorothy C. *Pastor and Laity in the Theology of Jean Gerson.* Cambridge, 1987.

Brown, Peter. *Authority and the Sacred: Aspects of the Christianization of the Roman World.* Cambridge, 1995.

———. *The Body and Society: Men, Women, and Sexual Renunciation in Early Christianity.* New York, 1988.

———. *The Cult of the Saints: Its Rise and Function in Latin Christianity.* Chicago, 1981.

———. "The Rise and Function of the Holy Man in Late Antiquity." *Journal of Roman Studies* 61 (1971): 80–101.

———. "Society and the Supernatural: A Medieval Change." *Daedalus* 104 (1975): 133–51.

Brundage, James A. *The Medieval Origins of the Legal Profession: Canonists, Civilians, and Courts.* Chicago, 2008.

———. "The Rise of Professional Canonists and Development of the *Ius Commune.*" *Zeitschrift der Savigny-Stiftung, kanonistische Abteilung* 112 (1995): 26–63.

Bryan, Lindsay. "Marriage and Morals in the Fourteenth Century: The Evidence of Bishop Hamo's Register." *English Historical Review* 121 (2006): 467–86.

Bynum, Caroline W. "The Blood of Christ in the Later Middle Ages." *Church History* 71 (2002): 685–714.

———. *Fragmentation and Redemption: Essays on Gender and the Human Body in Medieval Religion.* New York, 1992.

———. *Holy Feast and Holy Fast: The Religious Significance of Food to Medieval Women.* Berkeley, CA, 1987.

———. "Jesus as Mother and Abbot as Mother: Some Themes in Twelfth-Century Cistercian Writing." In *Jesus as Mother: Studies in the Spirituality of the High Middle Ages,* by Caroline W. Bynum, 110–69. Berkeley, CA, 1984.

———. *The Resurrection of the Body in Western Christianity, 200–1336.* New York, 1995.

———. *Wonderful Blood: Theology and Practice in Late Medieval Northern Germany and Beyond.* Philadelphia, 2007.

Caciola, Nancy. *Discerning Spirits: Divine and Demonic Possession in the Middle Ages.* Ithaca, NY, 2003.

Cadden, Joan. *Meanings of Sex Difference in the Middle Ages: Medicine, Science, and Culture.* Cambridge, 1993.

Camille, Michael. "Mimetic Identification and Passion Devotion in the Later Middle Ages: A Double-Sided Panel by Meister Francke." In *The Broken Body: Passion Devotion in Late Medieval Culture,* edited by A. A. MacDonald, H. N. B. Ridderbos, and R. M. Schlusemann, 183–210. Medievalia Groningana 21. Groningen, 1998.

Carozzi, Claude. "Structure et fonction de la vision de Tnugdal." In *Faire croire: Modalités de la diffusion et de la réception des messages religieux du XIIe au XVe siècle,* 223–34. Collection de l'École française de Rome 51. Rome, 1981.

Casagrande, Carla. "Guglielmo d'Auvergne e il buon uso delle passioni nella penitenza." In *Autour de Guillaume d'Auvergne (d. 1249),* edited by Franco Morenzoni and Jean-Yves Tilliette, 189–201. Turnhout, 2005.

Cawsey, Kathy. "Tutivillus and the 'Kyrkchaterars': Strategies of Control in the Middle Ages." *Studies in Philology* 102 (2005): 434–51.

Chazelle, Celia. *The Crucified God in the Carolingian Era: Theology and Art of Christ's Passion.* Cambridge, 2001.

Cheyette, Fredric. "Suum cuique tribuere." *French Historical Studies* 6 (1970): 287–99.

Chiffoleau, Jacques. "Sur la pratique et la conjoncture de l'aveu judiciaire en France du XIIIᵉ au XVᵉ siècle." In *L'aveu: Antiquité et Moyen Âge; Actes de la table ronde organisée par l'École française de Rome, Rome, 28–30 mars 1984*, 341–80. Rome, 1986.

Clanchy, Michael T. *Abelard: A Medieval Life.* Oxford, 1997.

———. "Images of Ladies with Prayer Books: What Do They Signify?" *Studies in Church History* 38 (2004): 106–22.

Clark, Gillian. "Adam's Engendering: Augustine on Gender and Creation." In *Gender and Christian Religion*, edited by R. N. Swanson, 13–22. Studies in Church History 34. Woodbridge, UK, 1998.

Classen, Albrecht. "The Literary Treatment of the Ineffable: Mechthild von Magdeburg, Margaret Ebner, Agnes Blannbekin." *Studies in Spirituality* 8 (1998): 162–87.

Cohen, Esther. "The Animated Pain of the Body." *American Historical Review* 105 (2000): 36–68.

———. *The Crossroads of Justice: Law and Culture in Late Medieval France.* Brill's Studies in Intellectual History 36. Leiden, 1993.

———. "Inquiring Once More after the Inquisitorial Process." In *Die Entstehung des öffentlichen Strafrechts: Beiträge zu einer Bestandaufnahme*, edited by Dietmar Willoweit, 41–65. Cologne, 1999.

———. "Who Desecrated the Host?" In *De Sion exibit lex et verbum domini de Hierusalem: Essays on Medieval Law, Liturgy, and Literature in Honor of Amnon Linder*, edited by Yitzhak Hen, 197–210. Turnhout, 2001.

Cohen-HaNegbi, Naama. "Accidents of the Soul: Emotions and Their Treatment in Medicine and Confession, 12th–15th Centuries, Spain and Italy." Ph.D. diss., Hebrew University of Jerusalem, forthcoming.

Cohn, Norman. *Warrant for Genocide: The Myth of the Jewish World-Conspiracy and the "Protocols of the Elders of Zion."* London, 1967.

Colman, Rebecca V. "Reason and Unreason in Early Medieval Law." *Journal of Interdisciplinary History* 4 (1974): 571–91.

Constable, Giles. "Attitudes towards Self-Inflicted Suffering in the Middle Ages." In *Culture and Spirituality in Medieval Europe*, by Giles Constable. Aldershot, UK, 1996.

———. "The Ideal of the Imitation of Christ." In *Three Studies in Medieval Religious and Social Thought*, by Giles Constable, 143–248. Cambridge, 1995.

Conway, Charles A. *The Vita Christi of Ludolph of Saxony and Late Medieval Devotion Centred on the Incarnation: A Descriptive Analysis.* Analecta Cartusiana 34. Salzburg, 1976.

Conybeare, Catherine. "The Ambiguous Laughter of Saint Laurence." *Journal of Early Christian Studies* 10 (2002): 175–202.

Coon, Lynda L. *Sacred Fictions: Holy Women and Hagiography in Late Antiquity.* Philadelphia, 1997.

Crachiolo, Beth. "Seeing the Gendering of Violence: Female and Male Martyrs in the South English Legendary." In *"A Great Effusion of Blood"? Interpreting Medieval*

Violence, edited by Mark D. Meyerson, Daniel Thiery, and Oren Falk, 147–63. Toronto, 2004.

Crisciani, Chiara. "Histories, Stories, Exempla, and Anecdotes: Michele Savonarola from Latin to Vernacular." In *Historia: Empiricism and Erudition in Early Modern Europe*, edited by Gianna Pomata and Nancy G. Siraisi, 297–324. Cambridge, MA, 2005.

Dacheux, Léon. *Un réformateur catholique de la fin du XVᵉ siècle: Jean Geiler de Kaysersberg, prédicateur à la cathédrale de Strasbourg, 1478–1510.* Paris and Strasbourg, 1876.

Daems, Willem F. "Spongia somnifera: Philologische und pharmakologische Probleme." *Beiträge zur Geschichte der Pharmazie* 22 (1970): 25–26.

Davies, Wendy, and Paul Fouracre, eds. *The Settlement of Disputes in Early Medieval Europe.* Cambridge, 1986.

D'Avray, David L. "Method in the Study of Medieval Sermons." In *Modern Questions about Medieval Sermons*, edited by Nicole Bériou and David L. D'Avray, 3–30. Spoleto, 1994.

———. "Sermons to the Upper Bourgeoisie by a Thirteenth-Century Franciscan." *Studies in Church History* 16 (1979): 187–99.

Dean, Trevor. *Crime in Medieval Europe, 1200–1500.* Harlow, UK, 2001.

De Jong, Mayke. "Power and Humility in Carolingian Society: The Public Penance of Louis the Pious." *Early Medieval Europe* 1 (1992): 29–52.

Dekker, Rudolf, ed. *Egodocuments and History: Autobiographical Writing in Its Social Context since the Middle Ages.* Hilversum, Netherlands, 2002.

Delehaye, Hippolyte. *Les passions des martyrs et les genres littéraires.* Subsidia hagiographica 13B. Brussels, 1921.

———, ed. "Recherches sur le légendier romain." *Analecta Bollandiana* 51 (1933): 34–98.

Demaitre, Luke. "Medieval Notions of Cancer: Malignancy and Metaphor." *Bulletin of the History of Medicine* 72 (1998): 609–37.

De Mayo, Thomas B. *The Demonology of William of Auvergne: By Fire and Sword.* Lewiston, NY, 2007.

de Moulin, Daniel. *De heelkunde in de vroege Middeleeuwen.* Leiden, 1964.

———. "A Historical-Phenomenological Study of Bodily Pain in Western Man." *Bulletin of the History of Medicine* 48 (1974): 540–70.

Denomy, Alexander J. *The Old French Lives of Saint Agnes and Other Vernacular Versions of the Middle Ages.* Cambridge, 1938.

Diepgen, Paul. "Aus der Geschichte des Schmerzes und der Schmerzbehandlung." *Medizinische Mitteilungen* 8 (1936): 218–25.

Diller, Anthony. "Cross-cultural Pain Semantics." *Pain* 9 (1980): 9–26.

Dinzelbacher, Peter. *Revelationes.* TSMA 57. Turnhout, 1991.

———. *Vision und Visionsliteratur im Mittelalter.* Stuttgart, 1981.

———. "The Way to the Other World in Medieval Literature and Art." *Folklore* 97 (1986): 70–87.

Donahue, Charles, Jr. "Proof by Witnesses in the Church Courts of Medieval England: An Imperfect Reception of the Learned Law." In *On the Laws and Customs of England: Essays in Honor of Samuel E. Thorne*, edited by Morris S. Arnold, 127–58. Chapel Hill, NC, 1981.

Dronzek, Anna. "Gendered Theories of Education in Fifteenth-Century Conduct Books." In *Medieval Conduct*, edited by Kathleen Ashley and Robert L. A. Clark, 135–59. Medieval Cultures 29. Minneapolis, MN, 2001.

Dubois, Jacques, and Geneviève Renaud, eds. *Le martyrologe d'Adon: Ses deux familles, ses trois recensions*. Paris, 1984.

duBois, Page. *Torture and Truth*. London, 1991.

Duby, Georges. "Réflexions sur la douleur physique au Moyen Âge." In *Mâle Moyen Âge*, by Georges Duby, 203–9. Paris, 1988.

Eamon, William. *Science and the Secrets of Nature: Books of Secrets in Medieval and Early Modern Culture*. Princeton, NJ, 1996.

Easton, Martha. "Pain, Torture and Death in the Huntington Library *Legenda aurea*." In *Gender and Holiness: Men, Women and Saints in Late Medieval Europe*, edited by Samantha J. E. Riches and Sarah Salih, 49–64. Routledge Studies in Medieval Religion and Culture. London, 2002.

———. "Saint Agatha and the Sanctification of Sexual Violence." *Studies in Iconography* 16 (1994): 83–118.

Elias, Norbert. *The Civilizing Process*. Translated by Edmund Jephcott. 2 vols. Oxford, 1994.

Ellington, Donna S. "Impassioned Mother or Passive Icon: The Virgin's Role in Late Medieval and Early Modern Passion Sermons." *Renaissance Quarterly* 48 (1995): 227–61.

Elliott, Dyan. "Seeing Double: John Gerson, the Discernment of Spirits, and Joan of Arc." *American Historical Review* 107 (2002): 26–54.

Elsakkers, Marianne. "In Pain You Shall Bear Children (Gen 3:16): Medieval Prayers for a Safe Delivery." In *Women and Miracle Stories: A Multidisciplinary Exploration*, edited by Anne-Marie Korte, 179–209. Leiden, 2001.

Emerson, Jan S. "Harmony, Hierarchy, and the Senses in the Vision of Tundal." In *Imagining Heaven in the Middle Ages: A Book of Essays*, edited by Jan S. Emerson and Hugo Feiss, 3–46. New York, 2000.

Enders, Jody. *The Medieval Theater of Cruelty: Rhetoric, Memory, Violence*. Ithaca, NY, 1999.

Enenkel, Karl A. E. "Pain as Persuasion: The Petrarch Master Interpreting Petrarch's *De remediis*." In *The Sense of Suffering: Constructions of Physical Pain in Early Modern Culture*, edited by Jan Frans van Dijkhuizen and Karl A. E. Enenkel, 91–164. Leiden, 2009.

Esch, Arnold. "Tre sante ed il loro ambiente sociale a Roma: S. Francesca Romana, S. Brigida di Svezia e S. Caterina da Siena." In *Atti del simposio internazionale Cateriniano-Bernardiniano (Siena, 17–20 aprile 1980)*, edited by Domenico Maffei and Paolo Nardi, 89–120. Siena, 1982.

Eubel, Konrad. "Vom Zaubereiunwesen anfangs des 14. Jahrhunderts." *Historisches Jahrbuch* 18 (1897): 608–31.

Evans, Gillian. "*Mens Devota:* The Literary Community of the Devotional Works of John of Fécamp and St. Anselm." *Medium Aevum* 43 (1974): 105–15.

Farnhill, Ken. "Guilds, Purgatory and the Cult of Saints: Westlake Reconsidered." In *Christianity and Community in the West: Essays for John Bossy*, edited by Simon Ditchfield, 59–71. Aldershot, UK, 2001.

Finucane, Ronald C. *Miracles and Pilgrims: Popular Beliefs in Medieval England.* London, 1977.

Fiorelli, Piero. *La tortura giudiziaria nel diritto comune.* 2 vols. Milan, 1953–54.

Fleith, Barbara. "Le classement des quelque 1000 manuscrits de la *Legenda aurea* latine. . . ." In *Legenda aurea: Sept siècles de diffusion,* edited by Brenda Dunn-Lardeau, 19–24. Montreal, 1986.

Fontanella, Lucia. *Un volgarizzamento tardo duecentesco fiorentino dell'"Antidotarium Nicolai": Montréal, McGill University, Osler Library 7628.* Pluteus testi 3. Alessandria, 2000.

Foucault, Michel. *Discipline and Punish: The Birth of the Prison.* Translated by Alan Sheridan. London, 1977.

Fouracre, Paul. "Merovingian History and Merovingian Hagiography." *Past and Present* 127 (1990): 3–38.

Fraher, Richard M. "Conviction according to Conscience: The Medieval Jurists' Debate concerning Judicial Discretion and the Law of Proof." *Law and History Review* 7 (1989): 23–88.

———. "IV Lateran's Revolution in Criminal Procedure: The Birth of *Inquisitio,* the End of Ordeals, and Innocent III's Vision of Ecclesiastical Politics." In *Studia in honorem eminentissimi cardinalis Alphonsi M. Stickler,* edited by J. Rosalius and L. Castillo, 97–111. Studia et textus historiae iuris canonici 7. Rome, 1992.

———. "The Theoretical Justification for the New Criminal Law of the High Middle Ages: 'Rei Publicae Interest, Ne Crimina Remaneant Impunita.'" *University of Illinois Law Review* (1984): 577–95.

Franchi de' Cavalieri, Pio. "Assum est, versa et manduca." *Note agiografiche (Studi e testi 27)* 5 (1915): 65–81.

Frede, Michael. "On Aristotle's Conception of the Soul." In *Essays on Aristotle's "De anima,"* edited by Martha C. Nussbaum and Amélie O. Rorty, 93–107. Oxford, 1992.

Freeland, Cynthia. "Aristotle on the Sense of Touch." In *Essays on Aristotle's "De anima,"* edited by Martha C. Nussbaum and Amélie O. Rorty, 228–34. Oxford, 1992.

French, Roger. "Astrology in Medical Practice." In *Practical Medicine from Salerno to the Black Death,* edited by Luis García-Ballester et al., 30–59. Cambridge, 1994.

———. *Canonical Medicine: Gentile da Foligno and Scholasticism.* Leiden, 2001.

Fried, Johannes. "Wille, Freiwilligkeit und Geständnis um 1300." *Historisches Jahrbuch* 105 (1985): 388–425.

Friedlander, Alan. *The Hammer of the Inquisitors: Brother Bernard Délicieux and the Struggle against the Inquisition in Fourteenth-Century France.* Leiden, 2000.

Fulton, Rachel. *From Judgment to Passion: Devotion to Christ and the Virgin Mary, 800–1200.* New York, 2002.

Gaffuri, Laura. "Du texte au texte: Réflexions sur la première diffusion de la *Legenda aurea.*" In *De la sainteté à l'hagiographie: Genèse et usage de la "Légende dorée,"* edited by Barbara Fleith and Franco Morenzoni, 139–46. Publications romanes et françaises 229. Geneva, 2001.

García-Ballester, Luis. *La búsqueda de la salud: Sanadores y enfermos en la España medieval.* Barcelona, 2001.

García Herrero, María del Carmen. *Las mujeres en Zaragoza en el siglo XV.* 2 vols. Zaragoza, 1990.

Gasper, Giles. "'A Doctor in the House'? The Context for Anselm of Canterbury's Interest in Medicine with Reference to a Probable Case of Malaria." *Journal of Medieval History* 30 (2004): 245–61.

Geary, Patrick. "Judicial Violence and Torture in the Carolingian Empire." In *Law and the Illicit in Medieval Europe,* edited by Ruth Mazo Karras, Joel Kaye, and Ann E. Matter, 79–88. Philadelphia, 2008.

———. "Living with Conflicts in Stateless France: A Typology of Conflict Management Mechanisms, 1050–1200." In *Living with the Dead in the Middle Ages,* 125–60. Ithaca, NY, 1994.

Geremek, Bronisław. *La potence ou la pitié: L'Europe et les pauvres du Moyen Âge à nos jours.* Translated by Joanna Arnold-Moricet. Paris, 1987.

Getz, Faye M. *Medicine in the English Middle Ages.* Princeton, NJ, 1998.

Gibson, Joan. "Could Christ Have Been Born a Woman? A Medieval Debate." *Journal of Feminist Studies in Religion* 8 (1992): 65–82.

Gil-Sotres, Pedro. "Derivation and Revulsion: The Theory and Practice of Medieval Phlebotomy." In *Practical Medicine from Salerno to the Black Death,* edited by Luis García-Ballester et al., 110–55. Cambridge, 1994.

———. "Sangre y patología en la medicina bajomedieval: El substrato material de la flebotomía." *Asclepio* 38 (1986): 73–104.

Ginzburg, Carlo. "Clues: Roots of an Evidential Paradigm." In *Clues, Myths, and the Historical Method,* by Carlo Ginzburg. Translated by John Tedeschi and Anne Tedeschi, 96–126. Baltimore, MD, 1989.

Glorieux, Palémon. *La littérature quodlibétique de 1260 à 1320.* 2 vols. Bibliothèque Thomiste. Paris, 1925–35.

Glucklich, Ariel. *Sacred Pain: Hurting the Body for the Sake of the Soul.* Oxford, 2001.

Goltz, Dietlinde. *Mittelalterliche Pharmazie und Medizin, dargestellt an Geschichte und Inhalt des "Antidotarium Nicolai," mit einem Nachdruck der Druckfassung von 1471.* Edited by Wolfgang-Hagen Hein. Veröffentlichungen der Internationalen Gesellschaft für Geschichte der Pharmazie e.V., neue Folge, 44. Stuttgart, 1976.

Good, Mary-Jo DelVecchio, et al., eds. *Pain as Human Experience: An Anthropological Perspective.* Berkeley, CA, 1992.

Gottfried, Robert S. *Doctors and Medicine in Medieval England, 1340–1530.* Princeton, NJ, 1986.

Gragnolati, Manuele. *Experiencing the Afterlife: Soul and Body in Dante and Medieval Culture.* Notre Dame, IN, 2005.

———. "Gluttony and the Anthropology of Pain in Dante's *Inferno* and *Purgatorio*." In *History in the Comic Mode: Medieval Communities and the Matter of Person,* edited by Rachel Fulton and Bruce W. Holsinger, 238–50, 362–64. New York, 2007.

Grahek, Nikola. *Feeling Pain and Being in Pain.* 2nd ed. Cambridge, MA, 2007.

Grig, Lucy. "Torture and Truth in Late Antique Martyrology." *Early Medieval Europe* 11 (2002): 321–36.

Guérin, Isabelle. *La vie rurale en Sologne aux XIVe et XVe siècles.* Paris, 1960.

Guiance, Ariel. "La mort du roi: Sacralité et pouvoir politique dans la Castille médiévale." In *Der Tod des Mächtigen: Kult und Kultur des Todes spätmittelalterlicher Herrscher*, edited by Lothar Kolmer, 299–320. Paderborn, 1997.

Gy, Pierre-Marie. "Les définitions de la confession après le quatrième concile du Latran." In *L'aveu: Antiquité et Moyen Âge; Actes de la table ronde organisée par l'École française de Rome, Rome, 28–30 mars 1984*, 283–96. Rome, 1986.

Hale, Rosemary Drage. "Rocking the Cradle: Margaretha Ebner (Be)Holds the Divine." In *Performance and Transformation: New Approaches to Late Medieval Spirituality*, edited by Mary A. Suydam and Joanna E. Ziegler, 211–35. London, 1999.

Hamburger, Jeffrey F. "The Use of Images in the Pastoral Care of Nuns: The Case of Heinrich Suso and the Dominicans." *Art Bulletin* 71 (1989): 20–46.

Handerson, Henry E. *Gilbertus Anglicus: Medicine of the Thirteenth Century*. Cleveland, OH, 1918.

Himmelfarb, Martha. *Tours of Hell: An Apocalyptic Form in Jewish and Christian Literature*. Philadelphia, 1983.

Hobbins, Daniel. "The Schoolman as Public Intellectual: Jean Gerson and the Late Medieval Tract." *American Historical Review* 108 (2003): 1308–37.

Hollywood, Amy. "Beatrice of Nazareth and Her Hagiographer." In *Gendered Voices: Medieval Saints and Their Interpreters*, edited by Catherine M. Mooney, 78–117. Philadelphia, 1999.

———. *Sensible Ecstasy: Mysticism, Sexual Difference, and the Demands of History*. Chicago, 2002.

Horden, Peregrine. "Pain in Hippocratic Medicine." In *Religion, Health and Suffering*, edited by John R. Hinnells and Roy Porter, 295–315. London, 1999.

Horton-Smith Hartley, Percival, and Harold Richard Aldridge. *Johannes de Mirfeld of St. Bartholomew's, Smithfield: His Life and Works*. Cambridge, 1936.

Hughes, Kevin H. "Eschatological Union: The Mystical Dimension of History in Joachim of Fiore, Bonaventure, and Peter Olivi." *Collectanea Franciscana* 72 (2002): 105–43.

Huizinga, Johan. *The Autumn of the Middle Ages*. Translated by Rodney J. Payton and Ulrich Mammitzsch. Chicago, 1996.

Hundersmarck, Lawrence F. "Preaching the Passion: Late Medieval 'Lives of Christ' as Sermon Vehicles." In *De Ore Domini: Preachers and the Word in the Middle Ages*, edited by Thomas L. Amos, Eugene B. Green, and Beverly M. Keinzle, 147–67. Kalamazoo, MI, 1989.

Hunt, David. "Christianising the Roman Empire: The Evidence of the Code." In *The Theodosian Code*, edited by Jill Harries and I. N. Wood, 143–58. Ithaca, NY, 1993.

Hunt, Tony. *Popular Medicine in Thirteenth-Century England: Introduction and Texts*. Wolfeboro, NH, 1990.

Hyams, Paul. "Trial by Ordeal: The Key to Proof in the Early Common Law." In *On the Laws and Customs of England: Essays in Honor of Samuel E. Thorne*, edited by Morris S. Arnold, 90–126. Chapel Hill, NC, 1981.

Jackson, Jean E. *"Camp Pain": Talking with Chronic Pain Patients*. Philadelphia, 2000.

Jacquart, Danielle. "De crasis à complexio: Note sur le vocabulaire du tempérament en latin médiéval." In *La science médicale occidentale entre deux renaissances (XIIe s.–XVe s.)*, by Danielle Jacquart. Aldershot, UK, 1997.

———. "L'enseignement de la médecine: Quelques termes fondamentaux." In *La science médicale occidentale entre deux renaissances (XIIe s.–XVe s.)*, by Danielle Jacquart. Aldershot, UK, 1997.

———. "Hildegard et la physiologie de son temps." In *Hildegard of Bingen: The Context of Her Thought and Art*, edited by C. S. F. Burnett and Peter Dronke, 121–34. London, 1998.

———. *La médecine médiévale dans le cadre parisien: XIVe–XVe siècle*. Penser la médecine. Paris, 1998.

———. "La reception du Canon d'Avicenne: Comparaison entre Montpellier et Paris aux XIIIe et XIVe siècles." In *Histoire de l'école médicale de Montpellier*, 69–77. Paris, 1985.

———. "Le regard d'un medecin sur son temps: Jacques Despars (1380?–1458)." *Bibliothèque de l'École des chartes* 138 (1980): 35–86.

———. "'Theorica' et 'practica' dans l'enseignement de la médecine à Salerno au XIIe siècle." In *La science médicale occidentale entre deux renaissances (XIIe s.–XVe s.)*, by Danielle Jacquart. Aldershot, UK, 1997.

Jacquart, Danielle, and Claude Thomasset. *Sexualité et savoir médical au Moyen Âge*. Paris, 1985.

Jansen, Katherine L. *The Making of the Magdalen: Preaching and Popular Devotion in the Later Middle Ages*. Princeton, NJ, 2000.

Jarrett, Bede. *Social Theories of the Middle Ages*. New York, 1966.

Jennings, Margaret. "Tutivillus: The Literary Career of the Recording Demon." *Studies in Philology* 74 (1977): 1–93.

Jones, Peter Murray. *Medieval Medical Miniatures*. London, 1984.

Kantorowicz, Hermann. *Albertus Gandinus und das Strafrecht der Scholastik*. Vol. 1. Berlin and Leipzig, 1907.

———. "Studien zum altitalienischen Strafprozeß." In *Rechtshistorische Schriften*, edited by Helmut Coing and Gerhard Immel, 311–39. Karlsruhe, 1970.

Karl, L. "La vie de St. Jehan Paulus." *Revue des langues romaines* 56 (1913): 425–45.

Keil, Gundolf. "Zur Datierung des 'Antidotarium Nicolai.'" *Sudhoffs Archiv: Zeitschrift für Wissenschaftsgeschichte* 62, no. 2 (1978): 190–96.

Kelly, Henry A. "Inquisition and the Prosecution of Heresy: Misconceptions and Abuses." *Church History* 58 (1989): 439–51.

Kieckhefer, Richard. "Holiness and the Culture of Devotion: Remarks on Some Late Medieval Male Saints." In *Images of Sainthood in Medieval Europe*, edited by Renate Blumenfeld-Kosinski and Timea Szell, 288–305. Ithaca, NY, 1991.

———. "Major Currents in Late Medieval Devotion." In *Christian Spirituality: High Middle Ages and Reformation*, edited by Jill Raitt, 75–108. New York, 1987.

———. *Unquiet Souls: Fourteenth-Century Saints and Their Religious Milieu*. Chicago, 1984.

Kienzle, Beverly Mayne, ed. *The Sermon*. TSMA 81–83. Turnhout, 2000.

King, Helen. "The Early Anodynes: Pain in the Ancient World." In *The History of the Management of Pain*, edited by Ronald D. Mann, 51–62. Carnforth, Lancashire, 1988.

Kleinberg, Aviad M. *Prophets in Their Own Country: Living Saints and the Making of Sainthood in the Later Middle Ages*. Chicago, 1992.

Kleinman, Arthur, Paul E. Brodwin, Byron J. Good, and Mary-Jo DelVecchio Good. "Pain as a Human Experience: An Introduction." In *Pain as Human Experience: An Anthropological Perspective,* edited by Mary-Jo DelVecchio Good et al., 1–28. Berkeley, CA, 1992.

Kosztolnyik, Zoltan J. "Pelbartus of Temesvár: A Franciscan Preacher and Writer of the Late Middle Ages in Hungary." *Vivarium: A Journal for Mediaeval Philosophy and the Intellectual Life of the Middle Ages* 5, no. 2 (1967): 100–110.

Kunzle, David. "The Art of Pulling Teeth in the Seventeenth and Nineteenth Centuries: From Public Martyrdom to Private Nightmare and Political Struggle?" In *Fragments for a History of the Human Body,* edited by Michel Feher, Ramona Naddaff, and Nadia Tazi, 3:29–89. New York, 1989.

Kuttner, Stephan. *Kanonistische Schuldlehre von Gratian bis auf die Dekretalen Gregors IX.* Studi e testi 64. Vatican City, 1935.

———. "The Revival of Jurisprudence." In *Renaissance and Renewal in the Twelfth Century,* edited by Larry Benson and Giles Constable, 299–338. Oxford, 1982.

Langbein, John. *Torture and the Law of Proof.* Chicago, 1977.

Langlois, Charles-Victor. *La connaissance de la nature et du monde d'après des écrits français à l'usage des laïcs.* Paris, 1927.

Lea, Henry Charles. *Superstition and Force.* Philadelphia, 1870.

Le Goff, Jacques. *La naissance du purgatoire.* Paris, 1981.

———. "Le vocabulaire des exempla d'après l'Alphabetum narrationum (début XIVᵉ siècle)." In *La lexicographie du Latin médiéval: Colloque du CNRS,* 321–32. Paris, 1981.

Lepage, Yves. "Les versions françaises médiévales du récit apocryphe de la formation d'Adam." *Romania* 100, no. 2 (1979): 145–64.

Lindblom, U., et al. "Pain Terms: A Current List with Definitions and Notes on Usage." *Pain* 24, supplement 1 (1986): S215–S221.

Lipton, Sara. "'The Swet Lean of His Head': Writing about Looking at the Crucifix in the High Middle Ages." *Speculum* 80 (2005): 1172–1208.

Little, Lester K. "Les techniques de la confession et la confession comme technique." In *Faire croire: Modalités de la diffusion et de la réception des messages religieux du XIIᵉ au XVᵉ siècle,* 87–99. Collection de l'École française de Rome 51. Rome, 1981.

Lochrie, Karma. *Margery Kempe and Translations of the Flesh.* Philadelphia, 1991.

Longère, Jean. *La prédication médiévale.* Paris, 1983.

Lopez, Elisabeth. *Culture et sainteté: Colette de Corbie (1381–1447).* Saint-Etienne, 1994.

Lottin, Odon. *Psychologie et morale aux XIIᵉ et XIIIᵉ siècles.* 9 vols. Gembloux, 1948–60.

Loughlin, Stephen. "The Complexity and Importance of *Timor* in Aquinas' *Summa theologiae.*" In *Fear and Its Representations in the Middle Ages and Renaissance,* edited by Anne Scott and Synthia Kosso, 1–16. Turnhout, 2002.

Mackinney, Loren. *Medical Illustrations in Medieval Manuscripts.* Berkeley, CA, 1965.

Mâle, Émile. *L'art réligieux de la fin du Moyen Âge en France: Étude sur l'iconographie du Moyen Âge et sur ses sources d'inspiration.* 3rd ed. Paris, 1925.

Mansfield, Mary C. *The Humiliation of Sinners: Public Penance in Thirteenth-Century France.* Ithaca, NY, 1995.

Marrow, James. *Passion Iconography in Northern European Art of the Late Middle Ages and the Early Renaissance.* Kortrijk, Belgium, 1979.

Mazzuconi, D. "Pauca quedam de vita et miraculis beate Francisce de Pontianis: Tre bio-grafie quattrocentenesche di santa Francesca Romana." In *Una santa tutta romana: Saggi e ricerche nel VI centenario della nascità di Francesca Bussa dei Ponziani (1384-1984)*, edited by Giorgio Picasso, 95–199. Siena, 1984.

McNamara, Jo Ann. "The Need to Give: Suffering and Female Sanctity in the Middle Ages." In *Images of Sainthood in Medieval Europe*, edited by Renate Blumenfeld-Kosinski and Timea Szell, 199–221. Ithaca, NY, 1991.

McNamer, Sarah. "The Origins of the *Meditationes vitae Christi.*" *Speculum* 84 (2009): 905–56.

McVaugh, Michael R. "*Incantationes* in Late Medieval Surgery." In *Ratio et Superstitio: Essays in Honor of Graziella Federici Vescovini*, edited by Giancarlo Marchetti, Orsola Rignani, and Valeria Sorge, 319–45. Fédération internationale des Instituts d'études médiévales: Textes et études du Moyen Âge 24. Louvain-la-Neuve, 2003.

———. *The Rational Surgery of the Middle Ages.* Micrologus' Library 15. Florence, 2006.

McVaugh, Michael R., and Luis García-Ballester. "Therapeutic Method in the Later Middle Ages: Arnau de Vilanova on Medical Contingency." *Caduceus* 11 (1995): 73–86.

Meijers, E. M. "L'Université d'Orléans au XIIIᵉ siècle." In *Études d'histoire du droit*, edited by R. Feenstra and H. F. W. D. Vischer, 3:3–148. Leiden, 1976.

Melzack, Ronald. "The McGill Pain Questionnaire." In *Pain Measurement and Assessment*, edited by Ronald Melzack, 41–47. New York, 1983.

Merback, Mitchell B. *The Thief, the Cross, and the Wheel: Pain and the Spectacle of Punishment in Medieval and Renaissance Europe.* Chicago, 1999.

Meyer, Paul. "Recettes médicales en français publiées d'après le manuscrit BN Lat. 8654ᴮ." *Romania* 37 (1908): 358–73.

———. "Recettes médicales en français publiées d'après le manuscrit 23 d'Évreux." *Romania* 18 (1889): 571–77.

———. "Recettes médicales en provençal d'après le manuscrit R. 14.30 de Trinity College (Cambridge)." *Romania* 32 (1903): 268–99.

Mills, Robert. *Suspended Animation: Pain, Pleasure and Punishment in Medieval Culture.* London, 2005.

Minnis, Alastair J. "*De Impedimento Sexus:* Women's Bodies and Medieval Impediments to Female Ordination." In *Medieval Theology and the Natural Body*, edited by Peter Biller and Alastair J. Minnis, 109–39. York Studies in Medieval Theology 1. York, UK, 1997.

Moeller, Bernd. "Religious Life in Germany on the Eve of the Reformation." In *Pre-Reformation Germany*, edited by Gerald Strauss, 13–42. London, 1972.

Moore, R. I. *The Formation of a Persecuting Society: Power and Deviance in Western Europe, 950–1250.* New York, 1987.

Moreno Rodríguez, Rosa María, and Luis García-Ballester. "El dolor en la teoría y práctica médicas de Galeno." *Dynamis* 2 (1982): 3–24.

Morini, Carla. "La *passio S. Agathae:* La tradizione latina tardo antica e alto-medievale." *Cultura et scuola* 137 (1996): 94–105.

———. "La *passio S. Agathae:* La tradizione medievale inglese." *Rivista di cultura classica e medioevale* 42 (2000): 49–60.

Mormando, Franco. *The Preacher's Demons: Bernardino of Siena and the Social Underworld of Early Renaissance Italy.* Chicago, 1999.

Moroni, O. "Le visioni di S. Francesca Romana tra medioevo e umanesimo." *Studi romani* 21 (1973): 160–78.

Mowbray, Donald C. "A Community of Sufferers and the Authority of Masters: The Development of the Idea of *Limbo* by Masters of Theology at the University of Paris (c. 1230–c. 1300)." In *Authority and Community in the Middle Ages,* edited by Donald C. Mowbray, Rhiannon Purdie, and Ian P. Wei, 43–68. Stroud, UK, 1999.

Muchembled, Robert. *L'invention de l'homme moderne: Culture et sensibilités en France du XVᵉ au XVIIIᵉ siècle.* Paris, 1994.

Mueller, Janel M. "Autobiography of a New 'Creatur': Female Spirituality, Selfhood, and Authorship in *The Book of Margery Kempe.*" In *Women in the Middle Ages and the Renaissance: Literary and Historical Perspectives,* edited by Mary Beth Rose, 155–71. Syracuse, NY, 1986.

Mueller, Joan. "Clare of Assisi and the Agnes Legend: A Franciscan Citing of St. Agnes of Rome as *Mulier Sancta.*" *Studies in Spirituality* 8 (1998): 141–61.

Murray, Alexander. "Confession before 1215." *Transactions of the Royal Historical Society,* 6th ser., 3 (1993): 51–81.

Nagy, Piroska. *Le don de larmes au Moyen Âge: Un instrument spirituel en quête d'institution (Vᵉ–XIIIᵉ siècle).* Paris, 2000.

———. "Les larmes du Christ dans l'exégèse médiévale." *Médiévales* 27 (1994): 37–49.

Nasrallah, J. *Saint Jean de Damas.* Harissa, Lebanon, 1950.

Newman, Barbara. "Devout Women and Demoniacs in the World of Thomas of Cantimpré." In *New Trends in Feminine Spirituality: The Holy Women of Liège and Their Impact.* Edited by Juliette Dor, Lesley Johnson, and Jocelyn Wogan-Browne, 35–60. Turnhout, 1999.

———. *From Virile Woman to WomanChrist: Studies in Medieval Religion and Literature.* Philadelphia, 1995.

———. "Possessed by the Spirit: Devout Women, Demoniacs, and the Apostolic Life in the Thirteenth Century." *Speculum* 73 (1998): 733–70.

Niebyl, Feter H. "The Non-naturals." *Bulletin of the History of Medicine* 45 (1971): 486–92.

Oberman, Heiko. *The Harvest of Medieval Theology: Gabriel Biel and Late Medieval Nominalism.* Cambridge, 1963.

Ottosson, Per-Gunnar. *Scholastic Medicine and Philosophy: A Study of Commentaries on Galen's "Tegni" (ca. 1300–1450).* Naples, 1984.

Palmer, Anne-Marie. *Prudentius on the Martyrs.* Oxford, 1989.

Passenier, Anke E. "The Life of Christina Mirabilis: Miracles and the Construction of Marginality." In *Women and Miracle Stories: A Multidisciplinary Exploration,* edited by Anne-Marie Korte, 145–78. Leiden, 2001.

———. "The Suffering Body and the Freedom of the Soul: Medieval Women's Ways of Union with God." In *Begin with the Body: Corporeality, Religion, and Gender,* edited by Jonneke Bekkenkamp and Maaike de Haardt, 264–87. Leuven, 1998.

Pennington, Kenneth. "Learned Law, *Droit Savant, Gelehrtes Recht:* The Tyranny of a Concept." *Rivista internazionale di diritto comune* 5 (1994): 197–209.

Pepin, Ronald E. "*Nouem Species Poenae:* The Doctrine of Nine Torments in Honorius Augustodunensis, Alain de Lille, Pastoralia, and Bernard de Morlas (al. Morval)." *Latomus: Revue d'études latines* 47 (1988): 668–74.

Perkins, Judith. "The 'Self' as Sufferer." *Harvard Theological Review* 85 (1992): 245–72.

———. *The Suffering Self: Pain and Narrative Representation in the Early Christian Era.* London, 1995.

Peters, Edward. "Destruction of the Flesh—Salvation of the Spirit: The Paradoxes of Torture in Medieval Christian Society." In *The Devil, Heresy, and Witchcraft in the Middle Ages: Essays in Honor of Jeffrey B. Russell,* edited by Alberto Ferreiro, 131–48. Leiden, 1998.

———. *Torture.* Expanded ed. Philadelphia, 1996.

Petroff, Elizabeth Alvilda. *Body and Soul: Essays on Medieval Women and Mysticism.* New York, 1994.

Philippart, Guy. *Les légendiers latins et autres manuscrits hagiographiques.* TSMA 24–25. Turnhout, 1977.

Piro, Francesco. "Sensi interni e eziologia degli affetti: A proposito di due *Quaestiones* sul dolore di Enrico di Gand." In *Corpo e anima, sensi interni e intelletto dai secoli XIII–XIV ai post-Cartesiani e Spinoziani,* edited by Graziella Federici Vescovini, Valeria Sorge, and Carlo Vinti, 189–210. Textes et études du Moyen Âge 30. Turnhout, 2005.

Porro, Pasquale. "Fisica Aristotelica e escatologia cristiana: Il dolore dell'anima nel dibatitto scolastico del XIII secolo." In *Enosis kai filia—unione e amicizia: Omaggio a Francesco Romano,* 617–42. Catania, 2002.

Prügl, Thomas. "Tristitia: Zur Theologie der *Passiones Animae* bei Thomas von Aquin." In *Die Einheit der Person: Beiträge zur Anthropologie des Mittelalters; Richard Heinzmann zum 65. Geburtstag,* edited by Martin Thurner, 141–56. Stuttgart, 1998.

Pryds, Darleen. "Court as *Studium:* Royal Venues for Academic Preaching." In *Medieval Sermons and Society: Cloister, City, University,* edited by Jacqueline Hamesse et al., 343–56. Textes et études du Moyen Âge 9. Louvain-la-Neuve, 1998.

Quinto, Riccardo. "Per la storia del trattato tomistico *De passionibus animae:* Il *timor* nella letteratura teologica tra il 1200 e il 1230s." In *Thomistica,* edited by E. Manning, 35–87. Recherches de théologie ancienne et médiévale, Supplementa. Leuven, 1995.

Raby, F. J. E., ed. *The Oxford Book of Medieval Latin Verse.* Oxford, 1966.

Radding, Charles M. "Vatican Latin 1406, Mommsen's Ms. S, and the Reception of the Digest in the Middle Ages." *Zeitschrift der Savigny-Stiftung, romanistische Abteilung* 110 (1993): 501–51.

Rasmussen, Ann Marie. "Fathers to Think Back Through: The Middle High German Mother-Daughter and Father-Son Advice Forms Known as *Die Winsbeckin* and *Der Winsbecke.*" In *Medieval Conduct,* edited by Kathleen Ashley and Robert L. A. Clark, 106–34. Medieval Cultures 29. Minneapolis, MN, 2001.

Reames, Sherry L. *The "Legenda aurea": A Reexamination of Its Paradoxical History.* Madison, WI, 1985.

Reeves, Marjorie. *The Influence of Prophecy in the Later Middle Ages: A Study in Joachimism.* Oxford, 1969. Reprint, Oxford, 2000.

Rey, Roselyne. *The History of Pain.* Translated by Louise Elliott Wallace, J. A. Cadden, and S. W. Cadden. Cambridge, MA, 1995.

Riddle, John M. *Dioscorides on Pharmacy and Medicine.* Austin, TX, 1985.

———. "Theory and Practice in Medieval Medicine." *Viator* 5 (1974): 157–84.

Roberts, Michael. *Poetry and the Cult of the Martyrs: The "Liber Peristephanon" of Prudentius.* Ann Arbor, MI, 1993.

Rollason, D. W. "The Cult of Murdered Royal Saints in Anglo-Saxon England." *Anglo-Saxon England* 11 (1983): 1–22.

Rosenwein, Barbara H. *Emotional Communities in the Early Middle Ages.* Ithaca, NY, 2006.

Ross, Ellen M. *The Grief of God: Images of the Suffering Jesus in Late Medieval England.* Oxford, 1997.

———. "'She Wept and Cried Right Loud for Sorrow and for Pain': Suffering, the Spiritual Journey, and Women's Experience in Late Medieval Mysticism." In *Maps of Flesh and Light: The Religious Experience of Medieval Women Mystics,* edited by Ulrike Wiethaus, 45–59. Syracuse, NY, 1993.

Rubin, Miri. "Choosing Death? Experiences of Martyrdom in Late Medieval Europe." In *Martyrs and Martyrologies,* 153–83. Studies in Church History 30. Oxford, 1993.

———. *Corpus Christi: The Eucharist in Late Medieval Culture.* Cambridge, 1991.

Rublack, Uhlinka. "Female Spirituality and the Infant Jesus in Late Medieval Dominican Convents." *Gender and History* 6 (1994): 37–57.

———. "Pregnancy, Childbirth and the Female Body in Early Modern Germany." *Past and Present* 150 (1996): 84–110.

Ruggiero, Guido. "Excusable Murder: Insanity and Reason in Early Renaissance Venice." *Journal of Social History* (1982): 109–19.

Saffron, Morris H. "Maurus of Salerno: Twelfth-Century 'Optimus Physicus' with His Commentary on the Prognostics of Hippocrates." *Transactions of the American Philosophical Society,* n.s., 62, no. 1 (1972): 5–104.

Salisbury, Joyce E. *The Blood of Martyrs: Unintended Consequences of Ancient Violence.* London, 2004.

Salmón, Fernando. "Academic Discourse and Pain in Medical Scholasticism (Thirteenth–Fourteenth Centuries)." In *Medicine and Medical Ethics in Medieval and Early Modern Spain: An Intercultural Approach,* edited by Samuel S. Kottek and Luis García-Ballester, 136–53. Jerusalem, 1996.

———. "Pain and the Medieval Physician." *American Pain Society Bulletin* 10, no. 3 (2000).

Sbriccoli, Mario. "'Tormentum id est torquere mentem': Processo inquisitorio e interrogatorio per tortura nell'Italia communale." In *La parola all'accusato,* edited by Jean-Claude Maire Vigueur and Agostino Paravicini Bagliani, 17–32. Palermo, 1991.

Scarry, Elaine. *The Body in Pain: The Making and Unmaking of the World.* Oxford, 1985.

Schild, Wolfgang. "Das Strafrecht als Phänomen der Geistesgeschichte." In *Justiz in alter Zeit,* edited by Christoph Hinckeldey, 7–58. Rothenburg o.d.T., 1984.

Schirmer, Elizabeth. "Reading Lessons at Syon Abbey: The *Myroure of Oure Ladye,* and the Mandates of Vernacular Theology." In *Voices in Dialogue: Reading Women in the Middle Ages,* edited by Linda Olson and Kathryn Kerby-Fulton, 345–76. Notre Dame, IN, 2005.

Schmid, Peter. "Sterben-Tod-Leichenbegängnis König Maximilian I." In *Der Tod des Mächtigen: Kult und Kultur des Todes spätmittelalterlicher Herrscher*, edited by Lothar Kolmer, 185–215. Paderborn, 1997.

Schmitt, Jean-Claude. *Les revenants: Les vivants et les morts dans la société médiévale*. Bibliothèque des histoires. Paris, 1994.

Semeraro, Martino. "Osservazioni in margine al '*Tractatus de tormentis*': Attribuzione e circolazione dell'opera sulla base di alcuni manoscritti." *Initium: Revista catalana d'història del dret* 4 (1999): 479–99.

Shaw, Brent D. "Body/Power/Identity: Passions of the Martyrs." *Journal of Early Christianity* 4 (1996): 269–312.

———. "The Passion of Perpetua." *Past and Present* 139 (1993): 3–45.

Shennan, J. H. *The Parlement of Paris*. Ithaca, NY, 1968.

Shoemaker, Karl B. "Criminal Procedure in Medieval European Law: A Comparison between English and Roman-Canonical Developments after the IV Lateran Council." *Zeitschrift der Savigny-Stiftung, kanonistische Abteilung* 116 (1999): 174–202.

Sigerist, Henry E. *Studien und Texte zur frühmittelalterlichen Rezeptliteratur*. Edited by Karl Sudhoff. Studien zur Geschichte der Medizin 13. Leipzig, 1923. Reprint, Vaduz, 1977.

Sijen, G. P. "La passibilité du Christ chez Philippe de Harveng." *Analecta Praemonstratensia* 14 (1938): 189–208.

Silverman, Lisa. *Tortured Subjects: Pain, Truth, and the Body in Early Modern France*. Chicago, 2001.

Siraisi, Nancy G. *Medieval and Early Renaissance Medicine: An Introduction to Knowledge and Practice*. Chicago, 1990.

———. *Taddeo Alderotti and His Pupils: Two Generations of Italian Medical Learning*. Princeton, NJ, 1981.

Skemer, Don C. *Binding Words: Textual Amulets in the Middle Ages*. University Park, PA, 2006.

Somerset, Fiona. "Excitative Speech: Theories of Emotive Response from Richard Fitzralph to Margery Kempe." In *The Vernacular Spirit: Essays on Medieval Religious Literature*, edited by Renate Blumenfeld-Kosinski, Duncan Robertson, and Nancy Bradley Warren, 59–79. London, 2002.

Southern, Richard W. *Saint Anselm and His Biographer: A Study of Monastic Life and Thought, 1059–c. 1130*. Cambridge, 1966.

Spijker, Ineke van 't. *Fictions of the Inner Life: Religious Literature and Formation of the Self in the Eleventh and Twelfth Centuries*. Turnhout, 2004.

Stegmüller, Friedrich. *Repertorium commentariorum in sententias Petri Lombardi*. 2 vols. Würzburg, 1947.

Stoudt, Debra L. "The Production and Preservation of Letters by Fourteenth-Century Dominican Nuns." *Mediaeval Studies* 53 (1991): 309–26.

Strohmaier, Gotthard. "Constantine's Pseudo-classical Terminology and Its Survival." In *Constantine the African and 'Ali ibn al-'Abbas al-Maǧūsī: The "Pantegni" and Related Texts*, edited by Charles Burnett and Danielle Jacquart, 90–98. Studies in Ancient Medicine 10. Leiden, 1994.

Suydam, Mary A. "Writing Beguines: Ecstatic Performances." *Magistra* 2 (1996): 137–69.

Swanson, R. N. "Passion and Practice: The Social and Ecclesiastical Implications of Passion Devotion in the Late Middle Ages." In *The Broken Body: Passion Devotion in Late Medieval Culture*, edited by A. A. MacDonald, H. N. B. Ridderbos, and R. M. Schlusemann, 1–30. Medievalia Groningana 21. Groningen, 1998.

Sweet, Victoria. "Hildegard of Bingen and the Greening of Medieval Medicine." *Bulletin of the History of Medicine* 73 (1999): 381–403.

Sweetman, Robert. "Christine of Saint-Trond's Preaching Apostolate: Thomas of Cantimpré's Hagiographical Method Revisited." *Vox Benedictina* 9 (1992): 67–97.

Taylor, Robert. "Sermon anonyme sur sainte Agnès, texte du XIIIᵉ siècle." *Travaux de linguistique et de littérature* 7 (1969): 241–53.

Tenenti, Alberto. *La vie et la mort à travers l'art du XVᵉ siècle*. 2nd ed. Paris, 1983.

Tentler, Thomas. *Sin and Confession on the Eve of the Reformation*. Princeton, NJ, 1977.

Thomas, Yan, ed. *Du châtiment dans la cité: Supplices corporels et peine de mort dans le monde antique*. Rome, 1984.

Thompson, Anne B. "The Legend of St. Agnes: Improvisation and the Practice of Hagiography." *Exemplaria* 13 (2001): 355–97.

Tobin, Frank. "Henry Suso and Elsbeth Stagel: Was the *Vita* a Cooperative Effort?" In *Gendered Voices: Medieval Saints and Their Interpreters*, edited by Catherine M. Mooney, 118–35. Philadelphia, 1999.

Tovar, Claude de. "Contamination, interférences et tentatives de systematisation dans la tradition manuscrite des recéptaires medicaux français: Le recéptaire de Jean Sauvage." *Revue d'histoire des textes* 3–4 (1973–74): 115–91, 239–88.

Trembinski, Donna C. "Insensate Saints: Contextualizing Non-Suffering in Early Dominican Legendaries." *Florilegium* 23 (2007): 123–42.

———. "Narratives of (Non) Suffering in Dominican Legendaries: Explorations and Explanations." Ph.D. diss., University of Toronto, 2004.

———. [Pro] passio Doloris: Early Dominican Conceptions of Christ's Physical Pain." *Journal of Ecclesiastical History* 59 (2008): 630-56.

Trexler, Richard C. "Gendering Jesus Crucified." in *Iconography at the Crossroads*, edited by Brendan Cassidy, 107–20. Index of Christian Art Occasional Papers 2. Princeton, NJ, 1993.

Trusen, Winfried. "Der Inquisitionsprozeß: Seine historischen Grundlagen und frühen Formen." *Zeitschrift der Savigny-Stiftung, kanonistische Abteilung* 105 (1988): 168–230.

Tugwell, Simon. "Humbert de Romans's Material for Preachers." In *De Ore Domini: Preachers and the Word in the Middle Ages*, edited by Thomas L. Amos, Eugene B. Green, and Beverly M. Kienzle, 105–17. Kalamazoo, MI, 1989.

Ullmann, Walter. "Reflections on Medieval Torture." *Juridical Review* 56 (1944): 123–37.

———. "Some Medieval Principles of Criminal Procedure." In *Jurisprudence in the Middle Ages*, by Walter Ullmann. London, 1980.

Universidad de Zaragoza. *Homenaje al Profesor Emerito Antonio Ubieto Arteta*. Zaragoza, 1989.

Van Caeneghem, Raoul C. "The Law of Evidence in the Twelfth Century." In *Proceedings of the Second International Congress of Medieval Canon Law*, 297–310. Rome, 1965.

Van Dam, Raymond. *Saints and Their Miracles in Late Antique Gaul*. Princeton, NJ, 1993.

Van der Zanden, C. M. *Étude sur le "Purgatoire de saint Patrice."* Paris, 1927.

Verrando, Giovanni Nino. "Passio SS. Xysti Laurentii et Yppoliti: La trasmissione manoscritta delle varie recensioni della considetta *Passio vetus*." *Recherches augustiniennes* 25 (1991): 181–221.

Vincent, Catherine. "Discipline du corps et de l'esprit chez les flagellants au Moyen Âge." *Revue historique* 302 (2000): 593–614.

Vitz, Evelyn Birge. "Gender and Martyrdom." *Medievalia et humanistica*, n.s., 26 (1999): 79–99.

Voigts, Linda E., and Robert P. Hudson. "'A Drynke That Men Callen Dwale to Make a Man to Slepe Whyle Men Kerven Him': A Surgical Anesthetic from Late Medieval England." In *Health, Disease, and Healing in Medieval Culture*, edited by Sheila Campbell, Bert Hall, and David Klausner, 34–56. London, 1992.

Webb, Heather. "Catherine of Siena's Heart." *Speculum* 80 (2005): 802–17.

Wei, Ian P. "The Self-Image of the Masters of Theology at the University of Paris in the Late Thirteenth and Early Fourteenth Centuries." *Journal of Ecclesiastical History* 46 (1994): 398–431.

Weimar, Peter. "Zur Entstehung des sogenannten Tübinger Rechtsbuchs und der Exceptiones legum romanarum des Petrus." In *Studien zur europäischen Rechtsgeschichte*, edited by Walter Wilhelm, 1–24. Frankfurt a.M., 1972.

Weinhandl, Margarete, ed. *Deutsches Nonnenleben: Das Leben der Schwestern zu Töss und der Nonne von Engeltal Büchlein von der gnaden Überlast*. Munich, 1921.

White, Stephen D. "Proposing the Ordeal and Avoiding It: Strategy and Power in Western French Litigation, 1050 to 1110." In *Cultures of Power: Lordship, Status, and Process in Twelfth-Century Europe*, edited by Thomas N. Bisson, 89–123. Philadelphia, 1995.

Wickersheimer, Ernst. "Bénédiction des remèdes au Moyen Âge." *Lychnos* (1952): 96–101.

Wiethaus, Ulrike. "Thieves and Carnivals: Gender in German Dominican Literature of the Fourteenth Century." In *The Vernacular Spirit: Essays on Medieval Religious Literature*, edited by Renate Blumenfeld-Kosinski, Duncan Robertson, and Nancy Bradley Warren, 209–38. London, 2002.

Wippel, John F. "Quodlibetal Questions." In *Les questions disputées et les questions quodlibétiques dans les facultés de théologie, de droit et de médecine*, edited by Bernardo Bazàn, et al., 2:153–224. TSMA 44–45. Turnhout, 1985.

Zaleski, Carol. *Otherworld Journeys: Accounts of Near-Death Experience in Medieval and Modern Times*. Oxford, 1987.

Zanella, Gabrielle. "Italia, Francia e Germania: Una storiografia a confronto." In *La peste nera: Dati di una realtà ed elementi di una interpretazione; Atti del XXX convegno storico internazionale, Todi, 10–13 ottobre, 1993*, 49–136. Spoleto, 1994.

Zborowski, Mark. *People in Pain*. San Francisco, 1969.

Ziegler, Joseph. "Medicine and Immortality in Terrestrial Paradise." In *Religion and Medicine in the Middle Ages*, edited by Peter Biller and Joseph Ziegler, 201–42. York, UK, 2001.

———. *Medicine and Religion c. 1300: The Case of Arnau de Vilanova.* Oxford Historical Monographs. Oxford, 1998.

———. "Religion and Medicine in the Middle Ages." In *Religion and Medicine in the Middle Ages,* edited by Peter Biller and Joseph Ziegler, 3–14. York, UK, 2001.

———. "*Ut Dicunt Medici:* Medical Knowledge and Theological Debates in the Second Half of the Thirteenth Century." *Bulletin of the History of Medicine* 73 (1999): 208–37.

Zink, Michel. *La prédication en langue romane avant 1300.* Nouvelle bibliothèque du Moyen Âge 4. Paris, 1976.

INDEX

Names of people who lived and died before the year 1300 AD are alphabetized by first name (e.g., Peter Lombard), names of later figures by last name (e.g., Besserman, Lawrence).